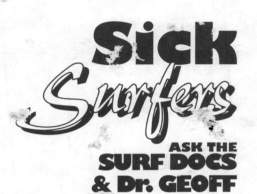

Sick Surfers

ASK THE SURF DOCS
& Dr. GEOFF

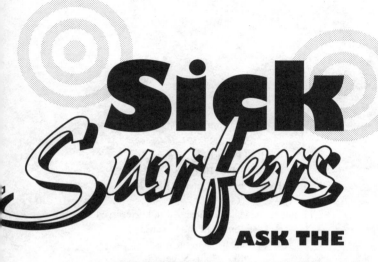

Sick Surfers

ASK THE

SURF DOCS
& Dr. GEOFF

Mark Renneker, M.D.

○

Kevin Starr, M.D.

○

Geoff Booth, M.D.

○

Copyright 1993 Bull Publishing Company
ISBN 0-923521-26-7
Bull Publishing Company
P.O. Box 208
Palo Alto, California 94302-0208
(415) 322-2855
Printed in the United States. All rights reserved
Distributed in the U.S. by:
Publishers Group West
4065 Hollis Street
Emeryville, CA 94608
Distributed in Australia/New Zealand by:
Ozzie Wholesale Book Co.
5/5 Kaleski Place
Moorebank, New South Wales
Australia 2170
Library of Congress Cataloging-in-Publication Data
Renneker, Mar. 1952-
Sick Surfers Ask the Surf Docs and Dr. Geoff / Mark Renneker, Kevin Starr,
Geoff Booth.
p.   cm.
Includes index.
ISBN 0-923521-26-7
1. Surfing—Health aspects. I. Starr, Kevin, M.D. II. Booth, Geoff, M.D. III.
Title.
RC1220.S77R46 1993
616'.008'87973—dc20   93-32172
CIP

Designed by: *Robb Pawlak*, Pawlak Design
Production Manager: *Helen O'Donnell*
Compositor: *Shadow Canyon Graphics*
Printer: *Diversified Printing*
Text and Display Type: *Gill Sans and Pepita*
Printed on recycled paper

Dedicated to . . .

Philip Dunne

Screenwriter and director, father and friend, a Malibu body-surfer who had his ears drilled back in the '50s! June 2, 1992.

Albert Booth

Dad to Geoff. June 29, 1993.

Rainer Arnhold, MD

Traveling light through a lifetime of service, he lives on in those he taught. July 13, 1993.

Steve Baser

Despite being a lawyer and a kneeborder (from LA yet!), he had no strikes against him. May 3, 1993.

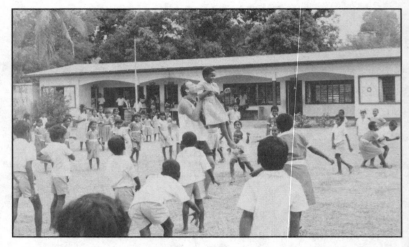

The authors and the publisher are donating a healthy chunk of the royalties to the **Steve Baser Memorial Fund**. Steve was an avid participant in the Surfer's Medical Association's on-going "Nabila Health Project." Nabila is the Fijian village closest to the famed surf destination, Tavarua.

Steve and the children of Nabila showed a special affinity for each other. This unique fund is designed to create sustainable disease prevention and health education programs for village children in Fiji and elsewhere.

Contents

Table of Contents

Sick *Surfers* ASK THE SURF DOCS & Dr. GEOFF

Table of Contents

Foreword

by
Fred Van Dyke

In 1968, an article that I wrote about surfers was featured on the cover of *Life* magazine in Australia, complete with a big wave surfing shot and the subtitle: "A Veteran Surfer Asks: Are Surfers Really Sick?" My article took up a different slant from what is covered in this book, *Sick Surfers*; I probed the behavioral questions of whether surfers are in a state of pre-adolescent arrested development, that perhaps they are male-bonded latent homosexuals, using a girl as something to show off to their fellow surfers at the beach, sticking her like a board in the sand and then going surfing.

Based on how the sparks flew on the North Shore that winter about what I'd written, you'd have to conclude I struck a sensitive nerve. Well, surfing and the people who do it have for the most part matured, but the question is still pertinent: "Are Surfers Really Sick?"

Surfing is in general a safe sport, but the way most surfers go about it isn't healthy. There's a big difference between pushing the limits with the wave—which is the excitement of surfing—and pushing the limits of your body. It's as if surfers are asking "How sunburnt, battered and scarred can I be, with weird bumps and growths popping out of my ears, eyes, skin, and knees, eating a lot of crap and never exercising except when I surf?"

On any given day in front of my house on the beach up from Pipeline, I see surfers limping along like zombies, with swollen arms, legs, and scratches from head to toe. Most let nature take its course, which many times means being forced to stop surfing for a few days, and, for some, an earlier-than-planned trip home to the mainland just to recover.

With what's in this book, surfers can become healthier than they ever thought possible.

Of course, when I was growing up as a surfer, back in the late '40s and early '50s, we didn't need a book like this. We surfed daily, in places like San Francisco, in raw sewage, with no pussy wetsuits or leashes, and no lifeguard facilities.

We built up resistance to every disease just by surfing in that raw shit. Actually, it was so thick at times that it helped to keep our bodies warm, and if that did not work, then we could always take a long piss into our bathing suits, savoring the hot-tub-like environment for a few seconds. Nowadays they even have Levi's that zip instead of button-up. Try buttoning your pants after a 5-hour session in 44° water with no wetsuit. It used to take hours before any of us knew that we had testicles, except for the uncomfortable choking in one's throat until they returned to where they belonged. We were raised thinking that the pungent smell of hydrogen sulfide, urine, feces, dead animals, and a few bait fish fragrances thrown in was the wonderful smell of the ocean. We savored it.

Penicillin was just coming into use by some of the more radical doctors. No tetracycline, crystacillin, anti-bacterial agents, as we know them now, and if you got a virus, which I am not even sure had been isolated at the time, you were on your own. You could compress, lance, soak in Epsom salts, pray, threaten the doctor, but essentially you were in the hands of your resistance build-ups.

Most of us probably had AIDS about 3 times a year, but dismissed it as a severe cold, survived, and didn't even stay out of the water with a fever of 104°. Hell, the cold water lowered the temperature in about 10 minutes, and by the time you swam to the beach after your 50th wipeout, you felt great, ready to go out and drink and make love all night.

So, aside from the fact that surfers today are doing things on waves that we only fantasized about, exploring untouched Northern California spots filled with White Sharks, and riding 25-foot waves that we thought unridable, you're still a bunch of pussy sissies.

You are all going to need this book.

Aloha,

Fred Van Dyke
Kailua, Hawaii

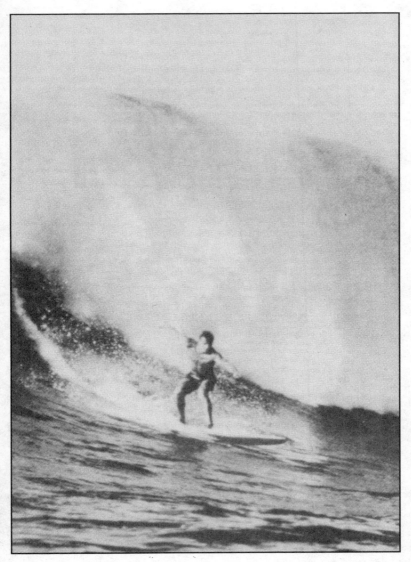

Fred Van Dyke, Waimea Bay in the pre-pussy days of surfing. *Photo courtesy of Fred Van Dyke.*

Commencement

The year I commenced residency, I found myself with money (but not much time) and so commenced an extended decade of Pacific Islands surf travels, commencing, naturally, with the great Hawaiian swell of December 1969.

Meeting surfers and traveling to some out of the way South Pacific islands led me to thinking about communicating medical information to lay people. Working with Aboriginal people in the Northern Territory taught me more about communication. It also gave me further insights into indigenous lifestyles.

In 1978, I floated the idea of a medical column in *Tracks* by the editor, Paul Holmes. He challenged me to do a piece for traveling surfers, and I responded with "Everything You Ever Wanted to Know about Staying Healthy While Travelling and Never Knew How to Ask in Swahili," which was the first Dr. Geoff column, in July 1978.

Letters flowed in from then on. My policy was to answer every letter, and leave it to the editor to decide which to publish. At that stage most *Tracks* readers were teenagers. Teenagers in Australia are only interested (indeed, fixated) on their sacral segments. This means that most letters concerned genitals and other body parts (skin, hair, physique, and such) that were (are) part of the "attracting" mechanism.

Disease, ailments, and injuries gradually evoked interest as surfing became more ferentic, more popular, more geographically dispersed (with mass travel and Indo opening up), and more open to all who wanted to try it. The older crew (that is, older than 25) were sticking with surfing longer, and things were going wrong with their bodies. Also, society was becoming more consumer-oriented as far as health was concerned, with people wanting to know and learn more about being in control.

When an old Torquay mate, Brian "Kanga" Lowdon rang me in early 1986 about "a surf-trip to Fiji with a group of medico surfers," I thought about it for two seconds, and said "yes," and immediately ordered a couple of new Mark Richards' boards for the trip.

Sick *Surfers* ASK THE SURF DOCS & Dr. GEOFF

That seminal September (1986) in the waves of Cloudbreak, Tavarua, and Wilkes, during the first ever medical conference on surfing, I met Mark Renneker, the organizer, and 18 other like-minded docs, health workers, and writers. The Surfer's Medical Association grew out of that meeting.

Less than a year later, Mark Renneker took the idea of a Dr. Geoff-like column to *Surfer* magazine's editor at that time—guess who—the very same Paul Holmes. "Surf Docs" was born, with Mark and then medical student Kevin Starr as Co-Editors, drawing on the consultative expertise of the ever expanding Surfer's Medical Association.

Dr. Geoff continued with added inspiration, including a mail-in questionnaire about surfing and disabilities, which added further impetus for Gary Blashke to get the Disabled Surfers' Association (DSA) up and running.

In October, 1989, I handed over the column to Dr. Bob. It continues to this day, and should be around for a long time to come, as should its American counterpart, Surf Docs. And just like the waves, the letters from sick surfers keep rolling in.

What you oh so lucky readers get in this book are some of the best columns (and baddest) from my eleven year tenure as Dr. Geoff. I've updated and spruced them up as needed, and, because this book will be read by Yank surfers as well, I've had to supply a number of Seppo translations (e.g., they have no idea what a "middie" is!).

You also get the pick of the crop from the Surf Docs columns. These are the complete, uncut "for space reasons" columns—all updated and buffed out. Plus, there are some things that *Surfer* magazine never dared to print. The Seppo's have always been less sex and genital-oriented (for obvious reasons), but we can't all be so unlucky.

So, get ready to open it up. Say ahh!

Dr. Geoff
Newcastle, New South Wales
Australia

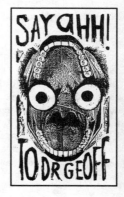

Preface

This book is intended for the self-care of surfers worldwide. It deals with the health and medical problems affecting surfers; the healthier the surfer, the less lost surf time. It's that simple.

It is written for surfers by surfers who also happen to be health professionals. For each of us, our first and foremost calling has been to surfing, the practice of medicine has followed.

Addressing the sub-culture that is surfing, including over five million surfers worldwide, this book is multi-cultural. By combining the best of the Dr. Geoff columns from *Tracks* (Australia's second oldest and largest surfing publication) with the best of the Surf Docs columns from *Surfer* magazine (America's oldest and largest surfing publication), this book readily bridges the American and Australian surfing sub-cultures. And, on the basis of our collective and (surf braggarts that we are) extensive foreign surf travels, this book should apply to surfers everywhere.

No such book exists for surfers. Non-surfing physicians and the non-surfing hoi polloi have no idea about most of the strange ailments that besiege surfers. Ear problems (Surfer's Ear—bony growths in their outer ear canals, called *exotoses*). Eye problems (fleshy growths on their eyes, called *pingueculae* and *pterygia*). Sinus problems (Surfer's Sinuses—sea water gushing forth hours after surfing). Cancer-like bumps and lumps from paddling (Surfer's Chest Knots—synovial cysts on the rib cage; Surfer's Knobbies—connective tissue overgrowths on the knees). The list of problems goes on and on.

And what about the more acute health problems faced by surfers when out in the surf or traveling to exotic places. Would you know how to rescue and resuscitate a drowning surfer? What would you do with a fracture or severe wound if you were hours or days away from the nearest doctor? How's your working knowledge of malaria?

About 95% of what afflicts surfers is covered in this book. For the less common ailments, the other 5%, the self-care approach which imbues this book should help the surfer get through it.

Surfers will do everything possible to avoid going to doctors. Often, when they've gone to a doctor with a surfing-related problem, they were simply told to stop surfing, and were sent a whopping bill. This book will help surfers determine where and when not to see a doctor. And if they do need to be seen, many times surfers have told us that showing the doctor a copy of one of our columns has served them both well.

We include the usual disclaimer, that the advice in this book is not meant to substitute for that of your doctors, but with the twist that what we are writing about—and teaching—is not comparable. We provide a series of case studies, a body of information and ideas. It is up to you (and, possibly, your doctor) to decide what applies in your particular situation. Every medical problem is unique. One case of Surfer's Ear is not the same as the next.

We also include the invitation to write to us care of the publisher as to what worked or didn't work for you about this book. Errors, suggestions, photos, your own cases. Hold forth, please! In general, though, if you have health questions, we would prefer you write care of *Surfer* magazine or *Tracks*.

There are occasional points of overlap and repetition among the various columns, left in because we wanted each column to stand alone and be complete. Plus, some facts are so important that they deserve repeating. Readers may note some contradictions between advice and facts given by Dr. Geoff and the Surf Docs; doctors are like waves, each is different.

As for the practical aspects of how best to use this book, look things up by consulting the Table of Contents or the Index in the back. Make note that the pieces are arranged alphabetically, and are in surfer's terminology versus medical talk.

This book is intended both as fun reading and as reference. Whether kept at home, read over standing in the surf shop, left in your van or stuffed in your backpack for surf trips, the book is meant to be used and to amuse.

Healthy surfing,

Mark Renneker, MD   Kevin Starr, MD   Geoff Booth, MD

Acknowledgments

Kevin

To my father, **Grover Starr**, who first took me down to the sea; to my mother, **Bonnie**, who supported everything even remotely worth supporting.

To **Bernie Tershy**, who taught me most of what I know about the ocean.

To **Jackie Feldman**, for love, support and countless pints of ice cream through the many days of "Surf Docs" and medical training.

To **Kate Linde**, whose creative medical school scheduling made "Surf Docs" possible, or at least a lot less of a hassle.

Geoff

My sincere thanks to **Paul Holmes** who had the foresight to allow "Dr. Geoff" to happen.

To **my parents** who took us holidaying on Torquay and introduced me to surfing. Vale Dad (29.6.93)

To my wife, **Narelle**, who did the typing for "Dr. Geoff." To our children, **Christian** and **Charles** who were neglected on the weekends of the *Tracks* deadlines.

To all my **surfing mates** (Torquay, Whale Beach, Avalon and Newcastle) who asked good questions, gave (and continue to give) me heaps, and continue to sponsor me ("Claw," "Sing-Ding," and Dennis).

To **Mark Richards**, who continues to inspire, both by his behaviors and surfboards.

Sick *Surfers* ASK THE SURF DOCS & Dr. GEOFF

Mark

To my father, **Richard**, a non-surfing psychiatrist, who supported me from day one in my quest to be many things, including surfer and doctor, and who was right there with me and Tres as we blazed down (and broke down) in pre-paved-road Baja, and many other Baja trips since, plus Fiji, and loads of other places.

To my mother, **Hanna,** a kindred soul though not a surfer, who taught me decisiveness and independence, and who some years back initiated the idea of she and me taking regular trips to the North Shore (a wonderful tradition!).

To sister **Toni** and her ex-surf rats, **Kevin** and **Paul,** now charging the rivers of Ohio!

To **Jessica**, who grew up in Malibu but never deigned to learn to surf (but she can boogie, oh can she boogie!). With me through an amazing 20 years, she has been to more incredible surf spots around the world than 99.9% of surfers.

To **Surfer** magazine, for sharing in the idea of bringing top-notch health information to surfers: Paul Holmes, Steve Pezman, Matt Warshaw, Steve Hawk, Ben Marcus, Steve Barilotti, Jeff Devine, Donna Oakley, Jody Kirk, and Lisa Boelter.

To the many consultants to the Surf Docs column. Some of you we call on often, others infrequently, some not yet, but we stand in absolute appreciation of your ongoing willingness to help when needed: Kim Bodkin, MS, Sports Medicine, Montara, CA; Geoff Booth, MB, Physical and Rehabilitation Medicine, Newcastle, Australia; Mark Bracker, MD, Wilderness and Sports Medicine, San Diego, CA; Chris Carver, MD, Neurosurgery, Salinas, CA; Robert Chatfield, DC, Chiropractic, Santa Cruz, CA; John Cherry, MD, General Surgery, La Jolla, CA; J. Grant Davis, MD, ENT, Santa Barbara, CA; James DiMarchi, MD, OB-GYN, Washington, DC; Dan Dworsky, MD, Internal Medicine, San Diego, CA; Randy Fulton, DC, Chiropractic, El Toro, CA; Shale Gordan, MD, Cardiology, Hermosa Beach, CA; Helmuth Jones, MD, Orthopedics, Chico, CA; Alex Kaliakin, DC, Chiropractic, Santa Monica, CA; Robert Lawson, MD, Environmental Health, Simi Valley, CA; Geoff Loman, MD, General Medicine, Ventura, CA; Paul Manchester, MD, Environmental Health, San Francisco, CA; Ricardo Mandojana, MD, Dermatology, Knoxville, TN; Gary Groth-Marnat, PhD, Health Psychology, Perth, Australia; Tom McLaughlin, PT, Physical Therapy, Duarte, CA; David McWaters, PharmD, Medications, San Francisco, CA; Richard Miller, PhD, Psychology, Malibu, CA; Anthony Moore, MD, Esoteric Medicine, La Jolla, CA; F. Ray Nickel, MD, Orthopedics, Ventura, CA; Andrew Nathanson, MD, Emergency/Marine Medicine, Los Angeles, CA; Mikele Nova, MD, PhD, Dermatopathology, La Jolla, CA; George Orbelian, Design Safety, San Francisco, CA; Rym Partridge, DDS, Dentistry, Santa Cruz, CA; William

Acknowledgments

Petersen, OD, Optometry, Dana Point, CA; Greg Raymond, MS, Environmental Health, San Francisco, CA: Margaret Ripley, MD, Orthopedics, Jacksonville, FL; William Rosenblatt, Ed.D., Psychology, Loch Arbour, NJ; Mike Rowbotham, MD, Neurology, San Francisco, CA; Ross Rudolph, MD, Plastic Surgery, La Jolla, CA; Robert Scott, MD, Surfer's Ear, Santa Cruz, CA; Daniel Sooy, MD, ENT, Santa Rosa, CA; Craig Swenson, MD, Orthopedics, La Jolla, CA; Craig Wilson, MD, Preventive Medicine, San Francisco, CA; Ethan Wilson, MD, Emergency Medicine, Corvalis, Oregon.

To the many, many people involved with the Surfer's Medical Association, whom in both major and subtle ways have helped shape and develop it, and in so doing added immeasurably to the Surf Docs column. Notably (and with some overlap with the above consultants), Jim Allen, Jack Attias, Doc Ball, Don Balch, Mike Baser, Andy Bennetts, Ron Bockhold, Mark Bracker, Jim Bradley, Ken Bradshaw, Chris Carver, Aaron Chang, Bob and Barb Chatfield, Dave and Jean Clark, George Cockle, Andrea Cohen, George Cromack, Craig and Lila Dawson, Neil Derechin, Paul Despas, Gary Deutsch, Peter and Sarah Dixon, Dragon, Marilyn Dougherty, Dan and Chris Dworsky, Michael Eurs, Mike Famularo, Rick Farley, Scott Funk, Paul Georghiou and Nabau, Darryl Genis, Mark Gillett, Huey Greenup, Dan Gribi, Gary Groth-Marnat, Bill Heick, Steve Heilig, Bill Hobi, Tony Jackson, Allston James, Helmuth Jones, Bill Jones, Alex Kaliakin, Greg Kennedy, Tom Kever, Tom Kirsop, Michael Kliks, Simon Leslie, Eliot Light, Elaine Light, Andy Lillestol, John Lindsey, Gerry Lopez, Brian Lowdon, Margaret Lowdon, Gary Lynch, Steve Mann, Mark Massara, Ula and Don McClelland, Linda McCrerey, Tom and Paula McLaughlin, David McWaters and Sandy Campbell, John Millard, Tony Moore, Tom Mulholland, Big Jone and Druku and the Village of Nabila, Richard and Laura O'Neil, George Orbelian, Rym and Winnie Partridge, Tony Peckham and Hilary Saner, Jeff Perkins, Rick Peters, Bill and Dianne Petersen, Jim Phillips, Terry Prince, John Przybyszewski, Greg Raymond, Randy Rockney, Bill Rosenblatt, Eddy Rubin, Gary Ryan, Hiroshi Sato, Robert Scott, Steve Shapiro, Ward and Paula and Maya Smith, Dan Sooy, Joel Steinman, Matthew Stevens, Nelson Swartley, Scott Thayer, Sedge Thomson, Bryan Thurmond, Fred Van Dyke, Norman Vinn, Don and Susan Wagner, Rick Williams, Alistair Wilson, Craig Wilson, Ethan Wilson, Candy Woodward, and Bank Wright. Full apologies to those not mentioned who should have been.

Finally, thanks to **David Bull** who invited us to do this book, and to **Helen O'Donnell** who put it all together.

About the Authors

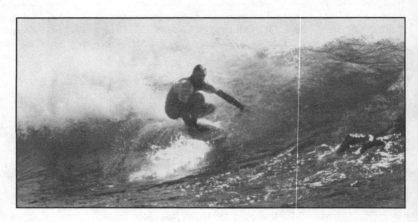

Dr. Geoff (aka Geoff Booth, MB, BS, DPRM, FAFRM (RACP), FACOM) is the Director of Rehabilitation Medicine at John Hunter and Royal Newcastle Hospitals in Newcastle, NSW, Australia. Geoff is a Founding and Lifetime Member of the Surfer's Medical Association and Co-Founder of Merewether Waterman's Club, and a member of Merewether Surfboard Club.

Geoff started surfing around Torquay, Victoria in 1960. His first board was a 10'3" triple stringer "Phil Edwards" design with balsa tail block. He has traveled extensively throughout the Pacific, "My first trip overseas was in November/December 1969 to Hawaii where I saw the biggest surf ever ridden—Greg Noll at Makaha. I now use surfboards by Mark Richards: 6'10", 6'11", 7'3" and 7'8". My favorite wave is long hollow left-hand wall in the 6-8' range. Some favorite Australian surf sports include Crackneck (Central Coast) and Mudjimba (Queensland)."

Geoff is a correspondent for *Surf Report,* an international monthly newsletter. Other publications include: "Surfing Fitness: What Can Happen and How to Prevent It" in *How to Surf: The Compete Guide to Surfing* (*Tracks*, 1992) and *Surfer* magazine's "A-Z of Traveller's Health" tips section.

Geoff is married and has two teenage sons, both of whom surf.

About the Authors

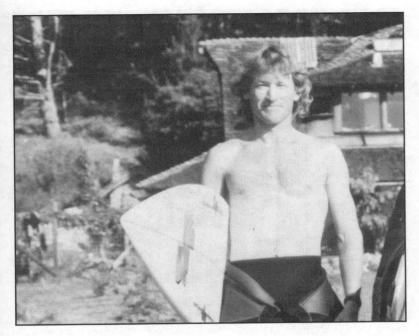

Surf Doc, Kevin Starr, MD, is a board certified family physician. He is a clinical instructor in the Department of Family and Community Medicine at the University of California, San Francisco. Kevin is a Lifetime Member of the Surfer's Medical Association, and is Founder and Director of the Cordilleras Project, a health education project in the Bolivian Andes.

Kevin has been surfing for 16 years, and has gotten himself drilled on big waves all over the Pacific. He is currently living out the back of his truck, which is usually parked on the North Coast (of California) during the winter and in the Sierra Nevada during the summer. He occasionally works and spends the rest of his time rummaging through boxes of climbing and surfing gear looking for stuff he's misplaced.

Most of Kevin's current projects involve educating people on ecological sustainability and the problems of the Third World. He's looking for the right place to start an "ecologically sound" health clinic. Kevin is quite happy and does not want to hear from any more job recruiters, investment brokers, or real estate agents.

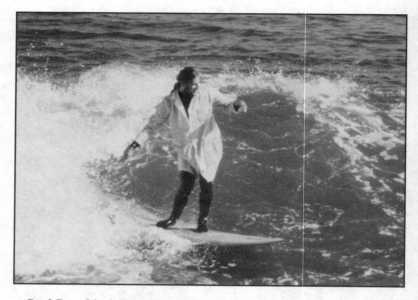

Surf Doc, Mark Renneker, MD (aka Doc Hazard). A surfer for 30 years, beginning in Santa Monica, then up to U.C. Santa Cruz for college, finally coming to live and take his medical training in San Francisco. He calculates that it took 29 years of schooling for him to finally become a board-certified family physician. His academic title is Assistant Clinical Professor, in the Department of Family and Community Medicine, at the University of California, San Francisco. Don't be too impressed by that, it just means that sometimes he volunteers his time to teach clinical preventive medicine to medical students and residents.

What he really does is live at Ocean Beach with Jessica and two iguanas, surf the biggest waves he can find, and when there are none, he works with diss'ed people: the disadvantaged and disallowed (at an inner-city clinic, The South of Market Health Center); the disabled and disregarded (at a geriatric and rehabilitation public institution, Laguna Honda Hospital); the disenfranchised and discalced (surfers); and the disheartened and dispossessed (as the Medical Equalizer, a cross-country telephone-based consulting and research service for people trapped in a medical nightmare and needing information and advocacy). He practices what he calls "optimistic medicine," that no matter how desperate or hopeless a situation may appear, there are always new things to try.

A twenty-year volunteer with the American Cancer Society, serving on umpteen committees and the Board of Directors in California, he has initiated and organized

About the Authors

over 20 conferences on cancer, and directed numerous cancer education projects, including a recent three-year national American Cancer Society $600,000 demonstration project that provided comprehensive cancer education and screening services to the poor of West Oakland.

He has authored or co-authored over 50 medical and lay articles and books, including *Understanding Cancer,* a popular university and community text on cancer (Bull Publishing, 4th edition due out in 1994). Over 100 articles have been written about his work, ranging from the *Wall Street Journal* to *The New Yorker,* plus numerous television pieces, including CBS "Street Stories."

He is a Founding and Lifetime Member of the Surfer's Medical Association, their first and only president (all bureaucratic structure was abandoned by the SMA in 1987), and the editor of *Surfing Medicine,* the journal of the Surfer's Medical Association. He is co-editor of the "Surf Docs" column, with Kevin Starr. He is on the Editorial Board of the Physician and Sportsmedicine. He was flattered to be included in *Surfing* magazine's 1993 list of all-time big-wave riders, but says he doesn't really deserve it. Aw, shucks!

His interest in all aspects of surfing has lead him to amass what is arguably the world's largest surf book and magazine collection, keep and continually replenish a stable of over twenty surfboards, (ranging from 6-foot small-wave boards to 12-foot big-wave guns), and sent him searching for waves throughout the world, including: Hawaii, western Canada, the entire West Coast as well as the Gulf and East Coasts of the U.S., the Caribbean, all of Mexico, Costa Rica, Ecuador and the Galapagos, Peru, Chile, Argentina, Brazil, Portugal, Scotland, Ireland, New Zealand, the east and west coasts of Australia, Bali, west and east Java, and, of course, Fiji. At present, his favorite surf spot is on the coastal Alaskan wilderness, only reachable by bush plane, at the foot of massive glaciated mountains, along a beach whose only footprints are from wolves and grizzlies, beneath a nest of bald eagles, where a perfect right peels off, and he alone has surfed.

About Face

Surfers Who Hate

"The world hates Americans,
Americans hate Californians,
Californians hate Southern Californians,
Southern Californians hate people from L.A.,
People in L.A. hate people from the Valley,
And people in the Valley hate kneeboarders."
– Holmes' Laws, circa 1973

Why do so many surfers hate each other? Why is there so much bigotry in our sport? What, in all innocence, you may wonder, am I referring to?

The most obvious example of surfing's bigotry is localism—a hatred of those who don't happen to live where you live or surf. At some surf spots, a non-local may be sworn at, chased out of the water, or punched out; the locals may even cheer if the non-local wipes out, loses his or her board, or gets hurt.

And then there's the widespread intolerance of "different" surfers—whether they be female ("chicks"), younger ("gremmies"), older ("old farts"), beginners ("kooks"), kneeboarders ("half-men"), bodyboarders ("spongers"), wave-skiiers ("goat-boaters"), or of a different race ("mokes" vs. "haoles," "Brazil nuts," etc.).

Overcrowding may be one factor. When the Surfer's Medical Association first began, with the goal of helping all surfers to become healthier, one member innocently spilled out, "but if less surfers are getting hurt, that means it will be more crowded!"

Our peculiar need not to be different is another ingredient. Horrible though it may sound, if you think about it, we generally look, dress, talk, and act alike—and, I suspect, we think alike. Witness how difficult it is for new surfboard designs to gain acceptance. But, finally, when the top guy gets into it, everyone follows.

True individualists are rare in surfing, and those that exist are heavily copied, e.g., Dora and Greenough. Others are distrusted. Consider poor Cheyne Horan, dragged through the muck for experimenting with different board and fin designs, life styles, and for exploring his sexuality.

Sociologists would tell us that our behavior is a result of being a sub-culture, that we're so different from the rest of society that we need to act and look alike to maintain our identity.

What does the future hold for us? If anything, hatred and bigotry in surfing is on the rise, given the ever increasing number of surfers and the resulting problems of overcrowding.

Despite being an optimist at heart, I think things will continue to get worse, until we collectively wake up to how we're behaving. Perhaps begin by taking stock of your intolerances. What are your peeves, dislikes, and hatreds of other surfers?

MARK RENNEKER, M.D.
Formerly a kneeboarder

Adrenalin

Rush Junkies

Dear Dr. GEOFF,

Much is made of the so-called adrenalin rush you get paddling out on good days or after riding a hot wave. Could you please explain what adrenalin is and is it really what you feel when you see a close-out set feathering on the horizon? Is it better described as straight-out of fear?

RICHARD
Auckland, New Zealand

■ ■ ■ ■ ■ ||||||

Dear Richard,

It is indeed some kind of omen when the best questions (at least in my opinion) ever addressed to me are from New Zealand.

Most surfers who've been around long enough have felt unbridled fear: heart pounding, dry mouth, cold clammy skin, funny tingling in the backside, dilated pupils and super alert

racing mind as that monster set starts to peak way outside. I liked Buzzy Trent's description (*Surfer*, Vol. 15, No. 1) of "Big waves are measured not in feet, but in increments of fear."

This statement, said to be made in 1964, clearly represents our own individual setting as surfers as to what really is a fear situation. It seems that many of the old time big wave greats were able to use fear in a constructive sense to overcome situations that would leave most of us in a dribbling mess.

Perched above each kidney like a schoolboy's cap is a special organ—the adrenal gland. An outer zone (cortex) is clearly separated from the inner zone (medulla). Adrenalin and to a lesser extent noradrenalin (also known as epinephrine and norepinephrine, respectively), are the chemicals produced by the adrenal medulla.

Both adrenalin and noradrenalin prepare the organism, in this case the surfer, to meet an emergency situation. Physiologists label this response to fear

3

as "flight or fight." In other words, fear becomes the stimulus that prepares the body for a maximum muscular effort.

Adrenalin is the chemical responsible for efficiently liberating and utilizing fuel. Noradrenalin is the chemical responsible for transmitting electrical impulses across part of the nervous system (the so called sympathetic nervous system).

To perform a maximum muscular effort requires skeletal muscle (mainly in the arms and legs) to:

1. **Be electrically set to achieve a series of super contractions—the functions of the nervous system.**

2. **Have delivered to it a rich fuel (oxygen and sugar) which can be efficiently converted into energy—the function of adrenalin.**

3. **Be supplied with enough blood (which carries the fuel) by an increased heart rate and force contractions as well as obtaining blood from less important areas (for example, the bowels). This shunting of blood from the skin explains why the skin feels cold in these situations.**

Clamminess, or increased sweating, is not noticed in the water, especially when an eight-foot-thick lip flicks thirty feet down towards a hapless surfer. Adrenalin also causes the blood supply of muscles to increase by enlarging the arteries. Clarity of thought, and a racing mind, are due to the direct effect of adrenalin and other chemicals on the brain.

Big waves are measured not in feet, but in increments of fear.

So to those of you who have successfully punched through an eight-foot-thick lip in the above situation, you'll be interested to know this incredible performance has been the end result of the above described changes. That is, altered muscle fibers are efficiently contracting all at once, fired by an adrenalin activated fuel source.

"Adrenalin rush" is merely journo jargo coined from the halcyon days of the sixties when speed was the principal consumer drug. It is basically the sense felt by a sudden large overdose (in comparison with natural amounts) of adrenalin.

4

Aggression

Clockwork Orange County

$\mathcal{D}$r. *Geoff saith:*

Man is the only "animal" on this planet whose deliberate acts of aggression are sewing his own seeds of destruction.

In surfing, this inevitable decline is already a living example in southern California. The original home of modern surfing—style, technology and development—is now a cesspool of mediocrity. Such is the end result of selfish man struggling aggressively to defend "his" history without any due thought to the consequences. Indignant aggressiveness, manifest by extreme, violent realism is the order for the day. The result: stagnation followed by decay.

Certain parts of Australia are, alas, exhibiting signs heralding a similar (perhaps inevitable?) decline.

Aggression, according to the Oxford Dictionary, is defined in terms of "beginning a quarrel, being offensive, being disposed to attack." It is the act of inflicting physical or, more subtly, psychological harm.

So what! "If that CB van-man, red-necked turkey scum . . . comes and surfs at *my* break, he just has to expect what's thrown at him." After all, aggro is what it's all about. I remember reading where Ian (Cairns) said, " . . . my approach is total aggro . . . "

SELF-AWARENESS

This type of thought would fairly sum up the mental approach of a large percentage of young surfers. It merely reflects the confused state many surfers find themselves in when they read journo drival about "Australian Aggro." Such confusion brought about by a total lack of understanding is the difference between "aggression" and "self-assertiveness." It also shows a complete lack of awareness of the underlying nature of aggression.

What Ian was really pointing out in his statement was his belief in himself. That is, his self-assertiveness in knowing (and over the years having proven) that he is able to move forward towards a goal without undue hesitation, self-doubt or fears. This is what many (but unfortunately not all) of the truly top surfers mean if they talk about "aggro." It really reflects a positive, self-assured approach based on true self-awareness.

With regret, it must also be pointed out that the dividing line between self-assertion and aggression is small. When self-assertion is thwarted, aggression may occur.

Aggressive behavior is the end product, the common confession of many different intentions. The intention of conducting harm because we are angry is not the only form of aggression. Aggressive behavior can also occur with the intention of "teaching" (read Jim Soutar's aggressive comments in "North Shore Injuries," *Surfer*, Vol. 20, No. 2, 1979), through defending one's life, in robbing a bank, or even an accident.

INSECURITIES

According to popular literature, aggression is "instinctive." What is meant by this is that aggression is a biologic drive—like hunger and sex—which constantly strives for discharge. If held back, it builds up, overflowing into a cataclysm of destructive violence.

This is simply not true. Aggression is merely a reaction to threat.

However, there are many people who are persistently aggressive—there being no apparent provocation. They are cruel and sadistic and enjoy violence. *Clockwork Orange* accurately portrayed such persons. Many seaside suburban breaks offer live-theater examples, ranging from Orange County to Manly.

How then does one explain the phenomena of surfing-provoked aggression. The surfer who must rant, scream and provoke a fight is reacting to a threat. However, the threat comes from *within*. This type of surfer has such deep-seated insecurities and fears, the only way he can cope is to show an aggressive exterior. Confident, self-assured surfers—although probably just as capable of reacting aggressively when their real interests are threatened—are much less outwardly aggressive than those who feel insecure.

Some psychologists use the term "benign" and "malignant" to distinguish these two forms of aggression.

Benign aggression is the angry response to a real threat and ceases when the threat ceases. This form of aggression is shared with the animal kingdom.

IRRESPONSIBLE RESPONSES

Malignant aggression occurs in an attempt to cover up inner fears about one's own powerlessness or insecurity, the threat being built-in within the personality. Rather than admit feeling hurt or vulnerable, the malignantly aggressive person reacts as if to say, "I'll show those bastards." Attack becomes the only form of defense. Malignant aggression is not shared with the animal kingdom. It makes us the only species capable of mass murder.

Gough Whitlam (an ex-Australian Prime Minister), certainly was appealing to the dark side of human nature when he stated to the populace "...maintain the rage...," after his dethroning.

Next time you're down at your favorite break, take time off to observe the various forms of behavior exhibited by the surfing pack.

The classical aggro-provoking stimulus is, of course, the drop-in. Most surfers get annoyed at being dropped-in on, but usually accept the situation—perhaps with a menacing glance or a quiet word when paddling back out.

The more insecure surfer will interpret being dropped-in on as some type of threat and react by yelling and threatening to "punch-in" the offenders head. This is a more exaggerated form of benign aggression.

However, the really insecure surfer—whose personality's only defense against his inner weakness is attack—will react to the "threat" with physical retaliation. "...I'll show that drop-in bastard, he won't get at me." Aggression becomes sustained and therefore malignant, and before long the situation ends in a fight, a deliberate attempt to hit the other guy with a board, or a "visit" from a few mates. Such malignant aggressive surfers are a menace by the very fact they *need* to prove something every time they surf.

SOCIAL FACTORS

Various social factors, such as overcrowding, money, peer recognition, sibling rivalry and the surfing media, all play their part in molding young minds. By constantly highlighting aggressiveness—and not defining the term properly—young surfers believe that causing harm to others is a natural way of life, and therefore, it is an expected behavior if one is to succeed. Such is not the case.

So what! One might feel that apart from being of minor nuisance value (a self-righteous belief, especially if you're not the one copping flak), surfing standards are pushed higher by aggression.

> **" . . . take time off to observe the various forms of behavior exhibited by the surfing pack."**

This is true in a limited extent only if aggression is used in a positive way to lift one's own performance, but not at the expense of someone else.

Total aggressive encapsulation was the main factor used to predict southern California's demise as a positive force in world surfing by that astute observer of human behavior, Mickey Dora, many years before the event. (For details read *Surfer*, Vol. 10, No. 4, 1969.) As an aside, I personally believe that, in fact, (by mainstreaming surfing into an "accepted, legit" sport) professionalism in surfing will become surfing's salvation rather than its demise—at least in Australia.

So next time something goes wrong in the water, stop and think before reacting. If you're incapable of this, get a friend to monitor your behavior while you're surfing. If, as a result, you find you're constantly screaming at and being physically aggressive to other surfers, you've got a problem. Not only that, whatever aspirations you have to get to the top can be forgotten. None of the top pros exhibit this behavior.

In other words, because the top surfers do not have a problem with inner insecurity they are able to channel *all* their energies into surfing. How about you?

AIDS

Too Serious to Joke About

Dear SURF DOCS,

I'll come right out and say it. I'm worried about AIDS. Do you have any information on AIDS for surfers?

**CHARLES
Seaside, Oregon**

▌▌▌▌▌▌▏▏▏

Dear Charles,

AIDS (Acquired Immunodeficiency Disease) is sometimes joked about by surfers, but it does affect them. The two largest risk groups for AIDS in the U.S. are homosexuals and intravenous drug users, and although it's never before been estimated how many surfers fall into those categories, the number is probably higher than you'd guess. Spend a minute and think of all the surfers you know who have ever shot drugs—they're at risk for AIDS (especially if they shared needles).

In macho (predominantly) male sports like surfing, bisexual and gay experiences are not uncommon—they're just seldom talked about. A few years ago one of the SMA Ear, Nose and Throat specialists diagnosed what may be the first AIDS case in a surfer. A gay male with AIDS consulted him for an ear problem (AIDS patients frequently have problems of the ear, nose and throat). Upon looking in the patient's ears, the telltale, bony growths characteristic of surfer's ear were noticed. After further questioning the patient revealed that, yes, he was an avid surfer.

When first contracted, the symptoms of HIV are just like the flu or mono: feeling very tired, achy, some fever, perhaps a rash, sore throat, dry cough and swollen lymph glands (especially in the neck). The full-blown infection of AIDS involves weight loss (generally more than 15 pounds), continually swollen glands in most places in the body (neck, underarm, elbow and groin), persistent fevers (often high), weeks of diarrhea,

9

profuse sweating at night, and unusual rashes or discolorations of the skin and inside the mouth. If you have any of the above symptoms, you should be seen by a doctor—whether or not it's AIDS, you're sick.

To lessen your chances of getting AIDS, don't use intravenous drugs (especially with dirty or shared needles, which can be safely disinfected by soaking in bleach for 10 minutes), and practice safe sex, using a condom. Unprotected intercourse with prostitutes—anywhere in the world—may expose you to the AIDS virus, as well as other sexually transmitted diseases.

There has been a great deal of concern over the apparent dumping of medical waste at sea, with used syringes turning up on beaches. What is the risk of AIDS from such a source? One study, in 1986, showed that the AIDS virus can survive in saline (i.e., salt water) for about 2 weeks! The risk is small and there are not yet any reported cases, but with zero medical waste dumping the risk would be zero.

AIDS is not spread by casual contact. For example, you couldn't get it from trying on a wetsuit or bathing suit that someone with AIDS has just tried on. If you think you may be at risk for AIDS, or just want to learn more about it, consider consulting a health or community resource (AIDS education group, physician, etc.), for further information.

Air
The Hypoxia High

Dr. Geoff saith:

Oxygen supply is a critical factor when you're held under water after a wipeout. Wiping out in big waves, such as at Sunset Beach, you may get hit twice: first, you get slammed against the surface of the wave, which forces all the air out of your lungs; second, you get pitched "over the falls" and pounded under water. Although you may be held under only 20 seconds, it seems like minutes because of the diminished air volume in your lungs, your anxiety level and the washing-machine thrashing you're getting.

You can increase your ability to hold your breath for such emergencies by training and conditioning your lungs. Try free diving during flat spells. Wearing mask, snorkle and fins, swim out to deep water—say, 20-30 feet (6-9 meters)—inhale a lungful of air and do a duck dive down to the bottom. Practice diving and pushing off from the bottom. Do these breathhold diving exercises every day for two weeks, and you'll be able to extend your underwater time on breathhold air. Then add to the difficulty of the training exercise: Swim along the bottom before coming up. Finally, add diving off the high diving board and swimming along the bottom of your local swimming pool for 25 yards (23 meters) or more.

In the open ocean, practice retrieving objects and bringing them to the surface. When you hit the surface, slide into a back float and breathe naturally.

You may feel spaced out after practicing free diving. This is why it's important to relax into a back float until your brain receives sufficient oxygen.

There are risks involved in this type of breathhold training. Conditioning yourself to hold your breath for a long time has nothing to do with using additional *alveoli* or lung sacs; it is simply an adaptation to overcoming the urge to breathe.

Breathhold (or free) diving is a risky practice because people get too proficient at it. This is why there aren't many spearfishing contests any more. Divers didn't feel the urge to breathe, so they stayed down too long, blacked out and drowned.

The problem is that the body has no warning signs of critically low oxygen levels. *Hypoxia,* or lack of oxygen, makes you feel giddy and high, not sick. The most critical stage of breathhold diving is starting up from the bottom—this is when you are most likely to black out. As you approach the surface, the oxygen level drops rapidly. Once you break the surface and breathe, your oxygen level quickly returns to normal.

Breathhold ability varies from one individual to another. Most people can dive safely to 20-30 feet (6-9 meters) for one minute. But diving 90-100 feet (27-30 meters) for three minutes is too dangerous. Many people who overcome their urge to breathe at that depth will black out and drown.

You may stay under water so long that you see stars, or lose sensation in your arms and legs, or black out momentarily. Known as "shallow-water blackout," this condition is a sign of severe oxygen deprivation to the brain. It can happen in two feet of water in a swimming pool. Remember breathholding training is DANGER-OUS and should be *practiced with caution* and *preferably with a friend,* so that you can watch over each other.

Amazingly, the human body can function even while deprived of oxygen. If you are successful in learning the breathhold diving exercise, you'll reach the surface as your lungs burn for air. Break the surface and float on your back a while to allow the sensations in your head and body to return to normal. A feeling of exhilaration and relaxation will envelop you—*the hypoxia high*—and you'll wonder why you were so scared down there.

Remember that when you push off the bottom at a depth of 30 feet, the water pressure feels heavy and you must work harder to reach the surface. But the higher up you swim, the less water pressure, and the easier your effort—which is fortunate, because by that time you're desperate for air.

One thing for sure, as you push your limits and stay underwater longer, you'll feel invincible.

But if you get too good at this exercise, if you blackout before reaching the surface, you won't feel anything ever again.

Alcohol, Alcoholism and Surfing

In the Drink

$\mathcal{D}$r. *Geoff saith:*

Let me offer a very clear warning: ALCOHOL AND SURFING DO NOT MIX.

The following facts need to be seriously considered:

● *Up to one-half of fatal drownings are alcohol-related.*

● *Alcohol is not a stimulant in terms of the central nervous system. In fact, it slows down or depresses electrical activity within the brain. So even though you might feel amped up, brain reflexes are in fact slowed down.*

● *The major effect of slowing down various brain reflexes is a reduced ability of the body to reflexly deal with unexpected situations or emergencies.*

● *These effects start to occur at blood alcohol levels (BAL) of 0.02, which is equivalent to about two glasses of beer in one hour, and dramatically increases at levels of 0.05 (three to four beers in one hour).*

● *0.05 is the level at which you will be arrested if you drive in New South Wales (it's 0.08 in California).*

● *Sudden cold water immersion after use of alcohol can alter body chemistry so much as to cause sudden death.*

I.D.ing ALCOHOLISM

There are differences among drinkers: the way they drink, the amount they drink, the length of time spent drinking, how often they drink, who they drink with, and what happens to them when they drink. Alcoholism is not a clear-cut disease entity. Among surfers there is a high incidence of problem drinking. How many surfers develop full-blown alcoholism is unknown. Surfer's drinking patterns (not to be confused with Surfaholics) place them at high risk for alcoholism and alcohol-related problems, such as falling off cliffs and auto accidents.

Probable alcoholism can be identified by truthfully answering the following "CAGE" questions (the more "yeses," the more probable):

1. Have you ever thought you should <u>C</u>ut down on your drinking?

2. Are you ever <u>A</u>nnoyed at others' complaints about your drinking?

3. Do you ever feel <u>G</u>uilty about your drinking?

4. Do you ever take morning "<u>E</u>ye openers"?

These are all symptoms of alcoholism.

Alcoholism is not defined only by quantities of alcohol consumed but by drinking patterns, development of tolerance, dependence, illness, and disruption of social functioning (such as fights and auto accidents). Alcoholism is not confined to skid-row people or to old folks. Teenage alcoholism is a major health concern.

Let me offer a very clear warning: ALCOHOL AND SURFING DO NOT MIX.

Alcohol, Alcoholism and Surfing

Alcohol is the major contributing factor in the cause of auto accidents. The highest rate of auto accidents is in the 15 to 24-year-old age group. High blood alcohol levels are found in more than half of all fatally injured drivers.

If you think you may have a drinking problem, chances are there's a local surfer who has been in recovery and can best assist you in getting some help and information. Seek him or her out and ask for help.

Another invaluable resource is the worldwide organization, Alcoholics Anonymous—better known as AA. Calling AA can be the first step to recovery. They will give you information on group meetings in every city, every day of the week. There are probably AA meetings just for surfers in some cities, as there are for doctors, gays, non-smokers, Spanish speakers, etc. If you yourself are not an alcoholic, but your parents are or you are involved with an alcoholic in any way, ALANON groups can give information and support. They will also be listed in any phone book, along with AA.

Why do you think Budweiser and the other alcohol companies like to sponsor California surf contests? Do you think it's because of their love of surfing? Or, is it to make the surfer wannabes think that drinking is healthy, just like the ocean and surfing. We've been had.

Alcohol and Memory

Gaily-Coloured Underthings

Dear DOCTOR WHATSISNAME,

I have a serious complaint that has been plaguing me for I can't remember how long. It is a constant source of annoyance to me and is threatening to befriend me with the lower echelons of society. My complaint is one of amnesia. Not your typical all-encompassing case of amnesia (I still have a 50% chance of remembering my name). Rather, mine is a periodical ailment affecting me unfailingly on Friday night and lasting approximately the weekend. Come Monday, I cannot recall out of the groggy reaches of my brain what, where, when, how, who or even how many has happened to me over the last two days.

A similar condition befuddles numerous acquaintances of mine who smile at my shoulder and say "Yoboyotty" almost at random.

However these people claim amnesia for mere twelve hour periods, invariably on a Friday or Saturday night. My only clues as to my movements over the weekends are my fetid, beer-stained clothes and the gaily-coloured undergarments that festoon my bedroom.

Please help me doc. I can't remember a bloody thing! On Mondays as I rejoin society I am left with a gaping hole where Saturday should have been and once again the question echoes through my skull: "Who owns the gaily-coloured underpants?" I've tried everything, even journeying north to the celibate guru's abode and there had vague recollections of an idyllic place called "The Hoey-Moey." But alas, on returning to the city, my weekends seem to elude me once again, and always the gaily-coloured under-things encroach on my personal freedom.

Alcohol and Memory

I would be pleased if you could prescribe something for my malady (a school girl taken twice daily with a little wine would be nice) as I am at my wit's end and awaiting your reply not only for my sake but for the sake of my peers.

My God, who owns the gaily-colored underthings!

D. VIATE
Coogee, New South Wales

██████||||

Dear Viate,

Recently, (and much against my better judgment) I joined the upper echelons of Newcastle society at the Mayfield (kind of equivalent to Redfern) Rugby Club at a smoko night. I met some most interesting people, in particular one person who, without a word of a lie looked like Yoda *(The Empire Strikes Back).*

This person was able to put away formidable amounts of alcohol with seemingly little effect. During the course of the night, I observed his various behavior patterns and also spoke to him at great length (mainly because he was a most interesting person). Towards the end of the night he pulled a small notebook from out of his hip pocket and read it. I asked what it was for and he said that it was a list of things he had to do the next day. After asking him if I could look at this book, I saw that in fact he had an incredible planning diary for every day. It listed all times, names, events, e.g., starting at 6:00 A.M. he had to pick up a number of people whose first names appeared in the diary together with a specific time. Later on in the day he had to catch a plane and the flight number, etc., was all there.

Now this technique is of course the standard one which those of us dealing with head injuries often teach patients to use when they have significant memory problems. The very sad part about most people who drink heavily is that they do not realize the gradual and insidious damage they do to various parts of their brain.

For practical purposes, the most easily identifiable problem which heavy drinkers have is "losing their memory." This is due to acute damage to an important area of the brain which lays down memory. The effect of this damage is that new memories are not layed down.

"The very sad part about most people who drink heavily is that they do not realize the gradual and insidious damage they do to various parts of their brain."

Probably of even more importance, but generally not recognized by doctors, is the damage done to the front part of the brain (frontal lobes) by alcohol. The frontal lobes are the highest center of evolutionary development and man arguably has the most highly developed frontal lobes of all living organisms (on earth at least).

This part of the brain is responsible for the formation of "stable plans and intentions capable of controlling subsequent conscious behavior."

What this essentially means is that our day-to-day planning, adjustment to change, new ideas, original thoughts, whether to go surfing at Angourie or Wreck Bay, is all related to whether our frontal lobes are intact or not.

Unfortunately, it is now being shown that alcohol permanently effects (unfortunately at a very early age) this important part of the brain. The end result being a mindless not very old vegetable essentially unresponsive to the environment or unable to adjust to it.

We've all seen just those types hanging out at the beach, or worse, out in the lineup, many wearing gaily-coloured undergarments.

Allergies

Snotty Surfers

Dear SURF DOCS,

My nose is always running these days, and I think I have an allergy. My question is what is an allergy, what causes it, and what can I do about it?

SNOTMAN
Orange County, California

▪▪▪▪▪▪▫▫▫▫

Dear Snotman,

One of our SMA consultants, Dr. Eliot Light, a family physician in Monterey, California, has a hypoallergenic reply for you.

Allergy, what is it, are they? What do they mean? Will they shorten my life? Will they go away? Excuse me while I blow my nose . . .

From a pain in the ass, to life threatening, allergies and allergic reactions

are extremely common conditions that affect certain persons when they are exposed to certain substances that are:

● *breathed in*

● *eaten*

● *injected*

● *touch the skin or mucous membranes*

Briefly, when the body experiences certain things that the body sees as foreign, the body produces *antibodies* or foreign-substance-fighting proteins that are produced to fight off the offending substance. This is good when the foreign thing is a virus or bacteria (which make you feel sick), but is a drag when it's your dog, Spot, or the wax on your surfboard.

All people have many of these little battles going on at any one time. Some people, however, put up a *big* battle— the people who have "allergies."

19

Allergic reactions, mild and severe, can include:

● *"Hayfever" (sinuses), with runny nose, sneezing, itchy or burning nose and eyes*

● *A wonderworld of rashes ranging from itchy and/or red skin to hives and eczema (a scaly, often reddish, possibly itchy patchy rash)*

● *Throat irritation or swelling; asthma, with difficulty breathing, coughing, wheezing*

● *Allergic shock (called anaphylactic shock), which can kill you (e.g., from a bee sting or allergy to penicillin)*

● *Diarrhea and other intestinal symptoms (especially in children)*

Some allergies are obvious, for instance violent sneezing and itchy eyes whenever a cat walks into the room. Others are subtle, their origins never fully known. Here's what you can do if you think you have allergies or have been diagnosed as having them.

WHAT TO DO

Become a detective. When you get symptoms, note where you are, what (or who . . .) is around. See if you can find a consistent trigger. Does it only happen at work, in a particular room, at one surf spot, but not another, a certain time of the year, or from one food?

Suspect an allergy if you have an illness that just won't go away. Symptoms that may mean allergy are frequent sneezing; stuffy, runny nose; watery, itchy eyes; sinus trouble; asthma; unexpected skin rashes; hives; headaches; earaches; coughing; dizziness; diarrhea; constipation; stomach ache; gas pains; or possibly frequent unexplained fatigue, depression, or mental problems.

As for specific allergies more common to surfers, the frontrunners are resins, catalysts, wax additives, and wetsuit materials causing contact allergy, usually a skin rash; or inhaled substances such as resin fumes and various particulates, including molds, in closed spaces like shaping rooms, surf shops, and especially cars that get cleaned every 12 months (or never).

Recent research indicates that respiratory allergies may actually be triggered by bacteria and molds growing in air conditioners, humidifiers, and drip pans of refrigerators. Clean these frequently and use a germicide.

A doctor can help identify environmental triggers. Certain skin and blood tests may help establish allergy as a diagnosis. Allergy specialists may test by adding small amounts of the *antigen* (the stuff that bugs you) and watching the reaction. Skin testing is done by scratching the surface of the skin under which a drop of the suspected substance is placed, and watching for redness and swelling. This has been shown to be somewhat accurate for molds, grasses, animals and pollens. Claims of accuracy for foods and other substances have yet to be substantiated. Don't be taken in by advertisements claiming to test your blood for all sorts of food allergies—medical research is spotty in that field.

Unless you have allergies, antihistamines are useless—don't take them for a cold.

TREATMENT

If you can't avoid or eliminate the trigger, one of the following may help.

Antihistamines

These medicines block effects of histamine and possibly other substances released by the activated cells that cause inflammation, itching and the watery stuff that comes from your nose and eyes. Most antihistamines are somewhat sedating, which is a polite way of saying that you may feel like you're strapped to a hammock on Venus. It is not usually described as a pleasurable downer sensation. Newer ones, available only with a prescription, have less of these effects but aren't always as effective.

There are many over-the-counter antihistamines to choose from, generally containing chemical names like chlorophene, triprolidine, or chloropheniramine maleate. The usual dose of these substances is 4 to 6 mgs, taken every 6 to 12 hours (but every person is different, requiring more or less.) They are not addicting, but at higher doses can interfere with physical functioning.

Many products add pseudoephedrine, a caffeine/adrenalin-like drug which counters the drowsiness from the antihistamines and shrinks mucous membranes. The usual dose of pseudoephedrine (Sudafed®) is 30 to 60 mg every 6 to 8 hours. Avoid combination drugs with aspirin, Tylenol®, decongestants, or other additives. These combination drugs cost more and clutter up your body. Unless you have allergies, antihistamines are useless—don't take them for a cold.

Topical (to put on skin) and Inhaled "Steroids" or "Cortisone"

Cortisone, a steriod, works at several sites to stop the allergic response and is available in topical form. This means that instead of taking them orally (prescription only—see below), they are applied directly to the problem area, the most common over-the-counter ones contain 0.5 to 1.0% hydrocortisone. There are forms that are inhaled through the nose for nasal allergies, drops for eyes, orally inhaled steroids for asthma, in addition to creams, ointments and lotions for the skin.

Cromolyn

Available largely as a spray or to be inhaled, this type of medicine can be very effective, and offers the distinct advantage of being almost devoid of side effects. They are definitely worth a try. They *prevent* allergy.

Oral or Injected Steroids

In severe allergic problems the only recourse is the "big guns." They are highly effective and are generally safe, but be sure to ask the doctor about potential side effects. The prescription tablets should only be taken for extreme allergic reactions, at the lowest dose possible, for the shortest period of time.

Foods and Nutrition

The universal symptoms of food allergy are *water retention* in the body: puffy eyes and face, and in women, their thighs. There are no nutritional supplements that have been definitely shown to alter the allergic response. There is, however, evidence that several types of oils and fatty acids may be helpful: fish oils such as cod liver oil contain substances called Omega-3 fatty acids which may alter some of the inflammatory substances involved. The same is true with evening primrose oil. They may be especially important in skin allergies and are worth a try.

Ankles

Benders and Sprains

Dear DOC,

You see, doc, my problem is my ankle, I keep tearing the same ligaments time and time again. Each time I do this is more severe than the previous time. I want to strengthen my ankle and prevent this half-yearly event from happening so easily. I can't get physio-therapy because I'm "doing time," and as long as I can walk, I'm OK by the docs in here (they don't doubt I need physio-treatment at the same time). Doc, is there something I can do along the lines of strengthening exercises myself, or am I doomed to this problem until I finish this sentence and get to the specialist and salt water to heal me?

MARK LEONARD
Goulburn, New South Wales

▮▮▮▮▮▮|||||

Dear Mark,

Firstly, it is important to figure out the cause (if possible) of consistently straining the one ankle.

Perhaps there are neurological reasons, such as a weaker leg on that side. Perhaps one leg is longer than the other. There are other reasons which should also be checked out.

Secondly, you are correct in that with each successive injury you *do* "weaken" the ankle. This is because the torn ligaments, instead of being made of nice healthy fibro-elastic material with plenty of proprioceptive (nervous system message to the brain to tell it where that part of the body is at the moment) feed-back to the protective muscles, become thickened with scar tissue which is less elastic and in which there are less proprioceptive nerve fibers.

Even without the benefits of a physiotherapist, you can undertake the following exercises which will help:

23

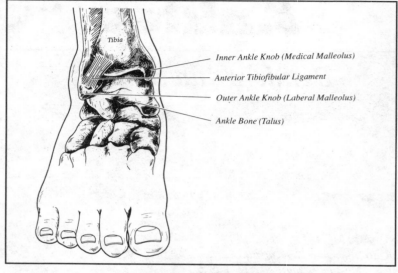

Tibia

Inner Ankle Knob (Medical Malleolus)

Anterior Tibiofibular Ligament

Outer Ankle Knob (Laberal Malleolus)

Ankle Bone (Talus)

Anatomy of the Ankle

● **Proprioceptive retraining:** This uses a balance board which could easily be constructed from a piece of wood fitted with a curved rocker bottom. By standing on either edge of the curve, practice keeping your balance and gently rock the board from side to side.

● **Isometric ankle exercises:** Stand with the outer border of your crook foot against an immovable object. Practice pushing the border of this foot against this object as if to push it over. Start off holding this push for 5 seconds and repeat 5 times (both ankles). Gradually build up to 10 seconds, hold and do 10 repeats.

● **Heel chord stretches:** Stand out from a wall so that your fingertips just touch that wall. Then put your palms flat on the wall, keeping your feet in the same position, and commence performing pushups into the wall. You will feel the heel chord and calf muscle stretch if you keep your legs and back still and straight.

Another way to do this is to stand on the edge of a step so that your heel stretches below the level of your toes.

Ankles: Benders and Sprains

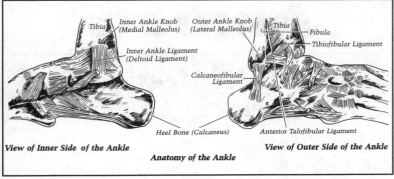

View of Inner Side of the Ankle

Tibia — Inner Ankle Knob (Medial Malleolus)

Inner Ankle Ligament (Deltoid Ligament)

Outer Ankle Knob (Lateral Malleolus)

Tibia — Fibula — Tibiofibular Ligament

Calcaneofibular Ligament

Heel Bone (Calcaneus)

Anterior Talofibular Ligament

View of Outer Side of the Ankle

Anatomy of the Ankle

● **Leg exercises***: Toe raises and heel walking are the two best forms of exercise.*

Toe raises *are commenced using body weight and standing on both feet. Perform 25 repetitions.*

When able to do this without difficulty, go to undertaking the same exercise but using one leg at a time. The final step is to do this exercise whilst carrying graded weights.

Heel walking *is undertaken keeping your toes off the ground and taking short "choppy" steps. Walk a distance of 30 meters (about 32 yards). When able to do this without difficulty, progress to walking on inclines and then using graded weights.*

If your ankle swells up, the use of ice can be undertaken. This needs to stay in place for around 15 to 20 minutes.

Bandaging can be used in the acute phase but this is probably not advisable in the chronic phase especially in ordinary circumstances. Athletic-type taping (including properly applied duct tape) or braces can be used in circumstances in which you know you will face some type of problem (e.g., surf over rough or uneven water (chop), etc.).

Anxiety

Big Surf is Measured in Increments of Excrement

Dear SURF DOCS,

Why is it that every time I get to the surf, while waxing up my stick and admiring the surge upon the reef, the one feeling that always comes over me is the urge to pinch a loaf?

RASCLOTT "THE BAKER"
Virgin Islands

■■■■■III|||

Dear Rasclott,

At a recent Surfer's Medical Association conference on Tavarua, Fiji, our group awoke one dawn to humongous, life-threatening looking surf, and before the sun had even risen, all the toilets were stopped up. And that wasn't the end of it. Out in the water, after the first set steam-rolled our whole group, one guy paddled quite a lot further outside than anyone else, rolled off his board, and acted like he was checking out his leash. But we all knew what was going on—that expression "shitting bricks" had come home to roost.

Part of the fight or flight response in all animals (including us) is that there is a massive outpouring of adrenalin, which hops up all body processes: heart rate, breathing, thinking, and shitting, to name a few. It's reasoned that, to fully be able to fight (or escape), your body needs to be lightened of its' load. So out it comes.

Perfectly natural, Rasclott. Try frequenting your toilet before heading down to the beach, unless you want to hold it in and truly enjoy your animal instincts.

Anxiety

Pre-Surf Jitters

Dear SURF DOCS,

I am a skateboarder who tried surfing last summer. Since then I've fallen in love with the sport/art. Although I'm not very good yet, I have tons of fun every time I go out. The problem is my nerves.

From the moment I wake up to the moment I get in the water, I feel sick. I get all jittery and nauseous, sometimes even vomiting one or two times. I always end up surfing on an empty stomach. The strange thing is, as soon as I start paddling out I feel great—amped up and ready to catch my first wave of the day.

My theory is that I'm so excited to go surfing my nerves can't handle it (I live an hour and a half away from the beach, so I can only go surfing three or four times a month.) Is there some kind of drug that could safely calm my nervous system? If not, is there anything else I can do? I really appreciate your help.

NEIL
San Francisco Bay Area

■ ■ ■ ■ ■ ||||||

Dear Neil,

We think your theory is absolutely correct. You're experiencing what psychologists call "anticipatory anxiety." In surfing terms, it's a case of pre-go-out psych-out. You are not alone in this. Most surfers, and, in fact, most all other athletes, frequently suffer from it.

So, what to do? Medications are rarely needed. Gaining insight and finding better ways to harness your mental energies is the answer.

Despite surfing's seemingly simple and laid-back nature, it is an incredibly complex and stressful activity. We're not talking about life-threatening giant Waimea or Pipeline—something that 99% of surfers will never deal with. And we're not talking about what the non-surfing world imagines are the dangers of surfing, drowning and shark-attacks—which, again, are exceedingly rare.

We're talking about the subtle and real stresses of surfing, many of which are peer-pressure related, and heightened for beginning and young surfers. These include worrying about how you'll look when you're surfing (from style down to the look of your wetsuit and board). Or worrying that by the time you get to the beach the swell will be gone or it will be onshore, and your friends will tell you that "you really missed it." Or, for a place like San Francisco, that you'll arrive to find that it's so big and gnarly that you chicken out (again, something made all the worse by being with friends—especially if they go out and you don't). Aside from the peer pressures of the sport, some surfers feel guilty . . . like they're "frittering their lives away" surfing . . . thinking, perhaps, they should instead be studying, working, or whatever. And there are thousands of other things to get anxious about as you head for the beach.

Unfortunately, you have a long drive to the beach—a lot of time in which to psych yourself out. Living closer to the beach would probably help a lot, but short of moving, here are some suggestions for psyching yourself up in a totally positive way:

● *First, when you're thinking about what the surf is going to be like or how you're going to perform,* *focus on remembering a recent go-out that went really well. Picture yourself feeling confident, paddling out in a strong manner, riding well, and think about how good you felt afterward. Play those memories over again and again, especially when you feel negative thoughts creeping in. As for worrying about the surf, if you've gotten a report that the swell is giant, begin thinking about a beach you can go to where you'll be able to handle it— don't even entertain the thought of trying to ride the hairiest, biggest spot.*

● *Practice simple relaxation methods, such as controlling your breathing. When you feel yourself psyching-out, try counting how many times per minute you're breathing. It will probably be upwards of 15 or more times per minute. Then begin slowing your breathing by taking longer and deeper breaths. Do it yoga style. Use your stomach muscles as you take air in. Pause at the top of your breath. Slowly release your air, and pause when it's all out. Get yourself back down to under 12 breaths per minute and you'll definitely feel more relaxed.*

● *Drive slower and more carefully. Surfers on the way to the surf are notoriously bad drivers, and you're going to be a real road haz-*

ard if your mind is occupied with a lot of negative thoughts. On the other hand, concentrating on driving safely and achieving superior control of your car will make you feel good, thus relaxing you.

● The way you eat and how much exercise you get can make a big difference. If you're eating well and working out (i.e., swimming, running, cycling, or surfing three or four times per week), you'll feel more confident about yourself, and be fit and ready for anything.

● Watch out for caffeine—coffee, tea, chocolate, most soft drinks. They can set off or worsen your psych-outs. Drugs like cigarettes or cocaine absolutely should be avoided. Their use alone can set off anxiety. Alcohol and marijuana will take the edge off of stress and anxiety (which is why most people use them), but then you're left with their less desirable effects: slowed thinking, impaired memory, and clumsiness. These same effects occur with prescribed anti-anxiety medications, such as Valium—and they're usually quite costly. All drug treatments for anxiety are imperfect solutions.

The keys to your dilemma are insight and confidence, Neil, which put you *in control*—control is where it's at when it comes to preventing anxiety.

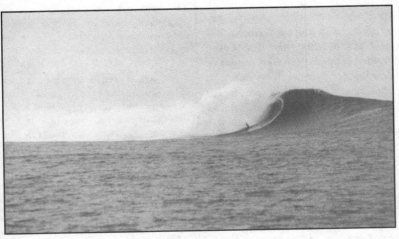

Dr. Renneker surfing 15-20 foot Cloudbreak, alone. Not a good time for the jitters. *Beach Photos.*

Arthritis: Aching Joints

The Courage to Paddle Out

Dear SURF DOCS,

I am 18-years-old and a victim of rheumatoid arthritis. For the past four years my physical condition has been going rapidly downhill. I was forced to stop all sports due to the severe pain and stiffness that I encountered. The affected areas included my ankles, knees, wrists and shoulders. The disease had progressed to quite a serious state, and the doctors said if I wasn't treated immediately there might be irreparable damage to my joints. At that time, which was in late June, I began gold injections, and I'm now happy to say that I have taken a turn for the better.

I am presently more mobile than I've been in a year, and I'm wondering if it would be okay if I tried to surf? I will, of course, ask my own rheumatologist this question, but I just wanted to get an opinion from a source close to the sport.

Thank you for making this option a possibility.

PER
Northern California

▌▌▌▌▌▌||||

Dear Per,

Your letter was the first we received after making the offer to answer surfers' health questions, and your letter alone makes it all worthwhile.

What you have is not the garden variety of arthritis that accompanies aging. A severe and often crippling disease, rheumatoid arthritis is when the body's immune system attacks the surfaces of joints, making joint motion very painful. Gold injections reduce the joint irritation, and are only useful for severe forms of arthritis.

Surfing may actually improve your arthritis (swimming is highly recommended for arthritis). Discuss your plans with your arthritis specialist

30

Arthritis: Aching Joints

(rheumatologist), but we say go for it—start surfing.

The first step is for you to get back in shape. Fitness and flexibility will be the most crucial elements of your surfing campaign. Build up gradually, though—over three to six months, maybe longer. Begin by swimming laps, with and without a bodyboard, and increasing the distance. You'll need to find your own ways to limber up your joints, but remember that you should be especially strong and flexible to make up for lost joint motion.

When you feel fit and strong, head out to the ocean. Start in calm water, then go out into the surf as your confidence increases. Pick a small, gentle wave. Work up to bigger surf when you feel ready. Work on developing a smooth, graceful style and avoid twisting, bone-crunching maneuvers. Consider kicking out early to avoid wiping out and hitting the bottom. Choose a board big enough to paddle easily, small enough to carry comfortably, and not so wide that it requires an unnatural shoulder motion to paddle.

Your joints will be less painful if you keep them warm. Wear a good quality, full wetsuit and booties. Come in if you get cold, don't try to tough it out. Expect some pain, but if your joint pains worsen you may have to stop. You know your condition best. Go gradually, and use common sense.

The SMA recommends that surfers become experts in their own health

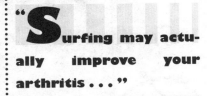

"**S**urfing may actually improve your arthritis . . ."

problems. The Arthritis Foundation (1314 Spring Street, NW, Atlanta, Georgia 30309, 404/872-7100; Arthritis Foundation of NSW, 66 Kippax Street, Surry Hills, NSW, 2010) is a good resource, and has a program called PACE—People with Arthritis Can Exercise. You could be their first (and best) surfer. Also, consider joining the Disabled Surfers' Association (P.O. Box A14, Enfield South, 2133, NSW, Australia), an Australia-based worldwide organization dedicated to helping surfers with disabilities keep surfing.

Per, your courage—in the face of what can be a terrible disease—is an inspiration to us all.

Asthma
Surfing as Cause and Cure

Dr. Geoff saith:

Surfing and asthma are compatible provided the surfer:

● *Understands his/her asthma*

● *Learns about his/her body's response to asthma*

● *Realizes that one "cause" of asthma is in fact exercise-induced asthma (EIA)*

ASTHMA

Asthma is defined as "hyperresponsiveness of airways to noxious stimuli."

In other words, various "irritants" float into the lungs via the air we breathe, land on the surface of the lung's airway tube (bronchi and bronchioles) and set up an irritative/inflammatory response which ultimately leads to spasm and narrowing of these airway tubes. This occurs in susceptible people, namely those with asthma.

"Irritants" include: air pollutants (sulphur dioxide and tobacco smoke), chemicals (including isocyanates such as those used in the surf industry), allergens (house dust, mites, pollens and animal dander), and changes in air temperature and humidity.

Asthma affects about 7-10% of people, most often in childhood. The number of people who surf and suffer asthma is not known. Dr. Geoff's disability survey showed that there was at least one person who contracted asthma and could no longer surf.

Similarly, the numbers of asthmatic surfers who actually develop EIA is not known.

Asthma

In the past, kids with asthma were not encouraged to play sports. Unfortunately, this led to a loss of general fitness, which in turn had its bad effects on the asthma sufferer. Nowadays fitness via sport is encouraged. In other words, it is important to be fit so that the heart and lungs can work efficiently to get oxygen from the air, get it into the blood stream via the lungs and, by pumping of the heart, deliver the oxygen into the exercising muscles.

With asthma, the airway tubes are narrowed and air (containing oxygen) can't move in *and especially out*, properly. A build-up of air occurs in the lungs. The air is actually trapped in the lungs, with greatly reduced turnover of new air and therefore very little new oxygen. There is less oxygen to get to the blood stream and therefore passed to the muscles. The muscles no longer work efficiently (from the aerobic point of view). The heart tries to pump harder. After a while the affected surfer feels distressed with wheezing, coughing, breathlessness, tightness in the chest, as well as a general tiredness and faint feeling.

Although tremendous gains have been made in the understanding and treatment of asthma, it is not a disease to be taken lightly. Today kids (and all asthmatic sufferers) have their "puffers" (inhalers) which deliver various chemicals directly to the linings of the lung airways. These puffers have been a tremendous help in allowing asthma sufferers greater freedom.

In general these puffers:

● *Prevent "irritable mast cells" from bursting open and releasing packets of chemicals. These chemicals (particularly histamine) act as irritants, causing swelling of the cell lining the breathing tubes as well as spasm of the muscles around the breathing tubes. The net effect is narrowing of the diameter of these tubes.*

Sodium Cromoglycate (called cromolyn or Intal®) is the chemical which "coats" the mast cells and stops them from bursting open and releasing histamine (as well as other chemicals).

● *Relax the tight muscles around the airways and allow the airways to "open up."*

These broncho-dilator aerosols contain chemicals similar to (but much more selectively-acting than) adrenalin. They act only on special chemical receptors found on smooth muscles encircling the airway tubes. (These chemicals stimulate the B2-adrenergic receptors causing the muscle to relax.) A number of different groups of these drugs are available. Selectivity of action, length of action and differing side effects provide a greater variety of treatment for different people. Commonly used B2 inhalers in Australia include Berotec, Bricanyl and Ventolin, and in the U.S., Alupent, Proventyl, and Ventolin.

● *Help to quiet down or reduce the effects of the inflammatory response. These are the aerosol steroids with brandnames like Aldecin and Berotide in Australia, and Azmacort in the U.S.*

Compelling research, largely from New Zealand, supports the idea of using steroid puffers over B2 puffers.

All asthmatic sufferers should make it their priority to work with their medical practitioner in developing the best possible treatment regime. This allows greatly improved quality of life with far less, if any, restrictions.

Mini-Wright peak flow meters for personal use are now available. This means the asthma sufferer can actually measure his/her degree of bronchial constriction. You can puff into the machine and see just how well your lungs are working. In turn this can help you to monitor how you feel against how well your lungs are actually working. It also shows you how well your aerosol sprayers (puffers) are working in controlling an attack of asthma. Nonetheless, even with this method, you must still not become complacent.

The Asthma Foundation of NSW, (Garden Mews, 82-86 Pacific Highway, St. Leonards, 2065, (02) 906-3233) is an excellent source of assistance to asthma sufferers (especially children) and their families. They provide various swimming programs, seminars, and disperse up-to-date information on the latest asthma management. In the U.S., contact: The Asthma and Allergy Foundation of America (1125 - 15th Street, NW, Washington DC 20005, 202-466-7643) or your local chapter of the American Lung Association.

EXERCISE INDUCED ASTHMA (EIA)

Probably about 80% of asthmatics at some time will have an attack of asthma during or after exercise.

This principally appears to be due to loss of water and heat from the airway tubes in the lungs. This occurs during exercise.

Asthma

You can observe the effect of this water and heat loss by standing in front of a mirror on a cold day after doing a few exercises and puffing deeply onto the glass. The mirror becomes "fogged up." Warm humidified air is being blown out from deep in your lungs and condenses on the glass.

When exercising, you need more air (oxygen). To supply this, your breathing becomes deeper and faster. Instead of breathing in and out between 5 and 10 liters of air per minute at rest, you now breathe between 50 and 100 liters of air per minute while exercising.

Air heating and humidification occurs mainly in the nose. When exercising you tend to breathe more through the mouth and the nasal humidification effect is lost (or at least greatly reduced). So not only are you breathing 10 times more air per minute, you are also not able to humidify (heat it and add water) as efficiently.

As a result the deeper airway tubes (bronchi and bronchioles) have to act as the air humidifiers. As a consequence they lose water and heat and the cells lining these tubes become "dry and cold." This makes them more susceptible to irritants in the air. In those unfortunate susceptible people, inhaling various irritants deep into the lungs leads to an attack of EIA.

The severity of such an attack depends a lot on:

● *How fit you are*

● *The temperature of the air and how moist it is (cold, dry air is particularly potent in cooling and drying the airways)*

● *How long and hard you've been exercising (the longer and harder the exercise, the more air is breathed in and out and therefore the drier the lungs become)*

● *The interval since your last attack of EIA*

Undoubtedly, surfing is a good sport from the point of view of being in a "moist" environment. Nonetheless, taking into account the factors above, there are problems such as:

● *Cold, dry winds—particularly in winter*

● *Offshore winds during the "hayfever" season (when lots of allergens are in the air)*

● *The need to sometimes have to paddle hard for long periods of time (particularly in big surf)*

● *The problems of being in a hypertonic (salty) environment*

In some people, breathing in air with a lot of salt can actually precipitate an attack of asthma itself. (As an interesting aside, this is used as a provocational test by the Navy to see whether its divers are susceptible to the problem). In surfing, especially after being buried by a heavy wipeout, it is possible to irritate the back of the throat (and in theory the lungs) with salt spray/foam.

How You Can Prevent an Attack of EIA from Coming on While Surfing

While it is not possible to guarantee that you won't get an attack of asthma or EIA while surfing, the following regime will at least significantly reduce the risks.

● *Surf regularly and keep up regular exercising (swimming, push-bike riding, jogging, although each of these activities themselves can cause EIA).*

● *Try and get into the habit of breathing through your nose more deeply during exercise. Make sure your nose is clear before exercise. Nasal steroids and cromolyn may prevent the nose from becoming blocked. Drixine or Tobi Spray (in Australia) or Afrin® (in the U.S.) will quickly open up an already blocked nose.*

● *Don't smoke (cigs, dope, or whatever) or inhale nonprescribed "stimulants" (petrol, coke, spray cans, etc.). As readers of Dr. Geoff's column know, these "don'ts" apply to everyone whether they have asthma or not.*

● *If you know from experience you're going to get EIA during a surf session, use your puffer beforehand. It's not possible to give an exact regime but in general terms: take two deep inhalations (puffs) of your bronchodilator aerosol (whichever you'd normally use, be it Bentolin, Berotec, etc.)*

or 2 to 4 inhalations of Intal or both. If you need to take both then take them in the order broncho-dilator first, Intal some 5 to 10 minutes later.

Remember Intal "coats" the mast cell and broncho-dilator aerosols keep the smooth muscle of the airway tubes relaxed. Some people only need Intal before exercise. Others only need a broncho-dilator. Some need both. You'll have to find out by trial and error.

Note that aerosol puffers must be taken immediately before exercise. If it's been 45 to 60 minutes since your last spray and you're going out for another session, you'll need to take a further dose of appropriate aerosol.

If you're already wheezy and want to surf, take two puffs of your broncho-dilator aerosol immediately before that session.

Try and regulate your surf sessions with your regular aerosol inhalation. Most people take their aerosols 4 to 6 times a day so it shouldn't be too hard to get 3 to 4 surf sessions to correspond with your regular aerosol inhalations.

Always take your broncho-dilator aerosol puffer out with you when you surf. Put it up your wetsuit sleeve or leg or sew in a suitable "pocket" (that won't rip open during a wipeout) into either your board shorts or wetsuit.

A controversial suggestion is that if you regularly have attacks of EIA, consider undertaking a 30 second sprint, 5 to 7 times with only short 15 second rests between each sprint. Do this 40 minutes before you go surfing. It may bring on an attack of EIA. Interestingly, about 50% or so of persons suffering EIA will "wear out" the response for a further attack for varying periods. However, the other 50% won't wear out the response. There is no way of really telling. However, it's an interesting concept and one worthwhile considering if you're a bit of an experimenter and you've got your own doc's okay.

What to Do if an Attack of EIA Occurs While Surfing

For safety, it is probably best to stop your session and paddle into shore (or boat).

Take one puff of your broncho-dilator aerosol. Wait 2 to 5 minutes and take another puff. Then paddle in slowly (if appropriate to the surf conditions). By waiting, the first puff will have helped to "open up" the airways and will allow the second puff to get deeper into the lungs.

Severe episodes of EIA could require 3 to 4 puffs of broncho-dilator. If you've stopped exercising, and have taken your puffer and still feel "breathless" after 20 minutes, it's best to seek medical help.

In general terms, if you are finding that in time your attacks of asthma and EIA are still difficult to control, the regular use of aerosol steroids (Becotide and Aldecin) can help make your other sprays work more effectively. Aerosol steroids *cannot* be used as a *pre-exercise* EIA blocker. They just *don't* work by this method.

If problems are still occurring despite all of this, you should discuss with your doctor referral to a Pulmonary Function or Respiratory Laboratory for more sophisticated lung function tests. It will help in working out a more effective regime of asthma management.

SURFING TO HELP ASTHMA

One of our SMA members, Brian Lowdon, participated in a fascinating study of teaching asthmatic children how to surf. The results: improved asthma, probably relating to their having gained still greater control over their breathing.

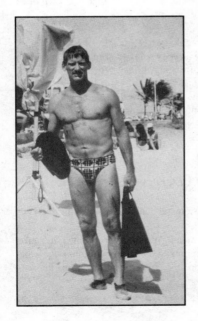

You need a good set of lungs to body-surf. A few scratches won't affect your breathing. Magic Mike, Oahu. *Photo courtesy of Dumpster Pete.*

Backs

Everything a Surfer Needs to Know

*D*rs. *Geoff* and *Renneker* (fellow back-suf-fers) saith:

Death, taxes and back pain are some of life's little unavoidable realities. Consider some interesting facts about back ailments:

● *90% of westernized industrial people (i.e., virtually all surfers) will experience at least one attack of back pain in their lifetime.*

● *Men and women are affected about equally.*

● *The great majority of back sufferers will get better in a short time (several days to several weeks).*

● *There are at least 30 different groups of people treating back ailments. Included are various physicians' groups, general practitioners, orthopedists, neurologists, neurosurgeons, osteopaths, physiatrists (physical medicine and rehabilitation specialists), rheumatologists; chiropractic groups, (of differing philosophies and techniques); as well as physical therapists, acupuncturists, naturopaths, posture and yoga teachers, rolfers, shiatsu therapists, cranial-sacral practitioners, and other body workers; and there are faith healers and many others. Differing philosophies and treatments abound. In the main, though, most sufferers get better regardless of which therapist treats them. Is it because of, or despite, treatment?*

● *Disc rupture with prolapse ("slipped or herniated disc") is **not** the most common cause of back pain.*

Sick *Surfers* ASK THE SURF DOCS & Dr. GEOFF

● *The richer the population, the greater the number of spinal operations performed. The U.S. has the highest rate of spinal surgery in the world. Interestingly, the coastal strips have the highest rate of surgery, with the west coast ahead of the east coast.*

● *The exact cause of back pain, even in this day and age, is extremely difficult to diagnose with any degree of accuracy.*

While all this controversy rages, the surfer with a back ailment is only interested in one thing: "Can I keep surfing with my bad back?"

Unfortunately, there are many surfers out there with chronic low back pain. In a study on chronic disability among Australian surfers, Dr. Geoff (*Tracks*, August, 1987) found that chronic back pain was the most common cause of disability (time out of water). 30% of the respondents suffered lower back pain. Age range was from 10 to 45 years. However, the good news is that 100% were able to return to surfing—even though 13% had to resort to other forms of surf-riding. Malibu's (longboards) were the surfcraft most commonly used as a vehicle to return to surfing.

The all important questions:

● *How can a surfer prevent himself from getting a bad back?*

● *If a surfer is unlucky enough to get a bad back, how can he get back to surfing and prevent it from ever recurring?*

Read through the following and you'll learn everything a surfer needs to know about backs:

● **Back Anatomy (pg. 41)**

● **Causes of Back Pain (pg. 43)**

● **Emergency Treatment (pg. 44)**

● **Prevention: Testing Yourself (pg. 47)**

● **Prevention: Exercises (pg. 50)**

● **Surfing with Chronic Low Back Pain (pg. 52)**

● **Special Back Tips for Surfers (pg. 53)**

40

BACK ANATOMY

To truly understand how to treat or prevent back problems, you need a basic understanding of the structure and functioning of the back. The "back" is in fact the lower part of the spine. It is called the *lumbar region*. Most people have 5 separate lumbar building blocks (vertebra).

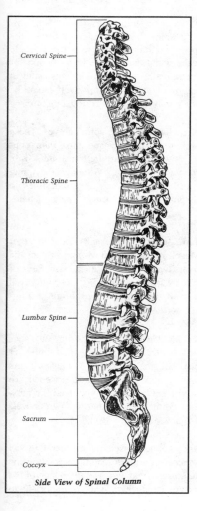

Cervical Spine

Thoracic Spine

Lumbar Spine

Sacrum

Coccyx

Side View of Spinal Column

Between each of these vertebra is a firm, semi-elastic shock absorber called a *disc*. Younger surfers' discs are 80% water. After the age of 25, discs tend to contain less fluid and be "stiffer."

The last lumbar disc (the L5/S1 disc) sits between the last lumbar vertebra (L5) and the sacrum (S1). The sacrum consists of five fused vertebrae without any discs between them. The very end of the sacrum is the coccyx (tailbone). The sacrum is joined to the pelvis on each side via the very strong sacro-iliac joints. The sacro-iliac joints dampen jarring forces from the legs below and body above.

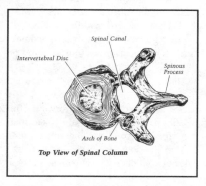

Spinal Canal

Intervertebral Disc

Spinous Process

Arch of Bone

Top View of Spinal Column

Reprinted by permission of The Putnam Publishing Group from *Sports Health* by William Southmayd and Marshall Hoffman. Copyright 1981 by Quickfox.

Behind each lumbar vertebra is an arch of bone, linked by joints to the arch of each vertebra above and below. These joints are called *facet joints*. Facet joints guide the lower back in bending forward (flexion) and backward (extension). Rotation is minimized by the facet joints. This is all to the better. Whereas discs allow a large degree of flexion and extension, they can only tolerate a limited degree of twisting (rotation).

A canal (the spinal canal) is formed by the bony arch of each vertebra. This allows the spinal cord to pass safely down the spine from the brain. However, the spinal cord ends between L1 and L2, (the upper two lumbar vertebrae). Most people who develop acute low back pain imagine the worst, being wheelchair-bound for the rest of their lives. Considering that the great majority of back ailments occur in the lowest part of the lumbar spine (from L3 down), the spinal cord itself cannot be injured, having ended at L1/L2, so lower body paralysis is *not* part of the picture.

Coming off the spinal cord at the level of each vertebra are spinal nerves. These electrical cables transmit signals from the brain to the muscles and make them contract. "Feeling" signals (temperature, touch, position and pain) are transmitted from the skin, muscles and joints via the spinal nerves to the brain. Although the spinal cord ends between L1 and L2, the spinal canal sends off large nerves destined to pass out through lower levels of the lumbar spine and also through 5 pairs of holes in the sacrum.

A complex interlinking of ligaments (short, strong fibrous bands) hold together and protect the joints (facets and discs). Muscles attach to, move and protect the joints and therefore the spine itself. Skin covers and protects all of the structures of the back (from surfboard fins, rocks and coral, for instance). The body is engineered to protect the back: skin absorbs and protects from direct blows, muscles protect ligaments, ligaments protect joints, joints protect bones.

The muscles important to the lower back include more than the obvious ones overlying the lower part of the back. Try to visualize the ways in which the lower back can move—bending forward (flexion), bending backward (extension) and twisting (rotation)—and you'll see that many groups of muscles are needed. To bend forward you need abdominal muscles, to bend backwards you need the muscles up and down the back, and to twist you need the muscles that wrap around the sides of your chest and abdomen and attach to the spine.

Also consider that if one muscle tightens up, another muscle must generally relax and allow itself to be stretched. So, for instance, in a prone paddling position the lower back muscles are tightened up and the muscles that attach to the inside of the spine and extend down through the pelvis are lengthened. This is important to understand because it explains the most common cause of back ache: straining muscles, either by over-tightening them or by over-stretching them.

Rotation seems to be a major source of lumbar disc damage but if the facet joints are sitting in a normal plane, they prevent excessive rotation (torque). Excessive torque can put a lot of stress on facet joints and the bony arch, leading to stress fractures. This condition (called *spondylolysis*) appears to be increasing among younger surfers. The exact reasons are not known but some theorize that shorter, wider-tailed multiple-fin boards demand a faster twisting style, generating more body torque and causing more stress on the lower back.

CAUSES OF BACK PAIN

Pain can arise from the skin, muscles, ligaments, bone, discs and nerves. A deep ache or throb is the most common type of pain experienced. "Stiffness" generally occurs because the muscles in the lower back are in spasm to prevent an injured part of the back from moving. Nature always tries to protect injured parts and muscle spasm is the natural way of immobilizing or splinting.

Irritation of spinal nerves causes a tingling, burning, pins and needles, shooting pain, or numbness down one or both legs. Any one of these symptoms is called *sciatica*. Usually this is felt in the back of the lower leg, great toe or outer part of the foot. Spinal nerves can be irritated in many ways—from being "pinched" by the vertebrae (what chiropractors call a subluxation) or discs, or from being stretched and pressured from swollen tissues around them.

Facet joint injury can also cause low back pain and referred leg pain. Sacro-iliac joint problems may also cause low back and buttock pain.

Muscle strains and sprains are probably the most common cause of low back pain. Most surfers can paddle in a typical prone, head up position for hours without cramping or pain in the lower back muscles—they're well conditioned. However, try holding yourself in a partial sit-up for just five minutes and your abdominal muscles will cramp and ache. Abdominal muscles in many surfers are poorly conditioned.

On the other hand, try sitting on the floor with one or both feet extended out in front of you and reach forward to your toes. Hold that position for as long as you can and keep bending forward—stretching your lower back and hamstring muscles. Then roll over in a prone position and pretend you're paddling. Feel that heavy,

cement-like ache in your lower back. That's from over-stretching the surfers' generally poorly conditioned lower back muscles. Conditioning means more than the
ability of a muscle to contract powerfully—the muscle should also be able to relax
easily and be stretched.

> " . . . the most common
> cause of back ache:
> straining muscles,
> either by over-tighten-
> ing or over-stretching
> them."

Pain can develop in the lower back as a result of a strain of any of the muscles
relating to the lower back. The body is not neurologically sophisticated when it
comes to the lower back. You can feel pain there even if the strained muscle is actually, say, in the butt or hip. Fortunately, muscle strain pain is usually short-lived
(hours to days) and usually just improves with rest (or preferably, light activity or
stretching).

Ligament strains or sprains, however, can lead to longer lasting pain (weeks) and
require an extended period of recovery.

One problem is that, usually, if one region of the back has been injured, the
resulting pain and spasm will immobilize it and force other regions of the back to
assume its function, leading to secondary strain and greater vulnerability to injury.

EMERGENCY TREATMENT

If you are dumped in the surf, land hard on your spine and can't move your legs, it
is best to remain flat. Do not let anyone manipulate you or "try to get you up and
about." Your surfboard could be used as a stretcher, especially in a wilderness surfing emergency. In other cases, once on the beach, stay flat on your back on the
sand, keep warm (leave wetsuit on) and await ambulance or medical help.

Backs: Everything a Surfer Needs to Know

Acute Back Pain Treatment

The following first-aid regime is for acute low back pain, provided the legs move and feeling in the legs is present.

● *Find a comfortable position. Don't try to stand up if it hurts too much. For sure, don't try to sit in a car. One or more of the following positions could be tried:*

   * *Lying flat on your back with or without support (a pillow, say) under the knees.*

   * *Lying on your side with your hips flexed and your knees pulled up to your chest (the fetal position), with a pillow behind your knees.*

   * *Lying in a bean bag with your legs in an elevated position.*

   * *Apply ice packs over the areas of pain or muscles that are in spasm. Leave in place for as long as is comfortable. Repeat frequently. When spasm/pain is reduced, very gentle spinal and hamstring muscle stretches can be commenced.*

● *Taking aspirin will help with the pain in the first few hours and then reduce inflammation and swelling over time. Take two aspirin every four hours around the clock, but beware if you have a sensitivity to aspirin. Other medicines may relieve you of severe pain (codeine-containing drugs, morphine-like drugs) but do not speed healing.*

● *Taking Valium-like drugs (benzodiazopines) may help relieve pain and spasm, but mainly seem to be effective in their ability to make you sleep and forget your misery.*

● *Taking N.S.A.I.D's (non-steroidal, anti-inflammatory drugs) like Motrin®, Advil®, Nuprin®, Naprosyn®, Voltaren®, Feldene® or other ibuprofen or ibuprofen-like drugs will help relieve pain and inflammation about as well as aspirin, but cost a great deal more. It isn't proven that any medication will speed healing.*

● *Use of a lightweight neoprene lumbar support may help.*

45

For most back pain episodes you don't need to see a health professional. Using the above methods and allowing your back to rest for the first 24-48 hours is all that is needed. Time heals. On the average, the pain will only be bad for three to five days, and you'll be moving around again fairly comfortably in one to two weeks.

However, you should seek medical help immediately if any of the following problems occur together with your back pain:

● *Low back pain which starts to spread to the buttocks and down the legs.*

● *Leg pain that gets worse with coughing, sneezing or going to the toilet.*

● *A change in bladder function (e.g., you can't pass urine or it starts to "dribble" out).*

● *A significant change in bowel habit, particularly if you lose control of your bowels.*

● *Numbness/pins and needles in the legs or around the anal (butthole) region.*

● *Leg weakness, or muscles atrophying (becoming thinner/smaller).*

● *Pain is getting worse, not better.*

A careful clinical examination will go a long way towards finding the cause of your back pain. A thorough examination by a health professional should include testing or evaluation of:

● *Posture/gait (walking, moving, standing, sitting)*

● *Range of movement, including trunk/hips and legs*

● *Testing muscle strength/tightness*

● *Manual testing of spinal segments (including reflexes and sensation in the legs)*

The health professional will then be in a position to decide what that problem is and whether other special tests such as x-rays are really going to be necessary. X-rays may be needed if disease or bone injury are suspected. For instance, it is possible to have an infection in a bone. Other special x-rays, including CT (computerized tomography) scans and MRI (magnetic resonance imaging studies), may be needed, but they should not be regarded as essential investigations in every case of back pain. They are expensive. (In the U.S., a CT costs almost $500, an MRI about $1,000.)

Very few cases of back pain lead to hospitalization. Unless surgery is needed, it has been shown that being in a hospital does not speed healing, but does cost thousand of dollars.

What few studies have been done comparing the results of different back specialists in helping back sufferers have shown that:

1. **General or family practice physicians are helpful only if they remain committed to helping and supporting the patient emotionally, rather than referring them to a specialist just to be rid of them, or simply handing out medication.**

2. **Orthopedists and chiropractors seem to be equally successful (or unsuccessful).**

3. **Neurosurgeons can be very helpful if the problem requires neurosurgery, but conceivably may make a person worse by operating.**

4. **Neurologists are seldom helpful.**

5. **Yoga, posture teachers and physical therapists can be helpful.**

6. **Physiatrists are the most helpful. Unfortunately, there are very few physiatrists in the world—it's a medical specialty in which no surgery is done, only physical and rehabilitative work.**

PREVENTION: TESTING YOURSELF

The basics of prevention of back ailments include good posture (during standing, sitting and dynamic activities like surfing), correct tone and strength of back-related muscles, normal body weight, safe work habits and knowing your limits (otherwise known as common sense). As far as posture is concerned, consider the following:

Sick $\mathcal{S}$ urfers ASK THE SURF DOCS & Dr. GEOFF

When looked at from behind, your head should sit squarely over your pelvis with the spine in a vertical line. The shoulders should be horizontal and parallel to the pelvis. Check yourself out in a mirror or by having someone observe you.

If a plumb line were used and a person stood side-on to the plumb line, the vertical line should pass through the ear hole, through the middle of the shoulder joint, through the hip bone, just to the front of the knee, and just in front of the large bony knob of the ankle.

When one is standing in an erect position, the spine is a series of curves in the neck, chest and low back. One way of testing the lower back curve is to stand against a wall with the heels, buttocks, shoulders and back of the head against the wall (although it is important to try and feel as natural as possible about standing like this). If the lower back curve is too great (*lumbar lordosis*), you will find you can put your fist between the wall and your lower back. If the curve is "normal," you will find that you can only fit your flattened hand between the wall and lower back.

During growth, many children go through stages in which there is quite a degree of lumbar lordosis present.

An optimal posture is one which puts the least amount of strain on ligaments and joints of the spine, pelvis and legs. It is a reflection of balance between curves of the spine, the degree of tightness versus slackness of ligaments/muscles and the degree of weakness versus strength of muscles.

The important muscles relating to the lower back include:

● *Trunk and abdominal*

● *Hip flexor/knee extensor muscles (iliopsoas and quadriceps)*

● *Hip extensor/knee flexor muscles (hamstrings)*

The are a number of methods available to test the degrees of muscle weakness, strength and tightness as well as ligament/joint flexibility relevant to the lower back. These include:

● *Sitting on the floor with your legs out and knees pushed onto the floor (feet at right angles to the floor). Try to touch your toes with your fingers.*

48

Backs: Everything a Surfer Needs to Know

This tests flexibility of spinal soft tissue, hip joints and hamstring muscles. Many surfers are unable to touch their toes this way. You can also do this test with only one leg out and the other tucked to the side—to avoid strain on the lower back, and to test which side is tighter.

● *Sit on the edge of a bed or table with your legs hanging loosely over the edge. Bring your head down and try to touch your knees. This tests the same tissues as above except the hamstring muscles are no longer included (because of the bent knees).*

● *Lie flat on your back. Flex your right knee up to your chest and keep your left leg resting completely against the floor. Now pull your right knee onto your chest and see if your left leg is able to lay flat on the floor without any movement. This tests the tightness of the hip flexor muscles.*

● *Lie flat on your back with your legs out straight. Try to lift up both legs at once while at the same time keeping your lower back firmly on the floor. This tests the strength of your abdominal muscles and the muscular control of your pelvis.*

● *Lie flat on your back on the floor, this time with your hips bent to 45 degrees, knees to 90 degrees and your feet flat on the floor. Grab your ear lobes and try to sit up without lifting your feet off the floor and without hooking your feet under anything, and without tearing your ears off (that is, don't pull yourself up by your ears). This tests the strength of your abdominal muscles.*

● *Lie squarely on your right side with your arms folded against your chest. Have someone hold down your ankles. Now lift the side of your body down to your hips off the floor. Don't rotate your trunk or legs. It must be a true side lift. Repeat this lying on the left side. This tests the strength of the side trunk and side leg muscles.*

● *Lie on your back on a long table with your buttocks on the edge of the table. Flex your left knee onto your chest and allow your right leg to lay over the edge of the table with knee and hip relaxed. The thighs should be at or below the horizontal. The knees should be bent at 90 degrees. This tests the tightness of the hip flexors as well as some of the thigh muscles.*

Try doing these tests alone and with other surfers, so you can compare results. If you perform poorly, you should be assessed by a qualified health professional so that an appropriate program of stretching/strengthening can be taught to you. If you develop back pain with any exercise, you should stop immediately.

Remember, it is possible to have excellent posture, strong "balanced" muscles and flexible joints but still have something wrong with your back due to birth defects and anatomical variations, infection, degenerative diseases, vascular disease, and even cancer.

PREVENTION: EXERCISES

Basic exercises all surfers should do are:

● *Abdominal strengthening*

● *Pelvic tilts*

● *Stretching your back muscles*

These exercises should be done every day if possible. Make it a habit. Some find it best doing them upon waking up, others before going to sleep—or in-between. Find your best time and stick to it. Make it as regular a habit as brushing your teeth, showering or surfing.

Abdominal Strengthening

These exercises should always be done with the hips and knees flexed. Sit-ups performed with the legs straight unfortunately strengthen the wrong muscles—the hip flexors. If these muscles become too strong and too tight, postural problems can occur which lead to back pain.

One way of doing abdominal strengthening exercises is to do curl-ups. Lie on your back on the floor with your arms folded on your chest. Hips and knees are flexed. Feet may be stabilized under a heavy object or someone can hold them, or they can just be placed flat on the ground. The lumbar spine is completely flattened so that it touches the floor.

Tighten (contract) the abdominal muscles to the point where your shoulders are lifted off the floor, without flexing your neck and upper back. Start by doing as many as you can and gradually increase the number each day. You should eventually be able to do at least 50, holding yourself up for about a second, or ten holding yourself up for five seconds. It is not recommended that you try to sit up fully (i.e., elbows or chin to knees). Full sit-ups can be harmful to the back and neck.

You can upgrade curl-ups by adding slope to the surface so that your head is lower than your hips, by holding the flexed position longer or by doing more. By flexing and, at the same time, rotating your trunk to each side you will build up all the abdominal muscles.

Lying straight on your side, doing side leg-lifts (lifting the upper leg skywards) will strengthen the muscles down the side of your abdomen. Try doing up to 50 per side per day. Not pointing your toes will intensify the conditioning.

Pelvic Tilts

Lie on your back on the floor. Hips and knees bent, this time with your heels closer to your buttocks. Contract the abdominal muscles and flatten the lumbar spine. Tighten the buttocks as if to pick up a marble. At the same time the buttocks are raised just off the floor. Be sure the lower back isn't raised. Hold this for 5 seconds and repeat at least 10 times. If you have trouble doing this, repeat it at least 3 times and build per day (maybe when you wake up, in the afternoon and before bed). As with all exercise, it's important to combine and balance your breathing in relation to what you are doing.

Stretching Exercises

Basic stretches:

● *Lie on a firm, flat surface, with one or both legs drawn up to the chest. Each knee should be pulled towards the corresponding armpit. This position is maintained for at least 5 seconds. Repeat at least 10 times or until you no longer feel your back being stretched.*

More advanced stretches (best done after someone experienced in back and lower back stretches has observed you doing them) include:

● **Hamstring and lower back stretch.** *Sit on the floor with one leg straight forward, with the foot pointing up and the knee straight. The other foot should be nestled in the inner thigh of the outstretched leg. Straighten your trunk into an erect position and slowly reach forward with your hands to the foot of the outstretched leg. As you feel your hamstrings tighten, try contracting them and they will begin to stretch out and allow you to bend* *further forward towards your foot. Eventually you should be able to rest your forehead on your knee. Switch and do the other leg.*

This is an advanced stretching method and should always be followed by:

● **Abdominal stretching (the Cobra).** *Roll on your stomach and place your hands flat on the ground next to your shoulders. Slowly raise your chin, then your head, then your neck, then your chest and finally raise your abdomen off the ground. Slowly return to the face down position. Time the stretch to last a full long breath: slow inhalation while raising up, and a full, slow exhalation while returning to prone. Do this five or more times.*

Specific additional exercises will depend on whether any specific problems were found during the self-testing regime outline above. Be inventive in finding ways to stretch. Individualize. Read, go to yoga classes, ask friends.

SURFING WITH CHRONIC LOW BACK PAIN

People suffering chronic lower back pain need to learn their limits. Even then, chronic lower back pain usually waxes and wanes over a day and it is best to try to learn this cycle of this pain. You will then know, or at least have a good idea, of the best times for you to surf. Later in the day is more favorable.

Unfortunately, there are no magic answers for chronic low back pain. Many problems are due to chronic strain (on a background of degeneration) of the lower lumbar discs and/or facet joints. A stretching/strengthening regime can help to some extent but mainly it is a case of learning to keep the spine "minimally" loaded. Learning to rise out of bed by rolling to your side and pushing yourself up with your elbows and hands, rather than sitting bolt upright, is important.

In surfing, sitting on your board, rotational movements during surfing and, on some occasions, paddling are primary aggravation factors. Actually, sitting in your car on the way to the beach is probably the worst.

In terms of pain, medications may help to some extent but the body can become habituated to them. Use of TENS (transcutaneous electrical neurostimulation) can often be very helpful. This is a machine which you can use whenever you want to without resorting to taking pills. As of 1993 there were no suitable waterproof TENS machines available for surfing but they can certainly be used before and after surf sessions. Heat before and ice after a surf may help, too.

Backs: Everything a Surfer Needs to Know

The most important thing, in the long run, is understanding your body, keeping yourself as fit as possible and "flowing with it." A positive attitude will do more to help you live with pain and disability than any medication.

SPECIAL BACK TIPS FOR SURFERS

Many surfers have back pain under the following circumstances:

● **Driving long distances.** *In this case, put a small pillow or rolled-up towel behind your lower back. Special pillows are made for this purpose (McKenzie Roll). Full seat lumbar support back-rests may not be effective. This will support and maintain your lumbar lordosis (or "back spring"). Break the long journey where possible (get out and stretch at stops). Don't sit longer than 90 minutes. It's hardest on the driver, so if you have a van or pick up, lie down when you're not driving.*

● **Plane trips.** *Put a pillow behind your back as above. Walk around the aisles or get up and stretch for 5 minutes every hour. If you're rich, travel business or first class. Break up the journey, if possible (this also helps jet lag).*

● **Putting on shoes, booties, and wetsuit.** *Every person with an acutely or chronically injured back has suffered the indignity of struggling to just get their shoes and socks on (sometimes it comes to having to ask someone else to do it for you); bending forward can be that painful (and that dangerous). However, if you instead lie down on your back, and bring your knees to your chest, you should be able to reach your feet painlessly. The same approach works with avoiding throwing your back out before (or after) surfing. Try putting on your wetsuit and booties while lying down. Don't be embarrassed to try this—it works!*

● **After surf backache.** *This is usually due to long periods spent in the prone position. Gentle back-stretches in flexion (laying flat on your back and bringing your knees up to your chest) as soon as possible after surfing will be helpful. A hot shower, hot tub or sauna may help. Lying down flat on your back with legs supported on pillows, couch or bean bag will be helpful.*

● **Surfing after spinal surgery.** *Your orthopedist or neurosurgeon will tell you when it is safe to resume activity. There are many people around* the world who have been able to resume surfing successfully after major back surgery.

After spinal surgery it can take between 3 and 6 months to get over the operation. During this time, you must keep yourself as fit as possible within your pain limitations. Swimming (if allowed by your doctor) is by far the best form of "fitness" as it does not jar the back. Water "running" can also be done.

As part of the build-up you could also practice paddling in still water. Gradually build up distance and power (alternating distance with fast strokes). Use of gym equipment such as Nautilus, Hydragym or Universal Gym can be very helpful to building up strength. Circuit training can also help build endurance (particularly the Hydragym). A waterproof back brace (neoprene, for instance) may help for the first few sessions as you regain your confidence.

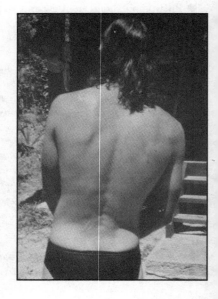

Severe lower back spasm in a very unhappy Dr. Renneker, on this Tavarua day unable to surf (much less stand up straight). It turned out to be a progressively degenerating L4-5 vertebral disc, which fully herniated three years later. The left lower back scars aren't related, just a record of having night-surfed Sunset Beach, Oahu. *Photo by Jessica Dunne.*

Backs: After Surgery

Take This Job and Shove It!

Dear SURF DOCS,

I'm 35-years-old, weigh 145 pounds, and have been surfing for over 20 years. Two years ago, I had a herniated disc in my back repaired (called a lumbar laminectomy, on the L5/S1 disc). Luckily, no fusion was required. Within six months I was back in the water, but needless to say it was not quite the same. Although I do back exercises and swim frequently, there is now enough pain to stop me from most outdoor activities, including surfing. Further tests (magnetic resonance imaging, MRI) have indicated no disc degeneration, so I know conditioning is the key.

The main culprit is my job. I'm in a pickup most of the day, and even though I'm using an orthopedic seat, gas shocks, and have a smooth riding truck, it remains the main cause of my continued back problems.

I realize I need to find another line of work to get me out of a pickup truck, but can you offer any advice on surfing and surfing styles with minimal back stress? I've been surfing a 6'2" or a 7'0" depending on wave size, but I'm considering going to a 7'6" to 8' pig-shaped board, thinking it may put less strain on my back, being more of a cruising shape.

CORY
Salinas, California

∎∎∎∎∎∎∥∥∥

Dear Cory,

To begin with, it may help to realize that you are not alone in facing a back problem. Eighty percent of all people will, at some point in their lives, have a back problem requiring them to seek professional care. In surfers it's probably even higher, maybe 90 to 95%. Such are the stresses to the back from surfing.

♪♪

Sick *Surfers* ASK THE SURF DOCS & Dr. GEOFF

Surf Docs is keeping track of the frequency and types of problems surfers write to us about, and, so far, back problems and surfer's ear are at the top of the list.

It's also interesting to realize that back problems are not, as most people would imagine, more common in older people. The age range most commonly affected is between 35 and 40. You're right in there, Cory.

Where you depart from the norm is in having had back surgery. Of all people who have back problems, very few end up requiring surgery: only 2 to 4% in the U.S., and 0.5% in Europe. The difference in the rate of surgery reflects two important facts:

1. **American surgeons are more cut-happy (this has been amply documented for practically all elective surgical procedures—back operations, hysterectomy, heart bypass, and others).**

2. **Non-surgical approaches, such as back exercises, posture training, yoga, and manipulation (i.e., chiropractic or osteopathic care), are quite effective in treating back problems. The simple combination of allowing enough time to heal and avoiding re-injury is often all that is required. Within six weeks, 80% of people will be well, regardless of what treatment method they pursue, including doing nothing but rest.**

"**T**hat brings us to the existential dilemma . . . what's more important, surfing or work?"

But some people do require surgery, and it appears you were one of them, assuming you weren't inappropriately pushed into it. At this point you have what is called a "post-laminectomy syndrome," a grab-bag term for the 50% or so of people who continue having back pain despite (and sometimes because of) having had surgery. Sometimes the surgery is done on the wrong disc(s), or is incomplete in removing or remodeling damaged tissue; sometimes the surgery damages previously healthy tissue, particularly nerves; sometimes the surgery leaves the area unstable, so that re-injury quickly occurs.

More often, it is something that no surgeon can be held accountable for: the reason for the back problem in the first place isn't corrected. You're probably right; your job, having to sit in a pickup all day, is almost certainly a major factor in your continuing back problems. We assume you can't work out of a vehicle with more back-efficient seating, like a van; and we assume you've explored with your boss the possibilities of doing other job tasks, ones that will be kinder to your back.

Backs: After Surgery

That brings us to the existential dilemma, one that all surfers face at some point in their lives: what's more important, surfing or work? Think on that seriously. Our advice to you is that if your job is interfering with your health and keeping you from surfing the way you want to surf (i.e., on a short board), then you should tell your boss "to take this job and shove it."

If you can't do that, or if you do, but continue to have back problems anyway, then, yes, changing to a longer, wider board will be easier on your back. A larger planing surface will allow you to glide more easily into waves, avoiding the kind of bent-forward, back-straining positions that are required to nurse a board into a wave (less of a problem in big and fast waves). Longer boards require different body mechanics to steer and turn them—less rotating, torquing, and twisting motions (which are hard on anyone's back) and more rail-to-rail weight shifts (infinitely easier on the back). A single-fin is probably better in that regard than a thruster; less pivoting motions are required with single-fins.

Lowering your center of gravity by squatting lower and letting your leg muscles do more of the work will put less strain on your back. Mark Richards, the four-time world champion, has been plagued by a bad back throughout his professional career. You'll notice that his surfing style has evolved to that which is most back-protective: his stance is low to the board, and he turns with his knees rather than by twisting his hips and back.

The timing of your surfing activities also makes a difference. Cracking it at dawn, when your back is less limber, makes less sense then going later in the day. Let your surf sessions be on days when you're well rested and have taken it easy up until you paddle out (i.e., not right after work, and not after driving a long distance).

Also, you should consider consulting other back specialists for treatment options and back-saving tips that your surgeon may not have presented to you. Try going to a physiatrist, a non-surgical physician specializing in back problems.

Backs: Back Pain in a Young Surfer

Dodging the Knife

Dear SURF DOCS,

I'm a 22-year-old surfer from Florida, and I've been surfing for about six years. About two months ago, while surfing, I noticed a slight pain in my lower back. I thought nothing of it, but that pain has continued to increase, and is now so unbearable that I can't surf, or skate, or do anything for that matter. I also have numbness running down my left leg, causing me to walk irregularly.

I went to the doctor, and he told me that I have a ruptured disc in my lower back. He said I needed surgery to remove the disc, and that if I had surgery I'd never surf again! Hearing that, I went to the chiropractor for four weeks. I felt exactly the same as before, so I stopped going. Now I'm again fac-ing surgery. Should I have it? Will I surf again? I'm getting really antsy!

CRAIG
Crabhole, Florida

■■■IIIIIIII

Dear Craig,

Let's cut to the punch line: Yes, the overwhelming probability is that you *will* surf again. Ninety percent of surfers will experience at least one attack of back pain in their lifetimes. The good news is, regardless of the type of treatment—or even having no treatment at all—the vast majority of back pain sufferers get better, even those with disc problems.

The back is mysterious terrain. Over 30 different health professional groups claim to know how to treat it best.

Backs: Back Pain in a Young Surfer

There is a bewildering array of theories as to what causes back pain, and how to treat it.

If you want to get some perspective on the whole back care field and how to approach solving your own back pain dilemma, check out a book titled, *Backache Relief*, by Arthur C. Klein and David Sobel, published in 1985 by Times Books. They surveyed almost 500 people who had been in your kind of situation—painful backs that the surgeons were sharpening their scalpels for—and found the following:

1. **The average back pain sufferer consults five or more back specialists.**

2. **From those various back specialists, the average back pain sufferer rarely receives the same diagnosis or explanation for what is wrong, or what to do about it.**

3. **The average back pain sufferer finally gets better by combining the best of all the recommendations.**

We asked three different SMA consultants to read your letter (neurosurgeon, orthopedist and chiropractor), and, given what we've just stated, we not surprisingly received three different sets of recommendations about what you should do. Here's our synthesis of that information:

1. **Hold off on surgery.**

2. **Give your back more time to heal, particularly by giving yourself a period of one to two weeks of absolute back rest (no work or exercise—not even a ride in the car).**

3. **Take charge of your situation, and explore other methods of back healing.**

It sounds too early to even consider surgery. Don't let the surgeon push you into it, especially with a "you'll never surf again" attitude, which is almost certainly wrong. Only rarely do ruptured or slipped discs require surgery. The only time surgery is usually needed is when the pressure on the nerves leading from the spine to the legs is causing more than just pain or numbness running down the leg. When the legs' reflexes are decreased and the legs' muscles are weaker and growing thinner, that's when you might need surgery.

Strict back rest means staying at home and babying your back. No lifting, no car rides anywhere, no going to work. Just rest for one to two weeks. During that time, try cycles of applying ice, on for 30 minutes, off for an hour. It should make a noticeable difference. No types of medications have ever been shown to speed back healing, they only help relieve discomfort.

As for nonsurgical treatment, real benefit can be had from chiropractic care, even though it didn't seem to help you. But, as with any doctor, knowledge and technique are everything. You don't say what your chiropractor did for you (what type of adjustment, by which technique), but the method we've heard of other disc-wrecked surfers being treated with successfully is called "flexion-distraction."

. . . the average back pain sufferer rarely receives the same diagnosis or explanation . . .

Going to a physical therapist is a good idea—they would have lots to teach you, and could expose you to some ingenious treatment methods. How about going to a physiatrist? No, not a *psychiatrist*. A *physiatrist* is a physician who specializes in physical and rehabilitative medicine. In the Klein and Sobel survey, physiatrists were found to be the single most successful back treatment specialists.

If you do end up having an operation—and we hope this letter reaches you before it's too late—the foremost goal of the surgeon should be to return you to surfing form. Any less effort and you should tell the surgeon to take a walk.

There are various operations to choose from. We'd recommend against fusion (fusing the injured bones together), as it can make returning to surfing more difficult. One of the newer types of back surgery—which is also the least invasive—is called *percutaneous aspiration discectomy*, or P.A.D. It's done under local anesthesia with just a needle, but only seems to work for certain types of disc injuries. There is also a new form of arthroscopic-like back surgery, such as is done commonly in knees and the large joints. It's called *micro-discectomy.*

And after your operation—or if you find ways to heal without one—we recommend swimming as a way to get back in shape for surfing.

Backs: Broken

The Man of Steel

Dear SURF DOCS,

In a boating accident in Ventura I broke my lower back, shattering the third lumbar vertebra [L3]. At the time of the accident I could not move my lower right leg. Surgery was performed, and metal rods were attached to L3 and L4, and an iliac bone graft was done.

I was told I would be able to walk again, but not seeing the long green wall again was my biggest fear. I've been surfing since I was 15-years-old, and I'm in good shape at 34. I've been in therapy for one month now, and I can walk a little, and it feels like one day I will surf again.

My questions are:

1. **Have you ever heard, good or bad, of any surfers having to overcome this fate, either with rods and all?**

2. **How much time did it take?**

3. **How did it affect their style?**

Any information would be greatly appreciated by both me (for the stoke) and my doctors (for the record). There are two other surfers in here, one from Newport and one from Maui, and we'd all just like to say "be careful out there, people, because you don't know what you've got til' it's gone." The words "keep surfing" now take on a different meaning.

JOHN
A patient in Rancho, Los Amigos Hospital, Downey, California

Note: The above letter was sent in to us typewritten, but just barely, as if by someone in their first day of typing class. There was a handwritten note attached to it that said: *"When I wrote this letter I failed to include that I also have a broken right hand—it took a long time to type it!"*

■■■■II||||

Dear John,

Fortunately, one of our orthopedic surf doc consultants did his training at your hospital, so he's well acquainted with just what you're going through. He said it sounds like you had a compression burst fracture, which basically means that your vertebra broke into many pieces. Luckily, it doesn't sound as if you suffered any permanent damage to the nerves that go to your lower body. The third lumbar vertebra is near the base of the spinal column, which means it needs to be quite strong, so that's why metal rods and bone grafts were used to reinforce it.

The rods hold it steady while the bone graft grows in, fusing the adjacent vertebra to the injured vertebra, making the area strong, but less flexible. The rods may sound radical, but they aren't. They're usually left in place and cause no pain. Sometimes they are surgically removed later. The graft, though, can cause pain for up to a year. In your case, shavings of bone were taken from your hip bone (the iliac crest) and grafted to each side of your injured vertebra, just as cement is placed between bricks to build a wall.

Many other surfers have had these kind of back-fusion surgeries, usually because of a ruptured disc (when the soft cushioning pad between vertebrae falls apart), but also for fractures such as yours. Most have been able to return to surfing. It does take time, though. In your case it will probably require at least three to four months of physical therapy after the surgery just to be able to walk well. That's when you can begin swimming and doing progressive stretching and strengthening exercises to get ready for surfing again.

Start with just paddling your board in calm water, in a bay for instance. It will be difficult at first: arching your back, as when paddling, will be quite difficult for some weeks. When you regain enough strength and flexibility to have a safe reunion with the ocean, start by just paddling on calm days (no waves). Finally, after what may take a full six months from the time of surgery, you should be about ready for your first waves.

Start in puppy surf and work up to your prior abilities very slowly, maybe begin by just belly riding in small surf. Your style for the first year may be slightly stiff, but eventually you'll be able to do it all: soul arches, crouching in the tube, and not feel completely vulnerable, as if your back could fall apart again. It won't, it should actually be stronger!

Our strongest advice, as you work towards that magical day of catching your first wave again, is to not rush yourself. Take it slowly and gently.

Baldness and Hair Loss

The Receding Tide

Dear SURF DOCS,

As I approach my late 20s, my surfing is on the increase but my hair is on the decrease. My hair is slowly but surely starting to totally thin out. I have looked into every so-called "miracle cure" and surgery technique. They either don't work or are too risky. A friend of mine just received a hair replacement system (a hairpiece) and it looks great. But he doesn't surf.

Do you know anyone with a hair replacement system that surfs, and if you do, can you tell me if it holds up in decent-sized waves?

I know this is an odd letter, but there must be a lot of other older, balding surfers wondering the same thing.

RIPPER
East Coast

∎∎∎∎∎∎∎∎||||

Dear Ripper,

Thank you for asking about something many surfers would be too embarrassed to bring up. Before addressing your specific questions, let's look at more general questions on how baldness relates to surfing.

Question: How many surfers are affected by balding?

Answer: A lot! Hair loss is strongly related to aging, and there is an undeniable "graying" trend in surfing (a 1982 *Surfer* survey found the average age of surfers to be 18.2 years, but a 1989 survey showed the age to have bumped up to 24.1 years). There are increasing numbers of balding surfers.

Question: At what age does balding usually begin?

Answer: Earlier than you might realize. It is perfectly normal for males (and females to a lesser degree) to begin losing some hair by about age 20 (it may not be noticeable except with a magnifying glass). By age 30, virtually all males will have some recession of their hairline near each temple.

Question: Would sun, heat, wind, or wipeouts have anything to do with it?

Answer: No. Those factors may cause hair-breakage, giving you a thinner head of hair, but they don't contribute to actual hair loss. Surfers don't bald earlier, faster, or more often than non-surfers.

Question: So what causes hair loss?

Answer: Genetics, mainly. But to understand that process, some background on normal hair growth is in order.

Hair is an inert substance, no more alive than the bristles on your hairbrush. It is made of a protein material called *keratin.* Each hair grows out of a hair follicle, a tiny pit lined with specialized cells and oil glands.

At birth, the hair follicles are under-developed—that's why a baby's hair is so fine. With age, the follicles enlarge and put out larger diameter hairs. The normal cycle of a hair follicle is to grow and shed many hairs through a lifetime. On any given day, year-round, it is perfectly normal to shed 30-100 hairs.

Whether you go on to actual baldness depends almost completely on genetics. Each hair follicle has a built-in genetic clock as to when and what degree it will begin to shrink and put out fewer, thinner, more brittle hairs, or no hairs at all.

In other words, you inherit the tendency to bald, and at present there is nothing you can do to alter your heredity. The genes can come from either side of your family (i.e., mother's or father's side). Baldness is an "autosomal dominant trait of varying degrees of penetrance," which is doctor-talk for if the gene is around, it is likely it will get passed on, but not a certainty. Just because your father or mother's father went bald doesn't mean that you will, too, but it is likely. Generally, your age of onset and pattern of hair loss will follow that of your relatives.

Question: Aren't there different types of hair loss?

Answer: Yes, but the only really important difference is whether it is normal or abnormal hair loss. Normal "male-pattern baldness," also called *anterior baldness*, is when hair is lost first from the front of the head, gradually working back towards the crown of the head. It is less common, but also normal, to start with a balding crown, and to lose hair from back-to-front. This is called *vertex baldness*. (This will not be on the mid-term, but is important to know when considering different types of treatment for baldness.)

The key to self-diagnosis of hair loss as normal or abnormal is whether it is symmetrical (equal on both sides of the head) and continuous (not in patches). Many things can cause abnormal, potentially reversible hair loss: scalp infections, skin diseases, malnutrition, toxins, hormone disorders, acute and chronic illness, and severe physical or

Baldness and Hair Loss

emotional stress (the hair loss is usually about three months after the event).

On any given day, year-round, it is perfectly normal to shed 30-100 hairs.

Some clues to abnormal balding include patchy, irregular loss; hair coming out in clumps (try the "tug test"—in various places on the scalp, try drawing together about ten hairs in a bunch and give a tug: loss of more than one or two hairs per tug may be abnormal); and chronic itching, crusting, or flaking of the scalp. If there's any doubt, see a doctor.

Question: What can be done about normal hair loss?

Answer: Until recently, there was little that could be done for hair loss. But now, as the television commercials state, "something can be done." The range of options is as follows:

● **Do Nothing, Accept It, Perhaps Enjoy It:** *Many cultures view baldness as a symbol of virility and maturity. You can even choose the Kojak and Midnight Oil Peter Garrett route and beat the follicles to the punch by shaving your head.*

If you choose this approach, or if nature has left you with scant hair, keep your head covered when in the sun and use sunscreen. Exposed scalp is highly susceptible to skin cancer. When out in the sun, use a waterproof, SPF15 (or higher) clear, alcohol-based sunscreen (it won't turn your remaining hair into a gummy furball!). Use a cap or hood when surfing to protect your scalp from the sun, and keep in mind that without an insulating layer of hair, you'll chill more quickly, so wear a neoprene hood when surfing in cold water.

● **Preserve What's Left:** *Preserve your natural hair oils by washing your hair less often, using a mild shampoo. Consider using a sunscreen-containing conditioner (but still wear a hat in the sun). Brush and comb gently, and avoid vigorous toweling and hair dryers on "high-hot." If you're heading for work right after surfing, maybe leave a little earlier so you don't have to do the old head-out-the-window-at-70-mph-surfer-hair-dry. Finally, there is no evidence that scalp massage or "100 brush strokes per night" will prevent hair loss or hair thinning.*

Sick *Surfers* ASK THE SURF DOCS & Dr. GEOFF

● **Rub Drugs on Your Head:** *A while back, doctors noticed that a blood pressure drug named minoxidil (Rogaine®) caused hair growth in both men and women. Some saw this as a nasty side effect, others saw it as a gold mine. It is now the only drug legally prescribed for male-pattern baldness.*

Minoxidil has been marketed as a drug to restore *hair growth in bald areas, but it only works for that purpose about 40% of the time. It's available in America and Australia and most other places in the world. However, in recent studies it is proving to be over 90% successful* **in preventing** *further hair loss in the early stages of baldness. Some doctors see it as a way of keeping their patients' hair follicles alive until a better treatment comes along.*

Interested? Here's how to use it (after seeing a doctor to get a prescription for it). It comes in a lotion, of which only a small amount (1 cc) is rubbed on the scalp twice daily (wait two hours after surfing). You must use it everyday. Stop and the balding process picks up where it left off. Side effects are minimal. It works best for vertex balding, and less so for anterior balding. The cost is about $50 per month, or roughly two surfboards per year.

● **Visit a Plastic Surgeon:** *This involves waiting until your hair loss has stabilized, and then going to a plastic surgeon for a hair transplant and/or scalp reduction. (In Australia, some hair clinics are run by specially-trained physicians, who are not plastic surgeons.) In a hair transplant, the surgeon uses a punch-like tool to take tiny bits of scalp from a still hairy area and plug them into the bald areas. It's hard to do large areas. It works best for receding hairlines.*

Scalp reduction is usually used for vertex baldness, and involves cutting out the bald area and stretching still hairy scalp over the opening.

Both techniques can work, but are expensive and may not look as good as you'd hope. Furthermore, the procedure may need to be repeated to keep up with ongoing baldness.

A word of caution: watch out for disreputable, non-board certified surgeons (i.e., not certified by the Board of Plastic Surgeons in the U.S.). Ask around and get the best. No matter what, don't let anyone implant any sort of artificial *hair in your scalp—it's like having a head full of splinters. No reputable surgeon would consider it.*

66

Baldness and Hair Loss

● **Have a Sex-Change Operation:** *As outrageous as this option sounds, we include it as a way of bringing out the fact that without testosterone—the male hormone produced by the testes—baldness is uncommon. That's one reason why women usually don't have much hair loss. And that's why you'll never see a bald eunuch, as was pointed out by a physician in eighteenth century Italy who noted full heads of hair in his male opera singer patients who had been castrated as children to maintain their soprano voices.*

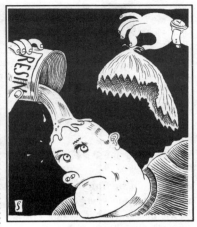

ILLUSTRATION: PETER SPACEK

● **Get a Hairpiece:** *The old shag-rug toupee is a thing of the past. The new hairpieces use color-matched human hair that is mounted on a breathable polyure-thane mesh and custom-molded to fit the contours of your scalp. The edges are woven into your hair to anchor it in place. Silicon adhesives are generally used to hold down edges not bordered by hair. On average, they cost about $2,000 (but can cost lots more). They can be so perfect you can fool yourself.*

Ripper, we do know of surfers who have hairpieces and they surf without any problems, even in large surf. The only thing you might have to be extra careful about is the unequal effect of the sun on the hairpiece versus your own hair. Consider wearing a neoprene hood or cap.

The hairpiece manufacturers we spoke with guaranteed their products in the surf, but get it in writing before shelling out any money. Call a dermatologist's office for the names of reputable hairpiece manufacturers and fitters.

Big Waves

Got What It Takes?

Dear Dr. GEOFF,

I have been surfing for a while and starting to ride some bigger waves. In the near future, I will be venturing down south to taste some southern juice. When surfing bigger waves I am having trouble conserving oxygen while underwater. I am reasonably fit, not overweight and don't smoke. I have heard of Cheyne Horan doing breathing exercises. Could you please give me some pointers on this subject?

Yours faithfully,
DROWNING

■ ■ ■ ■ ■ ||||||

Dear Drowning,

What an excellent question. First, I'll explain a little bit about the lungs and breathing.

The lungs are essentially a pair of elastic sponges sitting inside the chest cavity and actually "stuck" to the chest wall. The chest wall itself is made up of ribs, between which are muscles. At the base of the lungs is the very strong diaphragm muscle. By contracting and relaxing these muscles, and by also using abdominal muscles, the ribs move and the lungs passively follow. As the lungs expand, air is sucked in; as they contract, air is blown out.

Oxygen (O_2), the source of life, is the fuel in air used by the various body organs. Some organs can partly use metabolic pathways for energy not requiring oxygen to survive (e.g., muscles). However, the brain must always have oxygen to survive. Even a few seconds without it can be critical. Carbon dioxide (CO_2) is the by-product of the process of burning oxygen.

There are special centers inside the brain which control breathing. The act of breathing is an automatic process which we can control only up to a limit. This limit is dictated principally by the level of carbon dioxide in blood. The higher the level, the greater the stimulus to breathe. Conversely, the lower the CO_2, the less the stimulus to breathe. Similarly, the level of O_2 in the blood is important. The lower the O_2, the greater the stimulus to breathe; the higher the level, the less the stimulus.

Some free breathing divers (the not too bright ones) make use of these facts to allow them very deep dives. They breathe heavily for a while (hyperventilate). This blows off carbon dioxide in the lungs, lowering the CO_2. Also, the O_2 is increased. Thus, the stimulus for wanting to breathe (the level of CO_2) is lowered and they can therefore hold their breath longer. However, the risks of accident are very great and this method is condemned for surfers (and of course divers).

Let's look at the physiology of breathing for surfing (and surviving) big waves:

1. **Swimming underwater (i.e., getting deep quickly and getting back up to the surface) burns up a lot of oxygen. In some cases the O_2 level can become critically low. Remember, the brain must have oxygen to work and if there's not enough it becomes oxygen deprived. Unconsciousness can result.**

2. **If hyperventilation has already blown off a lot of carbon dioxide there will be reduced warning that the oxygen situation is getting critical. The level of CO_2 just can't get high enough to tell your brain you must breathe.**

Although low O_2 is a stimulus to breathing, it's nowhere near as powerful as high CO_2.

3. **The deeper the dive, the greater the problem. The greater the depth, the greater the water pressure against the chest. This makes the lung volume smaller. Relatively speaking, the level of oxygen in the lungs remains the same even though it's getting burnt up. However, as ascent to the surface starts, water pressure reduces and the chest volume increases making the relative oxygen level in the lungs suddenly very small. This further leads to a critical O_2 drop, leaving even less oxygen for the brain.**

4. **If arm and leg muscles fatigue and slow down, then blood is pooled in these muscles. Not enough is left to actually get back to the heart. As a result the amount of blood pumped by the heart (called *cardiac output*) is dropped. Oxygen is carried by the blood, so less blood means less oxygen for the brain.**

All these factors add up to cause *cerebral* (brain) *hypoxia* (lack of oxygen) with the risk of sudden unconsciousness.

Sensations of lightheadedness, dizziness or seeing stars (experienced when you get swallowed up and held down long enough by a big wave) are the warnings that significant cerebral hypoxia is not too far away.

Now if you put all this together, you'll see why surfing big waves is a critical act.

● *First, there's a degree of anxiousness (ranging from "mild apprehension" to "crying out for mother") which will cause hyperventilation to a lesser or greater extent. This lowers the CO_2.*

● *Second, if you get axed, it's usually in situations where you've burnt up quite a bit of oxygen anyway (scratching over set after set or clawing your way down the face of some monster). There's often not much time to take a really big breath after this either.*

● *Third, when you wipe out or have to struggle to get under a big wave, there's often an impact which knocks a fair bit of air out of your lungs before you even start to feel the effects of pressure from depth. Also, air in the nose and mouth is ripped out by the water turbulence. Less air means less oxygen available.*

● *Fourth, oxygen is used in the struggle to get out of or escape from the wave's underwater turbulence.*

This might mean diving down a long way (for details read Ace Cool's meeting with Outside Pipeline, diving down some 50 feet to escape a 30-foot closeout; Surfer, *April 1985).*

● *Fifth, when (if) you get up, the surface may be covered with foam so you can't get much breath. You also might be too weak to get much of a breath anyway.*

● *Sixth, the rest of the set keeps on hitting you on the head and the whole process is repeated.*

All the time the situation is getting more critical, as O_2 reduces, CO_2 is low and, of course, you're feeling weak and dizzy and the brain is getting more hypoxic.

Now, what I'm really getting at is that to be able to surf big waves means you *must* be fit. You must also be experienced, and you've got to want to surf big waves, more than anything else. Fitness for surfing can be helped along by full-on paddling and catching wave after wave, swimming, bike riding, etc., all in a flat-out mode. This produces aerobic fitness. The fitter you get, the more powerful the chest and diaphragm muscles become.

To learn breath control, activities such as swimming and yoga can be used. Wipeout techniques are important: quick wave penetration, avoidance of hitting the bottom (especially when it's coral), folding up and holding your nose and mouth to stop air from being ripped out, and flowing with the turbulence for as long as possible to quickly get out of the impact zone, being the major techniques that require practice.

> " . . . to surf big waves means you *must* be fit. You must also be experienced, and you've got to want to surf big waves, more than anything else."

Training yourself to dive deeply and quickly and be able to repeat the process, say, ten times (very, very difficult) is an important part of big wave riding fitness. (See *Air—The Hypoxia High*.)

From the medical point of view, some people biologically just don't have it, they can't develop very good levels of air entry into their lungs. Also, a number of medical conditions affecting muscles, joints (of the back and ribs) and the lungs themselves can "stiffen" the chest wall and lungs, preventing efficient breathing.

You say you're going down south; presumably you're from Queensland or New South Wales. Before you go into the cold water (which brings in a further set of problems), consider that there are plenty of big waves in "warm" waters in NSW. I'm sure you'd get more than enough challenge from big Forresters, Terrigal Haven, Queenscliff Bombora, Fairy Bower or Bare Island.

If you're serious about big wave riding (that is, waves over 15 feet), then all the best. We need a developing generation of big wave riding to continue the lines established by Joe Sweeney, Marcus Shaw, Brian Poynton, Bob Pike, Dave Jackman, John Monie (yes, the same ex-Parramatts coach), Ian Cairns, Simon Anderson, Gary Elkerton, Tom Carroll and Ross Clark-Jones. Without a doubt, big wave riding is the greatest challenge on this planet. There's really only a very small truly elite group of people capable of handling it, either physically or mentally. All the best.

Bones

Fracture Rehab

Dear Dr. GEOFF,

While playing soccer, in the tackle, the small end of the fibula was fractured, the tibula also had a hairline fracture. Because of the situation, I didn't feel the real pain of it until well after the game, although I knew I had done some damage.

Training soon commenced and training on it seemed the best idea, because the plaster seemed to tighten all the ligaments. The problem is my Achilles tendon, compared to my other leg, seemed to be a little thicker and tighter.

Could my Achilles have been ruptured? If so, what are treatments and alternatives? Also, could the small tendon connected to the end of the fibula have irreparably been damaged, or will it heal in time?

I have had ultrasound as well as stretches and have done small weights on the tip of my foot for therapy. My foot is fairly flexible, it's just the minute stretching feeling I get while running and turning.

Can it ever be as big as my other leg again?

The specialist said it was OK, just a little slow coming up.

Yours sincerely,
PELICAN

P.S. Walking up hills seems awkward.

∎∎∎∎∎∎∥∥∥

Dear Pelican,

In all bony injuries requiring immobilization in plaster, the soft tissues (skin, ligaments, muscles and linings of joints) undergo changes in which they stiffen up.

In the case of foreleg fractures (breaks) where the ankle is encased by

"Your broken leg will soon be as strong and big around as your good one . . . "**

tually (usually by six to twelve months, depending on how conscientious you are) your symptoms will completely disappear.

Your broken leg will soon be as strong and big around as your good one, especially if you exercise it consistently.

plaster, all the tendons and ligaments around the ankle stiffen up. Sometimes this can be a worse problem than the fracture itself. Often, quite a long period of gradual stretching of the muscles and tendons and remobilizing of the joints and surrounding ligaments is needed.

The thickening you describe in your Achilles tendon is part of this stiffening and tightening up process. You would not have been able to walk at all if it had been significantly ruptured, so I don't think this was a problem.

Treatment to date, consisting of ultrasound, stretches and weights, is quite reasonable. You should also add some balancing exercises (using a balance board). A mini-trampoline is sometimes also good. These can help reduce that stretching feeling you describe.

Walking up hills is awkward because of the tight Achilles tendon. Sometimes putting a small foam heel wedge between your heel and whatever shoe you wear will help this problem. Even-

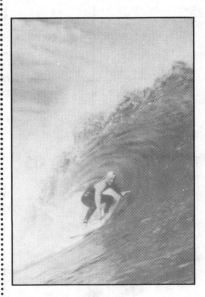

Stay healthy—stay tubed. *Photo by John Small.*

Bones

Broken Rym Bone

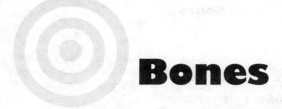

$\mathcal{S}$aith the *Rym Bone*, (Rym Partridge, DDS, from Santa
Cruz, California):

On his last day in Hawaii, a 38-year-old male dentist was surfing 12-15 foot Sunset,
did a late takeoff, wiped out and was struck in his right lower leg (probably by his
board). He noticed intense stinging in the heel area. Upon reaching shore he could
stand but had trouble walking up the beach. Looking at his right leg, there were two
small cuts on the right side of his ankle, with minimal bleeding.

Not really wanting to spend the money to go to an emergency room, and not thinking there was really much wrong, he went down the beach to have a friend of his, a
veterinarian, look at his leg. She cleaned it as well as possible and sutured the wound.

He flew home the next day, able to walk easily. Because of moderate swelling
and pain though, he began taking penicillin—hoping to avoid an infection. He was

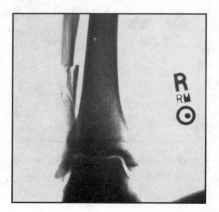

able to go to work, but noted sharp
pain whenever he put pressure on the
ball of his foot.

Three days later, the pain was
reduced, but still present. The wound
seemed to be healing well, with no
infection. Because the pain continued,
on the fourth day after the injury he
went and got it x-rayed.

Pause now, look at the x-ray taken
at that time and try to answer these
questions:

74

Bones

1. **What's the diagnosis?**

2. **What should he have done differently?**

With the x-ray in hand, he had the diagnosis—a compound, comminuted fracture of the fibula. *Comminuted* means that the bone was broken in more than one place, in fragments. *Compound* means that it was an open fracture, that the broken piece of the bone was sticking through the skin. The x-ray was read by the radiologist as also showing sand particles to be in the fracture site, and the orthopedic surgeon that was called in was concerned about possible *osteomyelitis* (infected bone).

Then the bones were properly set and cast for three months. He healed fine, and found himself surfing ten foot Bell's beach one week after the cast was removed.

Take-home message? He who has himself for a doctor has a fool for a patient? No, not really in this case. He did consult a fellow health professional, even though it was a veterinarian (maybe because this particular surfer has always been something of an animal). What this shows is that even health professionals can be fooled. If something doesn't look or feel right and what you're doing isn't making it better, have it checked out. For example, skin can be torn from underneath, by a broken bone, as was the case here.

By the by, in case you haven't guessed, the patient is yours truly, Rym Bone!

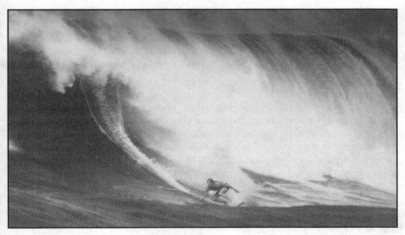

Rym Rides—looking at the lip on the "wave of dental health." *Photo by Winnie Partridge.*

Brain Surgery

Judging Breakthrough

*D*r. *Geoff saith:*

Arguments over the methods used to assess surfing ability and the quality of their style can never be settled while the human error factor exists. But now, thanks to an amazing technological breakthrough, we are able to make an exact measurement of the individual surfer's stoke level during his ride—surely the only true standard of measurement. Yes folks, modern medicine has once again come to the rescue. Dr. Geoff has been checking out the brain waves and is now prepared to reveal how a minor operation can put you on the road to surf stardom.

It has often been said that the greatest threat to the advancement of surfing has been the total lack of objective measurement of "good surfing." What is good surfing and how can it be measured when there are so many variables such as style and biased judging?

Two schools of thought have dominated the argument. Simple uncluttered surfing, in keeping with the classic Hawaiian cultural roots "the highest wave for the longest ride" is one. On the other hand there is the rip and tear, zig-zag, points for maneuvering, aggro consciousness, reflecting the guilt ridden, complicated, hung-up approach of today's complex society. Who knows which approach is valid? Can anyone ever be satisfied?

The answer my friends, to all these questions, as modern medicine has recently discovered, is a big resounding YES! Instead of frustration, with resulting aggression, it is now possible, with an exciting new operation, to promote tranquility. There is no longer any need to justify attitudinal jibing or even kick in the back door. What then is this new method?

Brain Surgery: Judging Breakthrough

THE PROBLEM

The basic fundamentals that need to be satisfied in order to measure an individual ride are: there must be no subjective element, the score must be visually instantaneous as the ride progresses, and the rider must agree with the score. The method of assessment must be reproducible, consistent, and easily understood by everyone (including Byron Bay hippies and Laurel Canyon trippies).

THE CLUE

A quick glance back through surfing magazines reveals a consistent groundswell of comment relating the effect of surfing on the mind:

> "While I was tubing it seemed like forever."

> "Everything changes, becoming slow and really intense inside the tube."

These are just two statements made on this radical change in perception which occurs when a surfer gets tubed. Luckily, a large amount of research has been performed over the last few years on brain waves, or if you like, the electrical rhythms of the nerve cells. So it was only natural that an attempt should be made to correlate the changes of consciousness when surfing with these electrical rhythms.

TECHNOLOGICAL ROOTS

During the '60s era of Californian dominance and Huntington Pier contests, secret experiments were performed. Surfing helmets were in fact secret brain wave receiver-transmitters. These basic experiments showed a highly evolved, specific area of the brain to be capable of forming "peak" shaped electrical discharges whenever the rider pulled off an outstanding maneuver. This was especially the case with tube rides, which of course were rare in those days.

Amazingly, this peak in brain wave activity of the rider corresponded exactly with the brain wave peaks among the spectators. The surfer was thus able to influence the audience. The better the performance, the purer the peak became—greater height (amplitude) and hanging around longer (time base). Another facet of this basic research revealed the tube ride to be the ultimate experience to rider and spectator alike. The larger the tube's dimensions, and the deeper the positioning within that spinning cone-like dream, the higher the brain wave peak and the longer it lasted.

Wow! What an amazing discovery! Brain waves and ocean waves in harmony! The order of the universe no less!

As space technology spin-offs were passed to the common man, the hopelessly inadequate helmet receiver-transmitters were replaced with micro-electrodes and micro-chip computers which were placed inside the brain.

After a few early mishaps, the operative technique improved and is now a simple and quick procedure. The only inconveniences are the initial two day hospital stay followed by a period of a few months waiting for the hair to grow back (the scalp hair must be shaved to avoid the likelihood of infection). Of course, with the present acceptance of shaved skulls (TV and rock musicians being the promotional media responsible for the phenomenon) many top surfers are now keeping the style; again reflecting surfing's ability to be an up-there trend setter.

JOCKO'S BIG DAY

Imagine the scenario. Pipeline absolutely smoking at its maximum tubing height, fifteen to eighteen foot emerald eyes! It's the final, only five surfers, no time limits, no hassles. The only rule is that a surfer must attain his best high within a five wave limit. Everyone is friendly, even casual.

Jocko paddles hard and drops in for his fourth wave, the last two inches of the inside rail just gripping as the board floats down into the abyss. Even though he's mentally relaxed, every muscle is straining to hold that edge at the same time as setting the critical first turn angle. Even as the board direction is set, the five-foot-thick lip is halfway down and folding about fifty feet along the wave.

On the beach, spectators, technicians, sponsors and reps are ashen faced with excitement. Even the folks back home in Mojave, in their Winnebagos are alive with excitement and expectation. The computer is clicking and chattering away while the oscilloscope is showing some electrical peaks. Jocko's weight and positioning are perfect. The board accurately responds to the three major forces: gravity, the suck of water up the face, and the frictional effects of the inside rail. As the green room assumes the shape of a perfect spinning cone with Jocko hanging near the apex, the emerald eye begins to wink. It is perfect positioning, and everyone knows it.

The tube's dimensions are 18 feet in diameter, 6 feet apex diameter, 55 feet in length! Never has such a wave been ridden by a mortal in such a position. He doesn't even bother to go for an in-the-tube spiral 360. Clatter, click, strobe, flash. A pure as can be brain wave peak flashes onto the screen. Amplitude 100 units. Total score = 100,000 units! The folks back home blink their eyes in disbelief, spectators stand slack-jawed. Jocko can't be seen, but there on the screen (and it can't lie folks) as the wave peels off is the biggest most sustained, purest brain wave ever seen. Intuitively everyone knows that with this wave Jocko has won, and they're right, as Jocko and board get spat out together with tons of spray 200 yards further down the line.

AFTERTHOUGHTS

After the event, Bazza is none too happy, as he also got one of the best rides of his life. Hurriedly the technicians set up a video replay with computer and oscillator print out. Bazza watches both his and Jocko's ride. The difference is small; same amplitude, but area underneath the peak is only 60,000 units. He just couldn't sustain the ride long enough. Like a true sportsman, he shakes Jocko's hand and after congratulating him, they walk off down Ke Nui Road as the sun slowly sets over Kaena point.

So my friends, medicine has again helped push the state-of-the-art a giant step forward. No more arguments! No more judges, (perhaps they can become electronics technicians). To all you up and coming Gilded Ockers, all it takes is a shaved head and a two day stay in hospital. Contact your nearest neurosurgeon and get ready for surfing in the '90s.

. . . The difference between us

is not very far.

Cruising for burgers

in daddy's new car.

My cerebral electrodes

bring me to

instantly

ecstasy.

(apologies to Frank Zappa)

Bumps and Lumps

Think of It as a Beauty Mark

Dear SURF DOCS,

Like all surfers, I've been hit by my surfboard. However, during a fun session at Nag's Head last fall, my board snapped back (thanks to my leash) and hit me in the forehead just below the hairline. It hit hard enough to draw blood, but wasn't serious enough to make me leave the water.

Anyway, I now have a small bump on my forehead that people keep asking about. It's not painful, but their questions prompted this letter. Should I seek medical attention for the bump? I never even noticed it until the last couple of months.

CHRIS
Virginia

∎∎∎∎∎∎∥∥∥∥

Dear Chris,

" . . . hard enough to draw blood, but not serious enough to leave the water . . ." Now, that's hardcore!

The bump on your head that's been such a conversation piece is probably just part of the normal healing process. When you get hit that hard, blood collects under the skin (that's what bruising is) and causes swelling. Much of the swelling goes away quickly, but the blood clots have to be reabsorbed by the body. Fibrous deposits are formed as part of the repair process—sort of an internal scar. In time, these are also broken down and reabsorbed by the body.

It can take months for your bump to go down completely. On a place like the forehead, where the skin is thin and tightly drawn over bone, even the smallest bump is visible.

If your bump doesn't appear to be getting smaller after six months, or if it becomes red and/or painful, perhaps

Bumps and Lumps

there's some kind of foreign debris inside that's slowing the healing process. When you get hit by your board there's always a good chance that fiberglass fragments could end up in the cut. If that happened, you may need to have a doctor open the bump and clean it out.

Getting hit by your surfboard is the most common surf injury, but you can cut down your chances of getting hurt again by following these recommendations:

● *Use a longer leash*

● *Sand the sharp trailing edges of your board's fins*

● *Put a safety tip on the nose of your board*

● *Avoid pointy tailed boards (pin-tails and swallow-tails)*

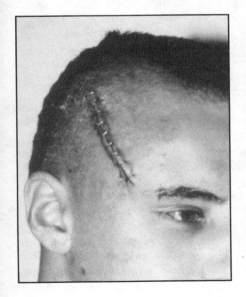

21-year-old surfer, brain laceration by surfboard. *Photo courtesy of Simon Leslie, MD.*

Bumps and Lumps

Surfer's Knots

Dear SURF DOCS,

When I read about the guy complaining of a bump where his big toe joins his foot, I just had to write. I developed a similar bump on my foot during my second year of surfing (last year), and I also had horrible ideas of it being a malignant tumor.

At first my orthopedist thought it might be fluid in the bone joints, or some other kind of soft-tissue growth. He stuck a needle in it to see if any fluid could be drawn out—this hurt like hell!

From my reaction, the absence of fluid in the syringe and the x-rays, the doctor decided it was probably a bone spur. He told me surgery was the only way to remove it, but that I could forego the operation if I could live with the situation.

Then, one day I was looking in the dictionary under "surfing," and I found the following:

> Surfer's knobs: tumorlike overgrowths of connective tissue just below the knees, on the tops of the feet and often on the toes, common among surfers who paddle in a kneeling position. Also called 'surfer's knee.' (*American Heritage Dictionary of the English Language, 1969.*)

I had been very conscious of dragging my back foot on take-off. My foot was often bruised, even cut on top, from the banging I subject it to. I am beginning to think this condition might not be as rare or freaky as I first thought.

Even though my take-offs are smoother now than when I was learning to surf, I find I must wear

Bumps and Lumps: Surfer's Knots

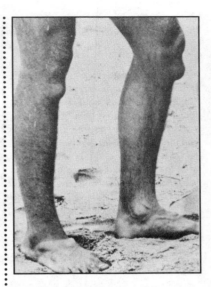

booties—even in mid-summer—to pad the bump from painful contact with my board. Also, sometimes when I walk my foot hurts, as though something is out of whack.

I found it interesting that an orthopedist-sports medicine specialist didn't really know what my problem was—yet, there it seems to be, right in my 1969 dictionary.

I hope the Surf Docs will decide this condition should be written up in your medical texts.

ROBERT
Dover, New Jersey

Dear Robert,

Congratulations, you've stumbled onto a favorite piece of surfing history: "surfer's knots." Also called "surfer's knobbies," these strange bumps (see picture) below surfer's knees and atop their feet attracted a great deal of attention in the early '60s when "surfing" was discovered by the American public. Along with Malibu and Gidget, bitchin' and stoked, jammies and baggies, there was, of course, surfer's knobbies.

Resulting from knee-paddling the longer boards of that era, and aggravated by epic applications of paraffin wax (hand impregnated by sand to rough it up), friction on the otherwise unpadded knees and feet (full wetsuits and booties didn't come into widespread use until the late 1960s) would lead to a heaping up of callous, cause the tissue under the skin to form into a soft pad, and sometimes irritate the underlying bone to form bone spurs.

They became the badge of *real* surfers, it was something to show off; the bigger your knots, the bigger the surfer. Newspapers and movies loved it, as did the medical profession. Medical journals in America, England, and France all carried reports on these surfer oddities. Fortunately, the knots proved to be largely harmless, seldom became infected, did not signify cancer, and usually would disappear if the surfer gave up knee paddling—which is just what happened in the late '60s when surfing shifted to the short-board. Thus endth the epidemic, except for the occasional surfer who drags their foot on standing up (as with you).

The recent resurgence of longboarding may lead to a return of surfer's knobbies, but it is unlikely. It wasn't longboarding per se that caused the knots, it was knee paddling, and knee paddling a longboard just isn't as popular as it once was, nor as necessary (it used to be a way to stay out of the cold water, but, now, with wetsuits, that's not an issue—plus, wetsuits provide padding). There are also chest knobbies, called *surfer's chest knots,* that can occur at the lower side of the rib cage. These are similar to the knee knots.

Dictionaries since the '60s have largely dropped the term. (Hey Robert, get a new dictionary if you want to get ahead in this world—you know, learn how to "prioritize" and "teleconference.")

As for educating doctors about problems unique to surfers (such as surfer's knots or surfer's ear), that is one of the goals of the Surfer's Medical Association. But don't hold out a lot of hope for us on that one; doctors are slow to learn. We find it far more effective to put the information in the hands of those that can best use it: surfers themselves. That's the reason we started this column.

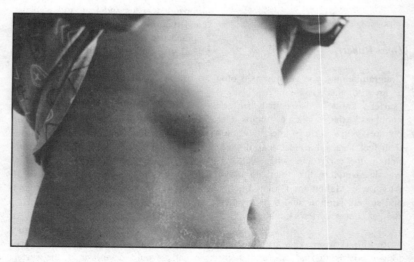

Those aren't breasts—they're *surfer's chest knots* (on "Beeper" Dave, just back from Baja. The knots are harmless, similar to the knobbies surfers get on their knees and feet. *Photo by Steve Heilig.*

Chest Pain

Heart Attack—NOT!

Dear SURF DOCS,

I'm a 16-year-old body boarder and I'm in the water quite a bit. For the past few months, I've experienced a pain in the center of my chest, right above my belly. The pain occurs around a half-hour after a long session. Whenever I inhale deeply, there is a sharp pain that lasts for a few seconds. This pain doesn't occur at any other time. I have had no problems in the past with breathing. Should I be worried about this?

NATHAN
Fernandina Beach, Florida

▌▌▌▌▐▐▌▏▏▏▏

Dear Nathan,

A pain in the chest should always be taken seriously, but it doesn't seem as if yours is something to worry about. But what is it? If approached logically ("thank you, Mr. Spock"), the cause of chest pain is usually easy to determine.

What you didn't mention, but we would guess it to be on your mind, as it would for most people who develop chest pains, is that you worry it may be a heart attack warning sign (angina). Worry not. Chest pain is very common from surfing, and, at some point, practically every surfer will think they're having a heart attack.

How can we be sure you're not having a heart problem? To begin with, heart attacks are very rare in people under 30. Secondly, heart pain is rarely made worse by taking a deep breath. So it must have to do with something else in your chest, which leaves your lungs or your rib cage as the possible culprits.

The fact that you mainly get it after long surf sessions would seem to indicate that it has to do with what you do with your chest. For instance your position when paddling, or particular maneuvers. Your lungs are completely enclosed by your rib cage, protecting them from outside pressures, so it seems unlikely that they are what's getting hurt.

" . . . at some point, practically every surfer will think they're having a heart attack."

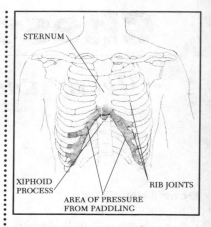

STERNUM

XIPHOID PROCESS

RIB JOINTS

AREA OF PRESSURE FROM PADDLING

That leaves the rib cage, which is made up of bones, muscles, ligaments, and joints—any one of which could be the problem. The centerpiece of the rib cage is the sternum (the breastbone), which runs straight down from your neck to your belly. At its lower edge, poking down into your stomach area, is a pointy knob called the *xiphoid process*. It is worth knowing about because sometimes, when feeling around their upper belly, people find their xiphoid process for the first time and are terrified, thinking that it might be a cancerous growth. Early in life the xiphoid is soft, but by about fifteen years of age it begins to harden and can be more easily felt. This hardening process continues until you are about forty.

There are also many joints in the front of the rib cage; between the xiphoid and the main body of the sternum, and between each rib where it attaches to the sternum. All of these joints move when you breathe, so if one

of them is injured, it will hurt when you take in a deep breath. As with every joint in the body, rib cage joints can become swollen and inflamed if battered and unnaturally used. That's our best guess for what's causing your pain: a battered rib cage joint(s). Doctors call it *costochondritis*.

It would be hard to say which of your rib cage joints is affected without examining you—but fortunately you can examine yourself and make the diagnosis. Lie down, let your chest relax, breathe slow and easy, and then, using one finger, begin pressing down hard over the area where you've been having pains. If pressing down brings out the same pain, you've got your diagnosis. Our guess, given what we've said about the xiphoid, is that the painful place will be between the xiphoid and sternum.

Treat it with daily aspirin or ibuprofen (Advil®) three or four times a day for a week or so, as well as daily icing of the painful area, to bring down the swelling and inflammation.

What is most important is to figure out how you've been injuring the area. The position of the chest when paddling a body board compared to a surfboard is slightly different, but in either case it depends on tightening your lower back muscles, causing your back to arch, raising your chest up off the board, which allows more leverage for the shoulders to drive your arms through the water. Try to notice how much of your rib cage is in contact with the board when you are paddling. That may be when you are doing the damage; it's better to use more of your belly as the platform from which to raise your chest. Try tightening your belly muscles to make the platform firmer. This will also take strain off the back from paddling.

Arm-paddling involves moving up onto your chest more, so in your case, try only kick-paddling (no arm-paddling) for the time you are treating your chest, allowing it time to heal. Also, begin to study the maneuvers you are doing for any that may be hard on your chest.

You'll heal, Nathan. After that, take two barrel rolls and don't call us in the morning.

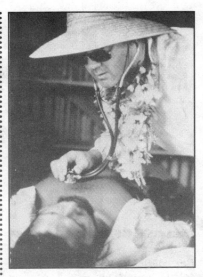

Beach Photos.

Cold Water: Hypothermia

Shivering and Shriveling

Dear SURF DOCS,

I'm cold! I've lived in California for the last eight years or so and have yet to be warm in the water. I'm 25-years-old, 5'11" and weigh about 155 lbs. Although I spent most of my younger surfing years in the paradise of the Hawaiian Islands, my shivering body and white finger tips are due to more than a mental hang-up with cold. My "coldness" stems beyond surfing. If I am exposed to any environment below 65°F (33°C), I turn into a human ice cube.

Over the years I have become accustomed to dressing for whatever condition confronts me: full-suit, booties, gloves, "dwid" lid for the early morning Blacks sessions, but they're a real bummer. Is there anything I can do besides bundling up to keep my blood moving?

LETTUCEMAN
Del Mar, California

▮▮▮▮▮▮▮▮▮▮

Dear Lettuceman,

Whether in winter or summer, Hawaii or California (or any other surf zone), cold is an ever present enemy of surfers. We referred your case to our hypothermia kahuna, Dr. Ethan Wilson, from Oregon, who drew together the cold facts.

Scientists have determined that the ideal environmental temperature for humans is 91.4°F (29.4°C). Prolonged exposure to any temperature below 85°F (53°C) can lead to hypothermia, particularly if you are wet (heat loss is 23 times higher in water than in air), exposed to wind (wind evaporation of water causes 30 times more heat to be lost), have little in the way of protective clothing (the more skin area exposed to the cold, the greater the heat loss), have

Cold Water: Hypothermia

a low percentage of body fat (15% is average for a college-aged male; elite athletes get down to about 5%), or haven't eaten much recently (metabolism—the burning of calories—is three times higher in the cold, and five times higher if you're shivering). Plus, breath-holding capability dramatically decreases as it gets colder, going from an average of 60 seconds (at room temperature) to 25 seconds in 59°F (27°C) water (if you have no protective covering).

Lettuceman, the correct application of the above facts should "cure" you. To begin with, we assume that you're a smart surfer and have made a good-faith effort to both physically and culturally acclimatize to California after coming from Hawaii. Surfers who wear only a t-shirt, shorts, and slaps when they go to the beach on cold winter mornings may look cool, but are sure to get colder quicker when they go out in the water. If you start cold, you'll stay cold—and surf worse. The surfers who know what's happening will deliberately over-dress for the cold: heavy jackets, sweat pants, Ugg boots. They're saving their calories for the surf.

It's best not to eat large amounts of food just before going surfing in cold water. This hasn't much to do with the old wives' tale of not eating before swimming, but relates to how much of your nice warm blood is diverted from your hands and feet to your stomach and intestine if you've eaten. So, eat well before you go out. Lots of complex carbohydrates are best. When it's cold you'll need calories to burn, otherwise you'll get colder and tire sooner. In truly

cold conditions, try short go-outs with a warm-up snack in between.

Also, drink lots of fluids (warmer = better) before going out in the cold. The body's natural response to cold is to shut down blood supply to the skin and direct it to the internal organs, (e.g., the kidneys), whose function it is to filter blood and make urine. So they'll produce up to three times more urine in the cold, which is why cold water surfers pee so much and get dehydrated so easily.

> " . . . heat loss is 23 times higher in water than in air . . . "

There are two basic ways to insulate yourself from cold water: a wetsuit and increased body fat, and one factor affects the other. In other words, thinner surfers need thicker wetsuits. A thin guy can lose up to ten times more heat than a fat guy! Lettuceman, your weight of 155 lbs. (69.7 kg.) is on the low side for your height (normal range for 5'11" is about 144-183 lbs (64-82 kg.), depending on your body frame). You might find that you'll be warmer simply by putting on 5 to 10 lbs. (2.25-4.5 kg.), perhaps just for wintertime.

As far as what kind of wetsuit to use, the wetsuit companies have done an underwhelming amount of scientific research on their products. We'd like to be able to precisely *prescribe* a wetsuit to a surfer, based on the key variables of body fat and body type, water and air temperatures, and wind factors—but, at best, we're left with hearsay and anecdotal information from the wetsuit manufacturers.

" **I**f you start cold, you'll stay cold—and surf worse."

In general, though, when it comes to wetsuits, thickness is less important than fit. Wetsuits work by keeping the water away from your skin, so the more skin you closely cover, the warmer you'll be. The function of the wetsuit is defeated if it is leaky or loose-fitting at the neck, wrists, or ankles. Consider the extra expense of taped seams and a dry zipper. Nylon on the outside (Nylon 2) makes a suit last longer, but significantly increases the amount of heat lost to wind evaporation. And don't forget that at least 30% of blood flow is to the head and neck, so a wetsuit with a high-neck is essential, as is a hood in low air temperatures or when surfing in the wind.

Smart surfers don't cut corners with their wetsuits, they buy the best one they can, make sure it's thick enough

for their needs, keep it in good repair, and replace it often (at least annually for the hard-cores). And they're knowledgeable about when to add in (and have them ready to use) booties, gloves, and a hood.

Finally, smart surfers have learned that if they're spending their sessions sitting on their boards and not riding or paddling, they'll get cold sooner. Paddling and wave-riding muscles pump heat into the body; it's the best way to get hot.

Cold Water: Ice Cream Headaches

Why We Don't Put Ice Cream on Our Heads

Dear SURF DOCS,

I just recently began to surf in the wintertime and I have some very simple questions: What are the risks of surfing in cold water? Are there any known long-term health effects of surfing in cold water? Finally, what causes "ice cream headaches?"

ADAM
Virginia Beach, Virginia

Dear Adam,

To your simple questions we can only provide complex answers, largely due to the fact that there is not a lot of research in this area.

The obvious immediate risk of surfing in cold water is hypothermia, a lowering of the body's temperature. It causes physical discoordination and disturbed mental abilities, which could lead to an accident or injury due to an error in judgment. However, wetsuits are now so well made and affordable that very few surfers venture into cold water without wearing one. These days, fatal or near-fatal hypothermia is a rare occurrence in surfing.

An argument could be made that hypothermia is more common in warm water surfing, due largely to the fact that most warm-water surfers don't have adequate wetsuit protection (if any at all) from wind-chill. Check out surfers getting out of the water in Hawaii, at Sunset on a typical tradewind day. Even some of the ones wearing vests are so cold they're blue!

The major long-term problem associated with cold water surfing is *surfer's ear,* which are bony growths in the ear canal. But, again, this condition may also occur in warm-water climes. It still isn't known just what causes surfer's ear, but it appears to be due to the combined irritative effects of water (whether cold or warm), wind, and possibly wave action, on the outer ear canal.

In cold-water regions, there is less intense and less frequent sunshine, which, combined with the wearing of wetsuits, would lead to less skin cancers and fewer problems from pterygia (growths on the eye).

. . . repeated exposure to cold water is not associated with a shortened life span, impotence or cancer . . .

If you're worried about more general health problems, rest assured that repeated exposure to cold water is not associated with a shortened life span, impotence (i.e., sexual problems), cancer, or any such condition.

"Ice cream headaches" can occur when water temperatures dip below 60°

F (28° C), and is due to cold water striking an unprotected scalp, causing an immediate reflex-reaction whereby the arteries in the brain first tighten up (constrict) and then relax (dilate). Our neurologist consultant feels that ice-cream headaches are more common in migraine sufferers. Ice-cream headaches are preventable by wearing a neoprene hood.

In balance, then, cold water surfing probably has no greater associated risk than warm water surfing, and both are low-risk compared to most other sports.

Cold Water: Arthritis

Joints and Stiffies

Dear SURF DOCS,

I recently heard that almost all the winter surfers (I mean dead of winter) have arthritis in their arms and legs. I'm only 14-years-old and have a five-millimeter wetsuit, booties, gloves and a hood. What is the truth in this matter?

PAT

"Arthritis isn't caused by cold at all, but is usually the result of accumulated wear-and-tear on the joints."

Dear Pat,

Arthritis refers to joints that have inflammation. An arthritic joint aches and is stiffer. Arthritis isn't caused by cold at all, but is usually the result of accumulated wear-and-tear on the joints. A full-on session in really cold conditions can sure make your arms and legs ache afterward, but it's not really arthritis, just muscle soreness. The reason people think cold water causes arthritis is that if you already have the condition, cold water can make it hurt worse.

You sound well-equipped for the cold. Consider, though, adding ear plugs to your equipment list, so as to protect yourself from *surfer's ear* and from the false rumors you've been hearing about arthritis in cold water surfers.

Cold Water Diuresis

Why Surfers Piss So Much

Dear SURF DOCS,

I am writing in regards to a friend who is too embarrassed to discuss his problem. I have been surfing with this buddy of mine for the past three years. In the last year, though, he has come down with a unique problem.

If the water is cold when we surf, when we head home or are changing out of our wetsuits, my friend slightly urinates without control. He claims that he can't feel it or stop it until it has run its course. The amount is enough to dampen the side of his shorts—quite embarrassing. He has opted to drive home with a towel between his legs as his predicament worsens.

Mind you, this condition only persists in cold water, so summers are fine. My friend is a medical student, plus his father is a doctor, but neither of them have found a reason or a cure. I figured that doctors who deal with surfers may have heard of such a case and could help.

CHAD
Laguna Beach, California

P.S. This is not intended as a joke.

■■■■■IIIIII

Dear Chad,

You are obviously not joking. This isn't the kind of story that is made up.

When someone loses control of their urine, scary things come to mind, like brain tumors and weird spinal cord diseases. But that seems unlikely in your friend's case. There is a pretty good

Cold Water Diuresis

explanation for it, and it's not really surprising that a medical student and doctor wouldn't know it. We're talking weird science here.

If you consult the *Undersea Biomedical Research* journal, Vol. 5, No. 4, December 1978, there is a research article by Rochelle and Horvath titled "Thermoregulation in Surfers and Non-surfers Immersed in Cold Water."

They showed that there are a number of ways in which surfers physically adapt to cold water immersion, including a blunting of the usual hypothermia response (less shivering), better maintenance of body temperature, and elevations of cortisol (i.e., cortisone).

They also discuss something called *cold diuresis,* which means that if you are exposed to cold temperatures you urinate more. The amount of urination varies from person to person, but can be quite significant. Some subjects imersed in cold water peed out almost 20% of their plasma volume (the plasma is the fluid part of blood).

This means that you'll pee more when in cold water than in warm water. It raises the dilemma that most wet-suited surfers frequently face: to pee or not too pee in their wet suit. If you try to hold it in, you'll experience the real proof of the phenomenon of cold diuresis. The urine is being produced so much quicker than normal, that your bladder's capacity will soon be exceeded, and a tremendous urgency to urinate will quickly set in. Our advice on the to-pee-or-not-to-pee issue is to pee. It's not good for your bladder if you're always pushing the limits.

" . . . to pee or not too pee . . . "

We mention the issue of peeing in your wetsuit because it's very possible that your friend does not, and that his bladder is so often past its limit that he doesn't notice the body's signals that it's time to go. We suggest that before going out he should always empty his bladder, and reduce the amount of liquids he drinks (especially tea, coffee, and soft drinks). And while surfing he should urinate as often as possible, and as soon as he gets out of the water.

That should put an end to his problem. However, if it persists, his bladder and urinary tract need to be studied by a urologist (and perhaps a neurologist), to see why he can't handle the extra amounts of urine being produced.

As an aside, it's not clear whether the thickness or quality of your wet suit makes a difference with cold diuresis. The response may occur just from a part of your body being immersed (feet, hands, or head).

Cold Water: Cold-Induced Angioedema

Winter Swells

Dear SURF DOCS,

I am a healthy 23-year-old with good circulation, and I'm a non-smoker. Last Christmas Day I went surfing for about two hours in the brisk, Northern California waters north of San Francisco. I wore a 3/2mm wetsuit and booties.

The problem occurred when I finished the session. My hands began to swell, and I was unable to bend them. It was hard to get dressed even! I also noticed that my knuckles had swollen to about a half-inch from the fingers. Two days later the swelling had gone down completely.

I was told the unusually cold water and my snug wetsuit had caused either hypothermia or frostbite. According to my description, *what's your opinion of what happened, and how can it be prevented in the future?*

JOE
Northern California

■■■■II||||

Dear Joe,

When you have to drive home with your fly undone because your hands are too stiff and numb to button things up— well, that sure seems like frostbite!

Actually, though, temperatures have to be below freezing (32°F; 0°C) to cause frostbite. Frostbite means that ice crystals have formed in the tissue. There can be swelling with frostbite, but it happens much later than yours did and is usually accompanied by a lot of pain.

Hypothermia (a drop in the body's core temperature) by itself wouldn't

96

Cold Water: Cold-Induced Angioedema

cause swelling either. In fact, it causes less blood to flow to peripheral areas like the hands and feet, such as in an attempt to avoid further cooling.

So, just what did happen to you out there? We don't know for sure, but what you describe may be something called *cold-induced angioedema,* an uncommon condition in which the blood vessels (*angio-*) react to cold by leaking fluid into and beneath the skin, causing swelling (*-edema*).

Cold-induced angioedema is similar to *cold urticaria,* which is an allergic welt-like reaction that typically affects the hands, feet and/or face. The swelling usually goes down in a day or so, as you describe. However, one thing you didn't mention is itching, and urticaria usually itches like crazy.

Attacks of cold-induced angioedema can also cause dizziness, nausea, even fainting—something you don't want to have happen in the water.

Try this test to find out if you're susceptible to cold-induced angioedema. Stick your hand in a bucket of ice water until it feels the way it did the day you got the swelling in your hand (don't overdo it), and see if the swelling recurs.

If you have the same reaction with that test, or if the swelling happens again while surfing, you should see a doctor. There are medications you can take, as well as other options (take this letter with you).

Here are some tips to help prevent the reaction, should it recur, as well as keeping your hands warm while surfing:

● *Wear neoprene gloves*

● *Wear a warmer, thicker wetsuit. Keeping your body warmer will increase the flow of warm blood to your hands. A snug wetsuit is desirable—it will keep you warmer.*

If—and we're not **certain** this was the case—you had an episode of cold-induced angioedema, it may have been a one-time deal, and perhaps won't happen again. These things can come and go in mysterious ways. If it does recur, work with your doctor to find safe ways for you to surf, and keep in mind that it usually goes away on its own.

We'd like to hear from any other surfers who may have had similar experiences. This is something we want to learn more about.

Cold Water Urticaria

Just Itching to Get in the Water

Dear SURF DOCS,

After three years of surfing, I've contracted what I consider a fatal disease. While surfing Salt Creek not long ago, I developed a rash that turned my skin bright red, and itched. I ignored it until I surfed the following weekend at Newport. Not only did I develop the rash again, but my hands and face became swollen. While walking back to my van I became dizzy and nearly passed out.

I went to several doctors, until one allergist diagnosed me as being allergic to cold surfaces. He proved this by taping an ice cube to my arm. I immediately developed the rash, and had itching that lasted about half-an-hour. The allergist then broke the news to me: There is no known cure. He even had the audacity to tell me to stay out of the water. Then he said, "Well, it could be worse." He prescribed an antihistamine three times a day. Please, may I have a second opinion?

HIGH-AND-DRY DOUG
Huntington Beach, California

■■■■III||||

Dear Doug,

What you've got sounds like *cold urticaria*, an allergic reaction to a drop in skin temperature. Symptoms may include hives, nausea, dizziness and even fainting. In most cases it's impossible to know why a person develops it, but it can be triggered by recent viral infections (such as mono or the flu), food allergies, other medicines or stress.

Hardcore surfers consider any illness that keeps them out of the water to be a "fatal disease," but people with cold urticaria have actually drowned from fainting in the water. You're right to take this seriously. Here are some ideas to get you safely back in the water as soon as possible:

1. Find out exactly how cold is too cold. Fill your sink with cool water, put your arm in it and add cold water until you get a reaction. At that point take the temperature of the water with a thermometer, and compare it with the water temperature in your area to see if it's safe to surf.

2. Try the medications from your doctor. They may prevent the reaction. Test them by taking cold baths at home first. If there's no reaction, you should be okay in the surf. If the antihistamine he prescribed doesn't work, ask your doctor to prescribe other allergy medicines. Remember, most allergy medicines may make you drowsy, so be careful driving and surfing. There are other treatments, such as ultraviolet light therapy and gradual desensitization, which have been successful in treating cold urticaria. Ask your allergist.

3. If you go surfing make sure you go with friends who know what's going on. They should know CPR and water rescue. (In fact, all surfers should know these techniques. Read over the CPR and Rescue techniques sections.)

4. Make sure your doctor has considered all possible causes for your condition (including those listed above, especially food allergies).

5. Learn about the disease. Sometimes you have to educate your doctor. A good book to read is *Urticaria*, by Beate M. Czarmetcki (Spinger-Verley, 1986). You can find it in medical libraries at universities.

Cold urticaria is not a life-long condition. Even without treatment it usually goes away permanently on its own. In the meantime, don't go surfing unless you and your doctor feel certain there's no danger of your passing out in the surf.

Colds

Surfing When Sick

*T*he Surf Docs saith:

One of the most common questions we hear is, "Do you think it's okay to go surfing when you're sick or have a cold?"

Generally, our answer is yes. If you feel like going surfing, you're probably well enough to do it. Will going surfing make you sicker? Probably not. In fact, it might make you better.

More specific guidelines aren't worth mentioning, because if the surf looks good, most surfers—sick or not—are going to go out no matter what a doctor says. However, if your fever is, say, over 101°F (69°C) you won't have much fun, and you'll probably surf lousy, too.

Be aware that when you're sick you won't have the same endurance, will get chilled and dehydrated more quickly, and may not have the same breathing capacity. On the other hand, if crowds are a problem, you've got the ideal deterrent: just hold off blowing your nose until you're out of the lineup, then let go with all the sticky green snot you can muster.

CPR for Surfers

*D*r. *Craig Wilson,* our public health minded Surf Doc, saith:

The ABC's on how to revive an unconscious surfer or any other person are **A**irway, **B**reathing and **C**irculation. You may save a life by learning Basic Life Support (BLS).

The main objectives in performing BLS are to prevent the arrest of breathing and circulation from airway obstruction, and to externally support breathing and circulation in a victim of cardiac or respiratory arrest by cardiopulmonary resuscitation (CPR).

Recommended procedures for doing CPR recently changed. What follows are the current (1993) recommendations from the American Heart Association.

AIRWAYS

Is this person or surfer in need of help? If you're in any doubt, find out. Anything which causes a decreased supply of oxygen or sugar to the brain, brain swelling, bleeding into the brain, or alteration of critical body chemistries can cause unconsciousness. Is he unconscious?

Shake and Shout

The best way to find out if the victim is conscious is to shake him and yell, "Are you okay?" If you think the victim has a broken neck, move him only if absolutely necessary, with his neck immobilized. Movement of the neck may cause paralysis. Suspect a neck injury in all unconscious surfers (over-the-falls face plants at beach breaks are common causes of broken necks.)

Call Out for Help

When someone responds, or if you're with a buddy, send that person to activate the Emergency Medical Services system—by dialing 911, in most communities.

Position the Victim

The victim must be on his back on a flat surface, with his head sloping down. The rescuer kneels to the side of the victim.

Open Airway

The most important action for successful resuscitation is the immediate opening of the airway. In the unconscious victim, the tongue may obstruct the throat and block the airway. Moving the lower jaw forward will move the tongue away from the back of the throat and open the airway. If foreign material is visible in the mouth (water, foam, sand or vomit), it should be wiped out. Excess time must not be taken to do this.

The head-tilt/chin-lift procedure is the most effective way to open the airway. One hand is placed on the victim's forehead, and two fingers from the other hand are placed under the chin. The forehead is then tilted back, and the jaw lifted upward.

BREATHING

Determine if the Victim is Breathing

Look at the victim's chest, listen for air escaping during exhalation, and feel for the flow of air. If the chest does not rise and no air is exhaled, the victim is breathless. If that is the case, perform rescue breathing.

Rescue Breathing

Mouth-to-mouth breathing can inflate the victim's lungs with sufficient oxygen with each breath, if done correctly.

Keep the airway open, pinch the victim's nose closed, take a deep breath, seal your mouth around the victim's mouth, and give two full breaths of 1-1½ seconds each. The rescuer should take a breath after each ventilation.

CPR for Surfers

Observe the chest expanding and air escaping during exhalation. If the victim's chest does not rise or allow air to escape, reposition his head and attempt to reestablish the airway.

Check for and remove any foreign material blocking the airway. The most common reason for difficulty with rescue breathing is improper chin and head positioning. The wetsuit may prevent the chest from rising. If help is available, instruct someone to cut off the wetsuit. *Do not take the time to do this yourself, and do not let this interfere with BLS.*

Since most drowning victims have very little (if any) water in their lungs, don't waste time trying to get it out.

CIRCULATION

Determine if the Victim's Heart is Beating

Check the carotid artery for a pulse (it's located at each side of the windpipe). Take 5-10 seconds to be sure. Maintain the head-tilt, and open the airway. If the pulse is present but there is no breathing, rescue breathing should be initiated at the rate of 12 times per minute (once every 5 seconds), after the initial 2 breaths. Check for a pulse every 30 seconds. If you have not already called for help, do so.

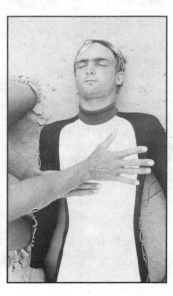

If no pulse is present, this is a *cardiac arrest* (a stopped heart). Brain death will occur within about five minutes. External chest compressions can produce circulation of the blood to the brain, if performed correctly, and prevent death.

Hand Position: Run two fingers up from the bottom of the ribs to the notch of the xiphoid—where the ribs form a "V" in the center of the body. Place the heel of the other hand two finger-breadths upward from the notch, so that the main force of compression is on the lower half of the sternum (breastbone).

Compression: With arms straight, the rescuer is positioned directly over his hands so that a squeezing force is directed straight down. Compress the victim's chest about 1-1½ inches, and then release the pressure. *Do not allow your hands to come off the victim's chest.* They must be repositioned if they come off, using the above method, so that the chest compressions are effective and do no harm to the victim. If you are doing the compressions correctly, the victim will have a pulse after each compression (if someone else has arrived on the scene, ask him to check).

If you're having trouble delivering proper compressions, because the surfer is lying on rocks or on soft sand, slide a surfboard under his back as a platform.

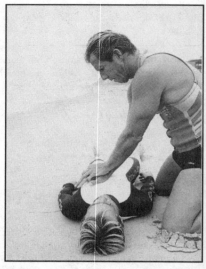

Jim Hogan (victim) and Richard Chew (rescuer) demonstrate CPR. *Photos: Tom Servais.*

Rescue breathing and cardiac compression must be combined for effective resuscitation by giving *15 compressions and two breaths, at a rate of 80 to 100 compressions per minute.*

After four cycles of compressions and breaths, check the pulse for five seconds. If the pulse is absent, resume CPR with two ventilations followed by the 15 compressions, and repeat this cycle until the victim breathes and has heartbeats on his own, help arrives, or you become too exhausted to continue. If the pulse is present, check the victim's breathing. If only breathing is absent, perform rescue breathing 12 times per minute, and monitor the pulse closely. **Do not interrupt CPR for more than seven seconds.**

If another rescuer is available at the scene, he should perform CPR when the first rescuer becomes fatigued—after checking to make sure that help is on the way.

Take a BLS/CPR class from the Red Cross, Heart Association, or at school. You can learn to save a fellow surfer's life.

Cramps

And Gramps

Dear Dr. GEOFF,

Well, I suffer from cramps in the calf muscle. It usually happens while I'm asleep and it wakes me up in the middle of the night. I don't suffer from them that often but when I do they kill.

In the surf when I duck dive or wipeout and I'm in a funny position, they start.

My grandfather reckons it's from lack of salt, or lack of stretching exercises before a surf.

Please help this hardcore surfer.

CECIL CRAMP

▮▮▮▮▮▮▮

Dear Cec,

I reckon your gramps may well be on the right track about cramps. Those old folk are nearly always right when it comes to health matters (it's often downright embarrassing).

The key ingredients of cramp prevention are diet, stretching exercises, cardio-respiratory fitness, staying warm and avoiding excessive fatigue.

The problem of surfing in cold weather is a very real one in terms of increasing the risk of cramps.

I certainly don't advocate the taking of added salt in your diet. Most people these days eat far too much salt. However, in terms of diet, giving your body a balance by supplying complex carbohydrates, vegetables, fruit, fiber, and small quantities of lean white meat (mainly fish) will guarantee optimal fuel for the muscles.

It is unnecessary, and undesirable medically, to add additional salt. It also destroys the subtle taste of most foodstuffs.

By getting fit in terms of supplying large amounts of oxygen to the muscles in an efficient fashion you will also help to reduce the risks of cramping. Running, bicycling, or swimming (using a rapid leg kicking technique) helps to get fit and build up muscular strength and endurance.

"The key ingredients of cramp prevention are diet, stretching exercises, cardio-respiratory fitness, staying warm and avoiding excessive fatigue."

Stretching certainly helps to reduce the risk of cramping. A pre-surf stretching session involving the quadriceps muscles (large muscles on the front of the thighs), hamstrings (muscles on the backs of the thighs), and various calf muscles is certainly worthwhile.

A simple calf muscle stretch is to stand on a stair or curb, with your heels and mid-foot hanging off the edge.

In cold water it is important to wear an appropriate well-designed wetsuit. Booties and surfing hood may well be necessary to complete protection against the cold. If the water is too cold you'll start to shiver and this will lead to earlier fatigue and increase the risks of cramping. Any postures involving awkward positions (such as constantly duck diving, etc) can also increase the risks.

Cramps are usually of nuisance value only, but under the wrong set of circumstances, especially if there is panic involved, could be a life or death situation. Follow the above advice and let's see what happens.

Cuts: Reef Cuts and Staph

Firing the Staph!!

Dear SURF DOCS,

About two months ago I returned from a primal tube jaunt to a lovely spattering of Pacific islands below the equator. The shallows there are consistently unforgiving, and I got more than my share of reef cuts.

This time—unlike many past excursions—a staph infection set in, and I—being tough and organically inclined—never filled the prescription from the doc. Instead, I used blood purifiers, herbal poultices and hot water soaks. It appeared that I'd conquered the infection, until it recently set up house-keeping in some cuts I had on my hands.

What's the best way to prevent and treat these persistent and apparently dangerous buggers of bacteria?

DANIEL
Santa Barbara, California

■■■IIIIIIII

Dear Daniel,

As most surfers can tell you, reef cuts have an amazing propensity to become infected. Just as reefs harbor fish and other marine life, they also teem with bacteria. Any cut you get in the tropics has a higher risk of infection because bacteria love warm, moist climates.

Staph infections are the most common types of wound infections. Staph (short for *Staphylococcus aureus*) are bacteria that can be found just about everywhere. They often cause abscesses (pus pockets) as the body tries to wall off the

107

infection. What's more, staph bacteria are often resistant to antibiotic drugs.

The best way to avoid a staph infection is to avoid getting cut. Since the feet are the most common site for reef cuts, using "Bali Boots" or wetsuit booties will save a lot of skin. It's probably best to wear ones that cover your ankles. A thin wetsuit is also a good idea, neoprene is a hell of a lot easier to repair than skin. Finally, avoiding shallow or exposed reefs and knowing what the bottom is like before you take off will minimize your chances of getting cut.

If you do get cut or scrapped, take care of the wound as soon as you get out of the water. It's critical that you get all reef and ocean debris out of it right away. Even if you can't see anything in the cut or scrape, and even if the water seemed crystal-clear, the wound is contaminated—guaranteed.

First, flush out the wound with fresh, clean water. **We are talking gallons here.** Use about three times as much as you think you'll need. Next, scrub the cut using warm, soapy water and a washcloth or soft brush. Ken Bradshaw advises, "Scrub it until it hurts as much, and is as red, as when you got it."

Remember, if you don't make absolutely sure that the sand and all other particles are out of the wound, they'll cause infection and slow the healing process.

Reef cuts are best left uncovered, wounds heal faster when exposed to air.

However, a cut should be covered if it can't be kept clean (e.g., when traveling) or if it rubs on clothing, in these cases use a nonadhesive dressing (such as a Telfa™ pad in the U.S.), and change it every couple of days or whenever it gets wet.

Saltwater can help healing, so going out in the water with a cut isn't out of the question. In fact, saltwater dressings are used in hospitals for daily wound care.

If you do go surfing, don't let the wound get sunburned and when you come out of the water wash the wound as carefully as you would a fresh one-- just don't scrub hard. Dry the wound carefully and apply an antibiotic ointment such as Bacitracin™ or Terramycin™.

The Surfer's Medical Association is studying other methods of wound care. For instance, Gerry Lopez's method is to scrub the wound clean, put Terramycin™ on it then cover it up with a completely impermeable dressing so no air can get to it (he uses one called Elastoplast™). He leaves the dressing in place for up to a week. Also there are newer more powerful antibiotic ointments on the market, one is called Bactroban™ (U.S.), requiring a prescription, that is specifically good for staph.

Good wound care will prevent most infections, but keep a close watch on all reef cuts. Early signs of infection are increased redness and tenderness, throbbing warmth and pus.

Cuts: Reef Cuts and Staph

Daniel, you were on the right track with the treatment of your infection: not all of them need antibiotics. Warm poultices and compresses or warm soaks (58-68°C; 90-100°F) are the first step. We recommend using them for 20 minutes, four times a day. Also, and this is important, keep the wound elevated above the level of your heart, allowing the infection to drain.

If the wound isn't getting any better or if you develop red streaks up the arm or leg, a fever or swollen painful glands (lymph nodes), then you should see a doctor. You may need to have the infection drained and/or take antibiotics such as erythromycin or dicloxicillin.

If you're going on a surf trip where you can't get to a doctor it's best to carry some basic medications with you and learn how to use them.

Occasionally, no matter what precautions are taken, staph infections just keep coming back. This can mean that a person is colonized with staph (the bacteria are holed up somewhere on or in the body and are constantly causing reinfection). The most common site of staph colonization is the inside of the nose. Anyone who keeps getting staph infections despite good wound care should be checked out by a doctor, sometimes it takes a combination of antibiotics as well as other measures to get rid of the buggers.

Rarely, a surfer with a reef cut may develop a pus-pocket caused by a *Vibrio bacteria.* This can be tricky to treat, and often requires surgical drainage.

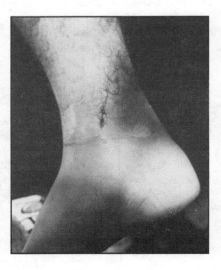

Laceration courtesy of Tavaruan coral, professionally sewn by the self-same surf doc, but on the flight home it began to swell horribly, red streaks began going up his leg, and a fever set in. He went straight to the hospital for intravenous antibiotics when he landed in San Francisco. *Beach Photos.*

Cuts

More on Cleaning 'Em

Dear SURF DOCS,

Regarding your advice and recommended treatment for reef cuts, I have found the use of a particular antiseptic detergent solution named Zephiran™, to be excellent benefit reef cuts and all manner of open-tissue wounds.

I first learned of Zephiran™ (in the U.S.) in Medicine for Mountaineering *(edited by James Wilkenson, MD and published by The Mountaineers, Seattle, WA), which proved to be an invaluable resource for both first aid and accurate, specific medical information:*

"Zephiran™ (benzalkonium chloride) is a detergent which kills bacteria without causing damage to the tissues, and can be used directly in the wound. Therefore, wounds should be rather generously rinsed with this solution after having been washed with soap and water."

> *. . .* **warm, soapy water may do just as good a job of clearing out bacteria as these more expensive solutions.**

Zephiran™ is available without prescription through local pharmacies in the recommended form of a 1:750 aqueous solution, to be diluted with water for direct use in open wounds.

DAVID
Florida

110

Cuts

Dear David,

Thanks for your letter. The search for the ideal reef cut treatment continues. Zephiran™ is great stuff, although fairly expensive. It works well when highly diluted. Just a squirt in a quart of water will do it. Diluted solutions of iodine-based antiseptics like Betadine™ also do an excellent job of killing bacteria, without damaging tissue.

It turns out, though, that warm, soapy water may do just as good a job of clearing out bacteria as these more expensive solutions. The trick is to use gallons of whatever cleansing solution you choose, making sure there isn't any residual dirt of other foreign material in the wound. That is the greatest single advantage of soapy water—it costs nothing, so you're more likely to do the job right. With the expensive iodine solutions, you might skimp--and short-change yourself in the long run.

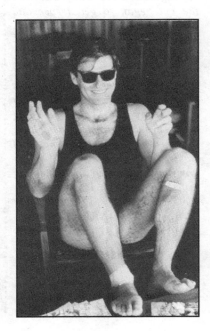

Reef encounter—he went for it, though! *Beach Photos.*

Cuts: Sea Ulcers

When Wounds Won't Heal

Dear SURF DOCS,

A while back I cut my foot really badly while surfing. The cut wasn't big, but it was really deep. At first I paid little attention to it and kept surfing almost every day, but soon the cut began to get deeper and deeper. Thinking I could outsmart it, I bandaged it every time I went surfing and wore a bootie on that foot.

So now, almost four months later, I've been forced to sit it out and let my cut heal. I'm going through hell right now, as I have the mentality of a grommet and surfing is all I think about. Is there any way I can speed up the healing process and still surf?

JAKE
El Cajon, California

■■■■IIIIIIIII

Dear Jake,

You've got what is called a *sea ulcer*, which is a common problem among surfers, sailors, and other seafarers. Sea ulcers typically develop in just the way you describe: first there is a cut, often a deep one; then, instead of healing shut like most wounds, it deepens and becomes encircled by a thick, rubbery kind of callous. And there it stays for weeks, months, even years, never looking particularly infected, but just never healing.

Sea ulcers are most common on the feet, ankles, and backs of the hands, which is a big clue as to why they develop. Ever notice how much a cut in the mouth will bleed, and then how fast it heals, compared to how little a cut on the ankle bleeds, and then how slowly it heals? Blood supply is the answer, and the foot region—even in completely healthy people—doesn't have very good circulation. For people with diabetes or circulation problems, poor wound healing is extremely common. One of the first signs of being a diabetic is that cuts on the feet never seem to heal. If you have a family history of diabetes, or this problem of poor healing recurs, you should be tested for diabetes.

112

Cuts: Sea Ulcers

As you have figured out, daily surf sessions won't help a sea ulcer to heal. It was wise to try to protect it from being rubbed or bumped, by wearing a bandage and bootie, but the real enemy is leaving the wound wet for extended periods of time. When a wound becomes wet, it loses its protective healing layers (scab, etc.), and is wide open for becoming infected from bacteria that may be around the wound or in the water.

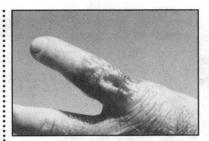

Coach Wright Photo.

The best strategy for getting a sea ulcer to heal is to keep it dry and clean (i.e., free from infection). Various goops and ointments, including the brand name medicines such as Neosporin®, Bacitracin®, Terramycin®, Bactroban®, Bactine®, Betadine®, Mercurochrome®, and other products such as aloe vera, vitamin E, cayenne pepper extracts, and gentian violet, have been tested to see which is best at wound healing. Let the truth be known that, none of them are real stand-outs over simply keeping the wound clean and dry. But, insofar as they help you do that, they are useful.

Probably the best antibiotic ointment for treating or preventing infection is Bactroban®, an expensive (about $10 a tube), prescription-only medication that is particularly good for staph infection. In Australia, Dr. Geoff reckons that any of the eye ointments containing chlormaphenicol are the best. The best drying agent is probably gentian violet, a messy purple liquid that costs about a dollar (ask for it at your drug store).

If you have a sea ulcer, stay out of the sea for a little while. It may take two weeks or longer to noticeably improve, but each *dry* day helps. If a classic swell comes, put antibiotic ointment on it, a well-padded bandage, and wear a bootie.

When you get out of the water, don't stand around wet, talking to your friends. Give immediate attention to your wound. Wash it thoroughly in fresh water, preferably *warm* water, which will increase circulation to the area. Get it meticulously clean. Then dry it, using the sun or a heat lamp. Perhaps top it off with a dab of gentian violet. Finally, cover it with a loose-fitting bandage that allows lots of air to reach it. Frequently check it during the day, and before going to bed to be sure it is clean and dry. Change your dressing often. Sometimes, taking an oral antibiotic (e.g., doxycycline) is necessary to knock out a deep-seated infection.

The best strategy for preventing sea ulcers is to not get cut in the first place, and if you do get a cut, to take care of it. Sometimes foreign material (fiberglass, coral, sand, etc.) gets in a wound, which if it isn't cleaned out, is a real set-up for a sea ulcer.

Cuts: Scrotal

Unraveling the Mystery

Dear SURF DOCS,

It was early A.M. at 1st Point Malibu on a somewhat sizable day in January of '64. I was wearing a short Farmer John wetsuit. I took off pretty deep on my first wave and ran to the nose of my 8'6" G&S. My fin snagged kelp and my board abruptly stopped. I grabbed for the nose of my surfboard, and over the falls we went. With the board submerged, it suddenly shot skyward with the fin slicing between my legs. I surfed a while longer, having a great session.

I had noticed a nagging pain in my groin area and headed back to shore. Opening the leg of my wetsuit to let the water out, my leg turned blood red! I ran to the bathroom to check it out. I peeled my suit down and to my SHOCK, my left testicle unraveled downward towards the ground!

It was like when you're a kid and you peel off all the white on a golf ball. The inside . . . FUCK, the inside was like rolled up FUCKING rubber bands. I was fourteen years old and tried to remain calm, but I FREAKED! I gathered up the bloody mess in a paper towel and literally held my future in my hands. WOW! What was I to do? Finally my buddy Ren comes in to see if I am all right. He sees my face white as a sheet, looks down and we both freak! He drives me to some Malibu emergency facility. It wasn't open, so we wait in his car, while I bleed. Well, after a lot of pain and five shots in my other nut, they fixed me as good as new. I really don't even have a scar since your balls are so wrinkled anyway. Funny thing my wetsuit wasn't even cut.

LARRY
Fort Point
San Francisco, California

P.S. Sometimes I wonder if I should invent a cup for surfing, considering today's boards have so many fins!

Dear Larry,

Glad you survived. A few points bear emphasizing:

1. Your wound was back in 1964, when the water at Malibu was presumably cleaner. Nowadays it appears that such wounds often become infected. Before you let any doctor sew up a surfing-related cut, be sure the wound is thoroughly flushed and cleaned. We'd recommend at least 5 minutes of flushing with a sterile solution (i.e., sterile water or an extremely diluted cleaning solution). Set your watch while they're doing it.

2. It is surprisingly common for wetsuits *not* to be sliced in such situations, but for the underlying skin to be cut. This is a testimonial to how flexible and resilient wetsuit material is compared to our skin. If you are struck hard through your wetsuit by a sharp or hard object while surfing, and the wetsuit doesn't seem damaged, peel it up and look under it to be sure you are okay.

3. The scrotum, the medical name for the wrinkly skin sack that contains the testes (balls), is nature's own "protective cup." But, as your case demonstrates, it sometimes isn't enough. We

> "**B**efore you let any doctor sew up a surfing-related cut, be sure the wound is thoroughly flushed and cleaned."

would recommend for male surfers to consider using any and all groin protection, especially if you are learning how to surf. This could range from the simple act of wearing Speedos® or trunks under your wetsuit to a jock strap or a protective cup (as is worn by athletes in many other sports). If not wearing a wetsuit, wear trunks that have some degree of protective support (or, consider a protective cup).

Cuts

Suture Yourself

I live in San Jose, Costa Rica, having come here to study and find incredible surf. All that ended abruptly with a grave injury to the heel of my foot, from the fin of the board of an out-of-control dude. Then a dude that wasn't a doctor put in two stitches, and then came the doctor to put in the other six.

Four-and-a-half months later I can't surf and can barely walk. I have an infection with **Staphylo-coccus aureus** *in the closed cut. I've been getting the run around with the wrong antibiotics. Now I've been on ciprofloxacin for two weeks.*

At this point, I'm very frustrated and the growing insanity of needing to get wet is devastating me. Please tell me what to take, do, or just what's up.

BUDDY
Costa Rica

▮▮▮▮▮▮|||||

Dear Buddy,

For every surfer who suffers a deep cut comes the inevitable question: to sew or not to sew? And underlying that question is the more fundamental one: what can I do with this cut so as to be back surfing as soon as possible? Buddy, you probably chose wisely in getting your cut sewn up; you just went about it wrong.

Your first mistake, as is true for most surfers who get cut, was that you evidently didn't clean it out well enough. All cuts, even those that obviously don't need stitching, should be scrubbed out and flushed with gallons of clean water. The ocean is teeming with bacteria, as is the surface of your skin—particularly with staph *(Staphococcal aureus)*. With every cut, bacteria is pushed into the body. Even the tiniest bit of residual scum, coral or fragment of fiberglass in a wound is a set up for an infection.

With all deep cuts you need to use a good strong light and a cotton swab (or clean chop-stick, etc.) to probe for damage to tendons, muscles, nerves, bone, and blood vessels. A cut tendon will look like cut rope; a sliced muscle like sliced steak; a mashed nerve like mashed spaghetti; crushed bone like crushed surfboard foam; and if a major blood vessel is involved, blood will pool where it is cut (five or so minutes of direct pressure can control virtually any bleeding vessel, even if a major artery has been cut).

" **The ocean is teeming with bacteria . . .** "

Assuming deep structures also haven't been injured, consider the following points in deciding whether to get stitched (sutured):

1. Compared to sutured wounds, wounds that are left open will heal slower and leave a bigger scar, but less often will become infected (suturing a wound that hasn't been well cleaned can seal in bacteria and led to infection).

2. Avoid suturing puncture wounds.

3. Even large cuts can be adequately closed with butterfly bandages (i.e., Steri-Strips®), particularly if tincture of benzoin (a sticky, smelly, brown liquid that can be bought over-the-counter) is used under the bandages to make them adhere better to the skin.

4. Even small cuts over joints are hard to keep closed with butterfly bandages and may require suturing.

5. Superglue® can be used to close small razor-like cuts (but watch carefully for signs of infection afterwards).

6. Sutured wounds can be surfed with (but try to wait 24-48 hours) if thoroughly cleaned and dried immediately after surfing, while butterfly bandaged wounds aren't as easy to surf with (the butterfly strips come off, and open wounds hurt more when exposed to the ocean).

7. If a cut is to be sutured, it should be done within six hours (up to twelve hours for cuts on the face), but a cut can be safely sutured even after a week if a technique is used known as delayed primary closure (done in an operating room, involving sterilization and surgical closure of the involved tissues, generally used only for major, gaping wounds).

8. **If you decide that you need suturing, the person who has the most experience will do the best job (i.e., full-time emergency physicians and surgeons, particularly plastic surgeons).**

9. **If you care about your good looks, consider having even small cuts on the face sutured: tiny sutures are used, they need only stay in for 3-4 days, and you'll end up with less of a scar.**

10. **Be sure you've had a tetanus booster within ten years.**

All cuts . . . should be scrubbed and flushed with gallons of clean water.

Although any surfer can learn to competently sew up skin cuts, they shouldn't try to sew up cut tendons, muscles, etc. You need a strong background in anatomy and a lot of experience before you take on that job.

We think that's the second place you went wrong, Buddy. We suspect the dude who put in those first stitches did not recognize (or know to look for) a cut or damaged Achilles tendon. That probably explains why you can barely walk. Fear not, though, a competent orthopedic surgeon should be able to repair it.

It also sounds as if you may have an abscess (pocket of pus), which should be surgically drained. Ciprofloxacin is a powerful antibiotic, but, as with most antibiotics, usually won't cure an abscess. The drug just can't get into the pus pocket.

Buddy, even though good waves and good medical care can be found in Costa Rica, at this point you're not scoring either of them. It might be time to come home.

N. B. This particular column had the dubious distinction of being picked out for reprinting in Harper's *magazine.*

Deaf Surfers

Sound Off

Dr. Geoff saith:

Surfing and deafness are perfectly compatible in most cases. The major problem facing a deaf surfer is one of social-communication during the act of surfing. As every surfer is aware, communication in the water is usually limited and is more of a series of territorial/power play "warnings," especially in the more crowded surfing zones.

Deafness should only really apply to persons whose hearing loss is so severe they cannot benefit from any type of amplifying device. However, it is not usually possible (and certainly not desirable) to wear amplifying devices in the water and so even a moderately deaf person (relying on an amplifying device on land) can effectively be completely deaf once out in the surf.

The following should be considered:

1. **Dropping in on someone that you didn't hear whistling, shouting or screaming at you.**

2. **Not realizing that a "friendly local" was talking to you. He, therefore, thinks you've got a bad attitude because you're "ignoring" him. This could lead to heavy vibes, especially if you're a stranger.**

3. **Ear protection should always be considered by everyone. For "deaf" surfers it is imperative to protect what hearing you've got left. Use of ear plugs, wetsuit hood and helmets for safety and to help reduce risk of exotosis is important. Avoidance of surfing in polluted areas where there is increased risk of ear infection also needs to be considered.**

4. **Where possible, surf with a friend who can act as your ears.**

119

5. If surfing a new spot for the first time, try to establish a positive relationship with the "locals." Smile a lot, act friendly, give the "thumbs up" or "V" sign when someone else gets a good ride.

6. If necessary, "communicate" to other surfers that you're hard of hearing or deaf.

7. Avoid dropping in. Develop a system of scanning up the line to make sure. If you do drop in, explain you're deaf. This is where having a non-deaf surfing friend helps to diffuse a potentially aggro situation.

8. Be on the lookout for changing conditions (rips, rocks and other hazards) when surfing a new spot. Pick up what the other locals seem to be doing. This particularly applies if you've not been able to "communicate" with the other surfers.

9. Carry an identity disc, card, bracelet, or necklace, alerting to the fact you have a hearing problem.

10. In the past, surf clubs for hearing impaired have been formed. For example, some years ago in Torquay, Victoria, Australia, a number of profoundly deaf surfers got together and formed their own club.

11. When surfing against non-hearing impaired surfers in competition, awareness of the starting/finishing horn can be a problem. Try to get the officials to use a flag system. Always wear a waterproof watch when surfing in competition and synchronize it to the official time.

12. With air travel, carry a disc or letter from your doctor, outlining the hearing problem. Let the chief flight steward or cabin attendant know about your hearing problem so that you don't miss out on in-flight goodies.

13. With foreign travel, and if a hearing aid is used, ascertain beforehand where repairs/service can be carried out in your country of destination. Always carry more spare batteries than you think you're going to need.

Dental

Emergencies and Treatment

Our esteemed dental kahuna,

Rym Partridge, DDS, of Santa Cruz, California prepared the following.

Surfers, blokes, mates, dudes, women and wet friends here's your chance to be a painless dentist for a friend in need, or yourself. Using some of the medications and simple tools we suggest you carry on a safari away from dental care, you can save a tooth. If you surf long enough, it's bound to happen that you'll be whacked in the mouth by your board. Suddenly you have a loose or broken tooth, or worse, a broken jaw. Read on . . .

First, let's talk about what tools you might need.

FIRST AID KIT FOR DENTAL EMERGENCIES

● **Toothbrush and Dental Floss:** *Use them often to keep those choppers clean and healthy.*

● **Oil of Clove (eugenol):** *For toothache and inflamed nerves. Buy at pharmacy, (no prescription needed), and at some health food stores.*

● **Tweezers:** *The longer the better. It's a many-use tool.*

● **Q-tips:** *For placing medicines, cleaning cuts. Not to be used in ears.*

● **3% Hydrogen Peroxide:** *For mouth and gum sores.*

● **Antibiotics:** *Have dentist or doctor give you a prescription for penicillin or erythromycin. Understand directions for use.*

● **Pain Killers:** *Ibuprofen for tooth emergency pain. Few side effects. Prescription from dentist or physician in 400, 600 or 800 mg tablets, or over-the-counter in a 200 mg tablet (Advil®). If no prescription, just take more of the 200 mg ones: four 200 mg tablets equals one 800 mg tablet.*

● **Benzocaine Ointment:** *A local anesthetic, sold as Orajel® in the U.S. (non-prescription).*

● **Cavit®:** *Temporary filling material, seals against heat and cold. Get from your dentist.*

● **Surf Wax:** *A last resort filling material.*

● **Goodies that Help:** *Dental mirror, flashlight (go first class and buy a Mini-Mag® type flashlight).*

Now, here's all the bad dental stuff that can happen to you.

BROKEN TOOTH

A broken tooth may or may not have an exposed nerve. If the nerve is exposed, you'll have pain from heat or cold, or exposure to the air going in and out of your mouth. If there's no serious discomfort, and if the tooth root stayed in, you may delay treatment until you can see a dentist.

If aching, place oil of clove (eugenol) on a Q-tip and swab it on the sore area. This will soothe and calm the aching.

If aching because of hot or cold air: seal out the air as best you can with Cavit®, or with surf wax (the stickier the better).

If a tooth is broken deep in the socket, let it bleed until a blood clot forms. The clot will cover the nerve and socket and protect the area. Don't rinse away the clot or you'll uncover the nerve ending.

If the broken tooth has a large cavity, fill the hole with Cavit® paste. You can press the paste in firmly with a Q-tip. Then bite down to push away the excess Cavit®. You now have a temporary filling that should last for a few days. *Lost or broken* fillings or missing crowns can be filled temporarily with Cavit®. Clean out hole first, then fill. Keep replacing as needed.

Dental: Emergencies and Treatment

LOST TOOTH

Teeth that are knocked out can be pushed back into place successfully if treatment is started *quickly*. If you can get to a dentist within 30 minutes, there is a 90% chance that the tooth can be successfully implanted. SAVE THAT TOOTH, OR ANY PART OF IT. If you're on a remote surf trip, you'll have to try to do it yourself.

Example: You've had a tooth knocked out. Handle the tooth by its crown, not the base, or you may damage the tiny nerve fibers. Attempt to place it back in the socket. Be sure your hands are clean to prevent infection. If the tooth won't go into the socket keep it in your mouth between cheek and gum. If that's not possible, keep the tooth moist in salt water, milk or a clean damp wash cloth or towel and get to proper help.

BLEEDING

To control bleeding in the mouth, pressure is the key. Keep pressing on the damaged area with gauze pads or a clean towel until major bleeding stops.

PAIN AND SWELLING

Ice packs on the damaged area prevent swelling and reduce pain. Use the cold treatment for *one day* only. Don't freeze the tissues. Take the ice away when the cold becomes uncomfortable.

TOOTHACHE

So, you've taken care of your teeth and just saw your dentist two weeks before your trip to Java or Tahiti and you still come down with a world pro-tour toothache which is really hurting. Here's possibly why: Old or new fillings and decay often come close to the tooth nerve and cause it to die at any time. This toothache may be of two types:

1. Toothache from live nerve (no infection, just severe aching): **The first symptom may be sensitivity to hot, cold, or just aching. If no swollen lymph glands under chin and no facial swelling, there is likely no infection present, and you have a live nerve toothache.**

Treatment: **If any cavity or cracks in the filling are present, swab with oil of clove (eugenol) from your dental kit with a cotton pellet or a Q-tip. If it is a large cavity, place Cavit® or surf wax over this. You** *may* see some improvement soon. In addition, take 600 mg of ibuprofen four times a day, for mild to moderate pain. This may quiet the nerve until you can return from the land of nice tubes and no dentists. Stronger pain medication, such as codeine with Tylenol® may be taken with the ibuprofen if pain persists; but try the ibuprofen first. You can surf and function better with this moderate pain reliever.

2. *Toothache from tooth with a dead nerve:* This type of toothache may not hurt as much but can be more dangerous to your health, due to the infection at the root tips. These teeth will not be sensitive to hot and cold, but they may cause facial swelling and/or swelling of lymph glands under the chin or along the neck.

Treatment: The only treatment (when you're in the outback) is to eliminate the infection with antibiotics. Take 500 mg of penicillin VK four times a day for five days (if allergic, take the same dosage of erythromycin). If facial swelling is just beginning, ice packs may alleviate the discomfort, but they won't heal the infection. The infection will usually run its course in four to five days, subside, and come back again in several weeks. Try to get back home (if possible) to get dental treatment as soon as you notice the infection.

Secondary dental treatment for both the dying live nerve and the dead nerve toothache is similar: either extraction or root canal treatment. If you're in a foreign country, call the U.S. Consulate for a recommended dentist if any major dental treatment is to be done.

For a moment of levity; if you are surfing in Panama, do you have the dentist do a Panama Canal? Or, if your roots are really in the Philippines should you ask for a Guadalcanal? Nah, nah, nah, nah! Just kidding!

GUM ABSCESSES AND GUM-FLAP ABSCESSES

If you get any type of food and bacteria lodged alongside of your tooth or underneath a gum flap of a wisdom tooth, you may be in for an infection similar to the dead nerve abscess just described. Yes, you should have had your wisdom teeth taken out years ago, but what to do now? The swelling may be in your face, jaw and glands, and be very painful.

Treatment: Take 500 mg of penicillin VK four times a day for five days (or erythromycin if you are allergic to penicillin). Take 600 mg of ibuprofen four times a day for pain. Rinse twice daily with 3% hydrogen peroxide with 50% water. Try to *brush* the solution down into infected areas of the gums as this may help remove any trapped food particles and bacteria. Have your dentist check the area to prevent this from recurring.

Note: Occasionally this kind of infection results in a small balloon of pus on the gums. If this small swelling is easily movable, you may pierce and drain it with a sterile pin, knife, or even the point of a Q-tip or toothpick. Drain it and rinse well. This same kind of draining can be done for a dead tooth abscess if it eventually becomes a fluctuant swelling (a balloon of pus—see you are quickly learning technical terms—read on).

TRENCH MOUTH, ANUG, VINCENT'S INFECTION— BASICALLY, SEVERELY INFECTED, SORE GUMS

This gum infection is so painful it seems like a toothache. The letters ANUG mean: Acute (real serious), Necrotic (dead skin), Ulcerative (ulcers in the dying skin), Gingivitis (gum infection). The gums in one or more areas of the mouth become sore, swollen and difficult to brush due to tenderness. You may look closely and notice a gray film of dead skin in the gum peaks between the teeth. They may also look eaten away. ANUG is the result of poor oral hygiene combined with fatigue and stress, especially during heavy travel.

Treatment: You *must* brush the sore areas of gums. If they are too sore, place benzocaine ointment on them before brushing. Rinse with 3% hydrogen peroxide in 50% water three times daily. Take 500 mg of vitamin C a day. Get lots of rest, remove stress factors, surf and hang loose! Things should clear up in three to five days.

CANKER SORES, COLD SORES (FEVER BLISTERS, HERPES BLISTERS)

These are extremely painful single or multiple ulcers in the mouth or on the lips. They are generally caused by sun exposure, stress, and/or fatigue (low resistance in the surfed-out surfer).

Treatment: Rinse daily with 3% hydrogen peroxide mixed 50-50 with water to prevent infection of the ulcer. If they are extremely painful, use benzocaine ointment to numb the pain temporarily. For open sores on your lips, you may want to use a thick layer of zinc oxide to prevent further sun exposure. These ulcers should clear up in a week.

Recent studies of an anti-herpes drug named *acyclovir* have shown it can prevent or shorten the course of herpes sores on the lips and mouth. It is a prescription drug, available in a cream or pill.

BROKEN JAW (FRACTURE AND JAW INJURIES)

If your board reshapes your face in the area of the lower jaw, you might find you can't bring your teeth together or chew. This condition may mean a jaw fracture or a dislocation.

The jaw will usually go back into place, but if the pain is extreme and you can't close your jaw, you probably have a fracture. This is serious and you should seek *immediate* help. Go to a hospital or oral surgeon.

First Aid for Jaw Injuries

Place ice packs on both jaw joints the first day to limit swelling. Second day, stop cold packs and use a moist hot towel on the jaw joints. Use pain medications as necessary.

First Aid for Jaw Fractures

1. **Begin taking 500 mg penicillin or 500 mg erythromycin four times a day as a precaution against infection. An infection in the lower jaw could actually result in a surgical loss of part of your face from a bone infection.**

2. **Stabilize the jaw with an ace bandage lightly wrapped under the jaw and around the head. Don't chew foods. Liquids only. Get treatment fast!**

3. **Remember, if your teeth do not meet properly you may have a fractured jaw. Another indication is a tear in your gums caused by movement of the broken bone.**

BLEEDING GUMS

OK, this is the most common and the easiest cured dental problem in the world! Factors which help cause bleeding gums are stress and lack of rest (very common for the traveling surfer or the student surfer who stayed up until 4 A.M. studying for finals).

Dental: Emergencies and Treatment

In any case, if they do bleed it means you have a mild gum infection and if present for days, weeks, months, or years, you will probably lose some teeth early in life.

The cure is simple. Brush and floss the areas that bleed vigorously (and all the other areas also) and the bleeding should cease in three to five days. I know, you say you *have* been brushing and flossing daily and they still bleed. That *can* happen, it just means your brushing and flossing technique isn't quite thorough enough. Let me provide some suggestions.

First, let's try a new technique in brushing! Brush first without toothpaste so that you will concentrate on reaching all areas of the teeth with the brush. Using toothpaste, we find that we foam at the mouth, spit twice, feel our tongue tingle, and declare to ourselves that we've finished cleaning our teeth. This foaming and tingling are not really a good indicator of how well we cleaned the food and plaque (bacteria) from our teeth and gums. So take your time, brush without paste, and when you're satisfied you really got them clean, you can finish up with toothpaste for a breath freshener and fluoride application.

Most Important: Before you go on that surf trip get checked out by a dentist. The cavity filled today won't keep you out of the water next month. Get on the wave of dental health.

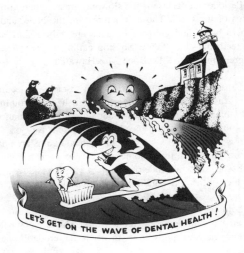

Dental

Periodontal Disease

More from da' Rym Bone

(Rym Partridge, DDS, in Santa Cruz, California):

First of all, congratulations, you are a surfer, a member of a group which seems to have a surprisingly *low* incidence of periodontal (gum) disease. Nevertheless, do you really want to be surfing in your forties with a complete or partial set of false teeth? That's right, mate, plastic choppers that fall out on good wipeouts; can you believe paddling to the beach with no teeth just in time to gum your breakfast? Well enough of these scare tactics, surfers really do have periodontal disease and many have lost a few, most, or all of their teeth.

Let's explain what periodontal disease is, and how to prevent or slow it down a bit. *Definition*: Periodontal disease is the slow, progressive deterioration of the supporting structures of the teeth. Those structures are the bone, and tooth ligament (attaching tooth to bone) and gums. The gums are only a skin *covering* of what really hold the teeth in—the BONE! So stop calling it *gum disease* because the main surf star here is the Bone ("Da Bone," for Hawaiians).

The first sign that you have some periodontal disease is bleeding of the gums when flossing or brushing. If you *never* floss or brush, well, you may *never* notice the bleeding. The bleeding signifies low grade chronic inflammation (infection) of the gums. If this inflammation and bleeding are present for 365 days a years for years at a time, this means these areas of your teeth and gums are not being properly cleaned by you for *years* at a time. Something has to happen, right? Well, the jaw bone holding the teeth starts to erode or dissolve. This is actually a gradual dissolving or disappearance of the upper and lower jawbones in your face.

As the bone holding your teeth erodes away (probably unknown by you), your gums may stay in the same position for a while. This creates periodontal (gum) pockets from the tip of your gums down to where the eroded bone attaches to the

Dental: Periodontal Disease

tooth. This gum pocket now traps food and plaque (bacteria), which decays and causes bad taste, smelly breath and even increases the rate of advancing periodontal disease with one loss. Great! And you never knew it was happening until it started getting bad.

The *main* cause of loss of teeth over the age of 25 is *not* decay but periodontal disease. You can lose the teeth without ever having a cavity in them. The way in which the otherwise healthy surfer loses his teeth is the *erosion* of tooth supporting bone until the teeth look ugly, and are now loose. Don't wait until then to start thinking about periodontal disease. Start your own home care oral hygiene program now and ask your dentist at your next six month check-up about the status of your periodontal disease and any gum pockets which you may have.

Surfers concerned with the overall health and appearance of their bodies will also have this same concern for their teeth and periodontal structures (again, that's bone, ligament, and gums).

So, let's get on the wave of dental health and keep surfing!

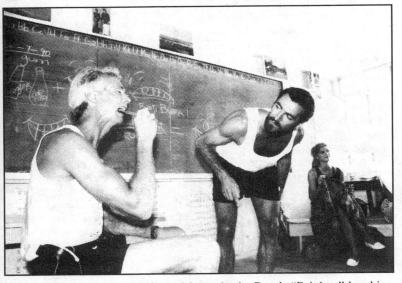

Fellow Santa Cruz dentist, Steve Mann checks Rym's "Painless" brushing technique at the Nabila school in Fiji. *Photo by Sandy Campbell.*

Depression

More Than a Wipeout

Dear Dr. GEOFF,

I have a problem of a psychological nature. To put it bluntly—I'm depressed.

I'm in my early twenties and I don't seem to know what I want out of life. I'm getting lazy and lack self-discipline and have no self-esteem. The only enjoyment I get is from surfing, bonging, and drinking.

Don't refer me to a shrink as I cannot afford one—just give me a little advice, please.

THANKS FROM NO-HOPE

P.S. I also have problems talking to chicks—so it's a vicious circle.

▊▊▊▊▊▊|||||

Dear No-Hope,

In a few short sentences you've covered an enormous amount of ground.

Surfing is a sport (lifestyle) which demands a lot of concentration and high levels of physical activity. It is thought (but not yet scientifically proven) that constant physical activity of an aerobic type (i.e., where the heart pumps forcibly for a prolonged period of time) has a protective effect on the mind. In other words, if you surf regularly, stress is better tolerated and the mind "feels more tuned up."

Most surfers can attest to this first hand.

On the other hand, bonging and grog both have the reverse effect on the brain. They are brain depressants in their own right—not to mention other unwanted effects in terms of memory disturbance, reduced concentration and brain cell death (certainly in cases of alcohol excess).

Depression

So you need to stop destroying your body (and negating the positive effects of surfing) from B & D (booze and dope).

Getting something *out* of life depends a lot on what you put *into* it. All of us change in our feelings of self-direction, life meanings, etc. I certainly can't give you a magical formula as I'm struggling with it as much as anyone else.

However, you should perhaps look at your talents, what you like doing (except B & D), the needs of others around you, and perhaps take a little time out to surf in less crowded conditions. Read a little and discover how some people "made it." You'll find that tolerance and love for humanity are common themes.

Self-esteem (feeling good about yourself) depends on past experiences, the way in which you were brought up in terms of parental models, development of true talents you might have and probably many others. Depression can have varying shades of gray and is certainly not a black and white emotion. Most of us feel low in mood or "blue" from time to time. Sometimes this can come on as a reaction to perceived failure in some type of situation.

However, of great seriousness is the very seductive form of depression which just creeps up and pervades all aspects of thinking and doing. This applies especially in cases of significant and prolonged depression. (Read *Darkness Visible*, a book by William Styron,

> " . . . constant physical activity of an aerobic type has a protective effect on the mind . . . stress is better tolerated and the mind feels more tuned up."

a particularly amazing account of his battle with depression.)

So my advice:

● *Go surfing!*

● *Stop the B & D forthwith and forever.*

● *Sit down and think about your positive talents. Then work on developing them.*

● *If you still feel overwhelmed by depression you should seek professional help. Preferably from a psychologist, social worker or psychiatrist skilled in these problems. Use of community health centers or similar services in Australia, at least, should be free and so the problem of cost shouldn't really enter into it.*

Diabetes and Surfing

Sweet Surfing

Dear SURF DOCS,

At certain times I have been afflicted with what can only be referred to as life-threatening occurrences. I am a Type I (insulin dependent) diabetic, and have had this illness for 15 years (I am now 20). Throughout the past 13 of those 15 years I have maintained super control over my diabetes. I have been surfing for about six years, and have been able to maintain good control as a result.

However, the last two years have been a little rough. For instance, I've experienced numerous insulin, exercise-induced hypoglycemic attacks after surfing that have left me unconscious, and I've had to be revived intravenously with dextrose administered by paramedics. Just recently I went surfing at the Ventura Marina and, afterward, I became incoherent (low blood sugar) while driving home and crashed my car. Luckily, nobody was hurt and damage was minimal, considering what could have happened. However, this incident has raised many questions about my diabetes.

When I know I'll be surfing intensely all day, I cut my insulin dosage in half and load up on both protein and simple, complex carbohydrates for breakfast. However, this does not seem to be enough, even with snacks in between.

My questions are these: Is there any sort of device I can wear while surfing that will indicate my blood glucose level and alert me when it's dropped below normal? Secondly, how can I prevent these occurrences from happening again?

I fear I may go comatose and inevitably die doing something I absolutely love—surfing. Your advice would be greatly appreciated by both myself and my family.

Diabetes and Surfing

JON
Glendale, California

▌▌▌▌▌|||||

Dear Jon,

Among the more than 10 million diabetics in the U.S. are athletes, and surfers. Most people, even diabetics and doctors, are mystified by this disease. So let's start at the beginning, and work up to what you need to know to successfully manage your diabetes, and continue to surf. If you carefully read the following, you'll have more practical information about diabetes than do most doctors.

A diabetic is a person with a disease called *diabetes* (persistent urination . . .) *mellitus* (. . . of sugar). It's a disease in which the body has trouble breaking down and using sugar (glucose), so that the blood begins to carry abnormally high levels of sugar, and the only way the body can dispose of it is via urine. A poor man's test for diabetes is to pee near an ant hill, and if the ants come running to check out the new candy store, it's time for you to run to the doctor—you've probably got diabetes.

Besides frequent urination, the other major symptoms of diabetes include: continual thirst despite drinking large volumes of water, weight loss and hunger, unexplained sensations and pains (often in the back). A morning (fasting) blood test to measure the level of glucose usually cinches the diagnosis if it is clearly above the normal range of 60 to 110 mg/dl.

"**A** poor man's test for diabetes is to pee near an ant hill, and if the ants come running to check out the new candy store, it's time for you to run to the doctor—you've probably got diabetes. "

There is no cure for diabetes, but it can be controlled by:

1. Limiting sugar intake (particularly simple carbohydrates, i.e., "junk food").

2. Maintaining normal fat stores (i.e., not being fat).

3. Avoiding dehydration, stress, and infections.

4. Taking sugar-lowering pills; or, if all of the above don't work, taking insulin injections. Among other abnormalities, diabetics don't produce enough insulin, a substance made by the pancreas that allows the body to break down and use sugar. Diabetics usually need to inject insulin twice daily.

Specialists in diabetes can't agree on how "tight" the blood sugar levels should be controlled. Some think that it should be held exactly within the normal range (say, 80 to 85 mg/dl), while others feel that "loose" control is safer, that otherwise there is too great a risk of taking too much insulin and developing *hypoglycemia* (low blood sugar, less than 60 mg/dl). As of 1993, though, the balance of evidence strongly points to *tight* control.

Hypoglycemia, as you have found, is a dangerous condition, that can lead to coma and death. It is usually preceded by a rapid pulse, feeling jittery, and having trouble concentrating. These warning signs give a diabetic the chance to pop some sugar in their mouth (most insulin-using diabetics always carry a packet of sugar or candy, just for that purpose). But some diabetics don't have these early warning signs, particularly if they have been diabetic for many years, as you have been. They may suddenly begin acting crazily, or lapse into a coma, and die. Without enough glucose, the brain becomes damaged within minutes.

Unfortunately a continual blood glucose monitoring feedback and alarm device is not yet perfected. So, when you go surfing it would make sense for you to stuff under the sleeve of your wetsuit, or in your trunks, a source of sugar that you could eat if you sensed an attack coming on, or, more logically, that you could take every thirty or so minutes to prevent an attack. Special glucose products are available for that purpose, in plastic tubes (Instant Glu-cose®. Or, be creative and create an in-water cuisine for yourself. Halloween treats are usually small and plastic shrink-wrapped (i.e., waterproof). PowerBars® (U.S.) slip easily up a wetsuit sleeve. Your biggest problem will be having to carry extras, for hungry and envious friends out in the water.

Yet, even with that precaution, you could get into trouble. Exercise causes the body to use up more sugar, meaning that diabetics should use less insulin if they are going to be physically active. The different types of insulin act slower or faster, depending upon if they are human (fastest), pork, or beef derived (this is in addition to the different lengths of action of insulins: short vs. intermediate vs. long-acting). Also, all types of insulin act erratically (usually quicker and stronger) if injected into a part of the body that is then heavily exercised. That means that a surfer shouldn't inject into the arms (paddling) or legs (standing and riding), choosing the belly instead.

> ❝ . . . you should teach your surfing buddies about what to do if you show symptoms of hypoglycemia. ❞

Diabetes and Surfing

Safest for a diabetic surfer, and this is what we'd recommend for you, would be not to take the dose of insulin that would normally cover the time during which you are surfing. Spending a few hours a day with a slightly higher than normal blood sugar ("loose" control) is not dangerous (aim for 125-175 mg/dl, or higher).

Be sure to wear a Medic-Alert bracelet or necklace at all times, especially when you are surfing. Because paramedics won't always be on hand, particularly if you surf remote places, you should teach your surfing buddies about what to do if you show symptoms of hypoglycemia. If you are conscious, they should give you glucose by mouth (fruit juice or soda pop will work fine); if you are unconscious, they can inject you with glucagon, which works opposite of insulin.

Ask your doctor to prescribe you a "Glucagon Emergency Kit for Diabetic Insulin Reaction." It comes with instructions, and is simple to use. Keep it in your car or with your beach stuff. Injecting glucose under your skin would work, too—if you were to keep a vial of it available, along with a needle and syringe, and instructions.

Preparation and prevention is the key. Eat and drink plenty before going out, and make yourself come in for more of the same once an hour (set your watch). The spontaneous "go for it" attitude in surfing doesn't apply to caring for diabetes. But having diabetes doesn't mean that all you'll end up doing in surfing is perfecting the "coffin" maneuver. Stay loose (sugar level-wise) and you shouldn't have any more problems.

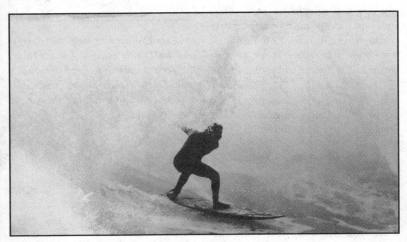

Western Oz. *Photo by John Small.*

Disability

Leg Lost to Cancer

Dear SURF DOCS,

I am a 21-year-old student living in Toronto, Canada. Seven-and-a-half years ago I lost my left leg to cancer. As a boy I always loved the water and dreamed of learning to surf. What I want to know is this: Would surfing be possible for me now?

I am a very athletic individual, and am involved in many sports throughout the year. This last winter I won the Ontario Ski Championships, and came in second in the Eastern Canadian Ski Championships (single leg category). My sense of balance is excellent, as well as my ability to swim.

Surfing on one leg seems pretty impossible, but I have designed a board that just might work. (See figure at right.)

Do you know of any company that would be willing to take the

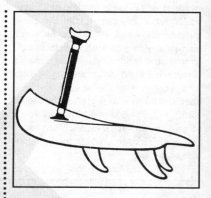

time and money to help me design and build this board? I want to be the first amputee to surf. I think it would prove that people with disabilities can do anything they want to do.

Sincerely,

JOHN
Toronto, Canada

136

Disability

Dear John,

What a stoker it was to get your letter! The answer is yes, you can *definitely* learn to surf, and your disability should not present much of a barrier to your becoming an accomplished surfer. But—sorry to take some of the wind out of your sails—you won't be the first amputee surfer. In *Surfer* magazine there was an article on a one-legged surfer in Volume 23, #3. Apparently the person was able to stand-up surf using his regular prosthesis (artificial leg), meaning he probably had a below-the-knee amputation. Australia's *Tracks* also had a fantastic article (September 1988) about a one-legged South African surfer, named Patrick Sparg.

As you know, John, there is a huge difference between below-the-knee and above-the-knee amputees, as to the degree of function and support provided by a prosthesis. In your case, it sounds like you had an above-the-knee amputation, which is sometimes what's done for cancer in the leg.

Here's what we recommend (in this order):

1. **Become an accomplished swimmer in the ocean, and begin logging time in the waves—that means you'll need to spend extended periods on the coast, away from Toronto.**

2. **Start bodysurfing, with a good swim fin on your one leg and not a prosthesis.**

3. **Advance to bodyboarding. At this point, you may find it so satisfying—as many people do—that you'll never get around to trying stand-up surfing.**

4. **Try kneeboarding or wave-skiing, where you ride a board sitting down, and your amputation won't make any difference.**

5. **If you still want to go on to stand-up surfing, get yourself a soft, 8'-or-longer surfboard. Try using it with your prosthesis in the forward foot position, not as your back/pivot foot (one-legged stand-up surfing without a prosthesis would be possible, but you would not be able to turn the board—you would have to go straight).**

6. **If the previous suggestion worked, get yourself a regular surfboard and go for it! If it did not work, *then* begin experimenting with the board designs you included with your letter.**

Your designs are ingenious, and if it turns out to be the only way for you to be able to stand-up surf, we will personally find a surfboard maker to do the job for you. However, at this point we're a bit apprehensive about the plan.

To begin with, how will you go from the prone position to the standing position on take-off and be able to place your stump into the socket? If, on the other hand, the socket is designed so that it's tethered to your stump at all times, what happens when you wipeout? How will you get free from your board?

One way around these problems would be to place the stump-socket in the middle of the board as a forward foot. If it didn't interfere with paddling it would be much easier to take-off, stand up one-legged and place your stump into the socket. In surfing the front foot is used more for leaning and controlling trim—something your mounted prosthesis-socket would more easily accomplish.

Finally, be sure to write to: The Disabled Surfer's Association, P.O. Box A14, Enfield South, NSW Australia 2133 or call 011-61-2-642-7243.

Keep us posted on your progress!

Surf Doc Follow-up:

John came to visit us in San Francisco. Blowing the minds of everyone on the beach, he dumped his artificial leg on the sand, hopped down to the water and paddled out with us.

Like any first-time surfer, he got tumbled and trashed, but finally caught a wave and was totally stoked. Sitting on the beach, John talked about his future in surfing. It seemed that bodyboarding—not stand-up surfing—was the answer. John's combination of guts, creativity and innate athletic ability would allow him to be a full-on bodyboard surfer, while stand-up surfing would

probably always involve clumsy equipment and high frustration levels.

Surfer's Design Forum editor, George Orbelian (a San Francisco local), also spent time with John, further brainstorming on ways for John to overcome his handicap. Bob Wise, SF surf shop owner extraordinaire, ended up happily donating a bodyboard to John.

Since John's letter appeared in this column, we've gotten many letters from surfers sending him encouragement and ideas. U.S. Manufacturing Company, the largest maker of artificial limbs in the U.S., offered to help in any way they could, and an LA prosthetic specialist called with an offer to help develop a board and prosthesis. It's great to see the surf community pull together to help someone like John attain his dream.

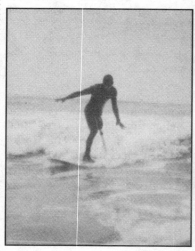

Disability

Spinal Cord Injuries

Dr. Geoff saith:

West Australian, Craig Brent-White's life was changed by one little tube—the one that broke his neck when it ground him head-first into bare rock. Craig was lucky; thanks to quick thinking from fellow surfers and the nature of his injury, he'll walk again.

It has been considered to be almost bad mannered to discuss spinal cord injuries or shark attacks with surfers, particularly the "go for it" type. But it is senseless not to be aware of the likelihood of injury and prepared to deal with it. Here, Craig recounts his experiences and Tracks medical correspondent, Dr. Geoff, includes advice for anyone unfortunate enough to suffer or witness a serious spinal injury.

Craig's Story

"With the sun making its presence felt on distant trees and the familiar offshore easterly brushing the bush that sloped to the coast, the day was bright with expectation. We gave breakfast a miss, despite the general post-bong numbness, and made the beach by 6:30 to find Big Rock doing it at six feet, clean and hollow and we had it all to ourselves, baby.

"We didn't let the fact that the tide was a bit low stop us from heading straight into the line-up, even though this place really jacks up out of deep water, damn that shifting peak. Ah, here's one . . . looks good, down the face . . . turning under the lip . . . hanging in there, Fuck! The ledge and then crunch!

"I'm a bit blurry about the sequence of events after that. The head-on collision with the reef was erased from my memory. I was struggling to stay alive or afloat or something and wondering what the hell had happened. Why was I so stiff, and why couldn't I move properly?

"I was groaning away in the water until Drew heard me and carefully dragged me to the beach. Thank God my brother had the presence of mind to ignore my pleas to try and adjust my back so I could get back in the water. Where was my mind? Placing me flat on my back on my board they carried me up between the rocks and the dunes to the site.

"The chiropractor was the first stop. By this stage I was freaking. Why couldn't I move and why was there so much pain? He examined me and then said, "I'm not touching him, I think he's badly hurt. Let me ring the hospital and book him in for x-rays." The prints showed twisted dislocation and fractures in a couple of vertebrae with a broken facet bone (wing-like bones that extend from the spinal column). The resident doctor said the injury was serious and that I was lucky to be able to move my legs.

"Because of the unstable nature of the injury I was immediately flown to Royal Perth Hospital where calipers were inserted in the skull for traction. I lay on a table under bright lights while my head was shaved. Then a course of attack was planned across my skull with what felt like a felt pen and they went to work on me. The sight of a hand brace being drilled into my skull was most disturbing. The next 48 hours was spent in a pethidine haze. I was in unbelievable pain and was unable to move for five days.

"They turned me over every two hours and drained my bladder four times a day. Then I started to think, what if it's permanent? My poor cock; I couldn't stand having a dirty tube stuck down my John Thomas for the rest of my days.

"I had to ask someone. The doctor explained that it wasn't permanent, and added that I was lucky to have the slightest movement. Each vertebra is associated with different areas of the body and my levels of injury, if the break had been completed, would have left me a quadriplegic. The difference between walking and being crippled was a fraction of a millimeter.

"The doctor impressed upon me my good fortune in having someone there like my brother to make sure I was flat at all times. Many people's injuries are compounded as a result of incorrect handling after the accident. Last year Perth's spinal unit treated 68 spinal injuries, of which 50% are fully quadriplegic, and 30% are paraplegic. The remaining few have various disabilities. So you can see the odds aren't in your favor if you suffer a spinal injury.

"For the very few of us who have come into contact with the world of paraplegics and quadriplegics there is no need to describe what it means to lose the ability to walk and perform even the most basic tasks.

Disability: Spinal Cord Injuries

"So what do you do if you have an accident while surfing? Yes, old buddy, it could actually be you that gets nailed. If you don't like that idea, then how about this one. You're a bystander when someone is dragged out of the water unconscious or paralyzed. What do you do?"

Dr. Geoff replies:

Spinal injuries are not common in the relatively safe sport of surfing. However, there is a definite trend towards what appears to be a kamikaze attitude. (It would be interesting to speculate the reasons for this.) This unthinking and uncaring "go for it" attitude will certainly lead to an increase as more young immortals with neither sufficient experience (say 5 years), nor respect, put themselves into irreversible situations.

It's a long way between surfing 3-4' beach breaks and 10' Pacific or Indian Ocean coral reef tubes.

STATISTICS

Australia has one of the highest incidences of spinal cord injuries in the world. There are about 19 new cases per million population every year. Of these 276 persons, about 80% are males. Nearly 50% are aged between 16 and 25.

Whereas many spinal injuries are associated with car accidents, a significant percentage of serious neck injuries (resulting in quadriplegia) are associated with water accidents—diving into shallow water, water skiing and surfing.

Once injured, the spinal cord does not regenerate. Most people with spinal cord injuries will remain in a wheelchair for the rest of their lives, with or without the use of their arms. Nowadays most spinal injured people have almost a normal length of life span. A spinal cord injury at 20 means about 50 years of life in a wheelchair.

ANATOMY

Thirty-one individual blocks (vertebrae) make up the bony organ called the spine and give the trunk its amazing mobility (mobility for el mysteriosos and snapbacks). Each vertebra is joined to the next by a system of ligaments, discs and muscles, to give this range of movement.

At the same time, the vertebrae surround and protect the spinal cord. Electrical impulses travel up and down this organ—down from the brain to make various muscles work, up from the skin and various organs to tell the brain what's happening.

This spinal cord is the essential relay pathway for all sensation, movement, and control of various organs concerned with the bowel, bladder and sexual functions. Nerves pass from the spinal cord out through holes in the vertebrae and pass to the skin, muscles and organs.

If the spinal cord is destroyed around the level of the 4th cervical vertebra, no movement of the arms or legs can take place—true quadriplegia.

Between the 5th and 7th cervical vertebrae, varying amounts of upper limb movements remain. The lower the level, the more function remains. Quadriplegia is still the term used if some upper limb function is lost.

When spinal injury occurs in the chest and upper lumbar region, movements are either fully or partly lost—paraplegia is then used to describe the situation.

At all levels, if the spinal cord is destroyed, loss of normal bowel, bladder and sexual functions occurs. Rehabilitation techniques can restore a part of these lost functions. However, it is a poor second best when compared with normal functioning.

INJURIES

At the moment of impact between body and ocean floor (rock, coral or sand), the exact amount of damage to the spine will depend on:

1. **How much force is applied.**

2. **The type of force, whether it is compression, rotation or flexion/extension.**

3. **The site of impact.**

Obviously the amount of force occurring at the moment of impact is directly proportional to the size of the wave. However, other factors include wave shape (hollow, spitting cylinders vs. flat rollers), wave speed, and depth of water. For example, inside Pipeline at 10' is far more dangerous that Bells at 15'. This is because of differences in wave power and water depth (as well as shape).

Considerations of the type of force often explains why a particular injury has (or has not) occurred.

Head-first dives, with the neck slightly bent forward and looking to one side, will produce the perfect scenario for disaster. Just put your own neck in this position and imagine jumping off an 8' wave and hitting your head on the bottom!

Serious neck injuries are associated with these forces because the cervical spine is so mobile (and relatively weak) that the vertebrae become dislocated and rip into the spinal cord.

AVOIDANCE

Shallow-water surfing demands practice in the art of wiping out (as well as the ability to make instantaneous decisions). At the same time it requires a great amount of experience and the ability to keep inside the framework of one's own limitations. Very few people have the surfing abilities of the top surfers, despite what the media has to say. Just in the same way an average motorist would crash within the first few minutes of the Formula 5000 event, the average surfer would be drowned in giant Sunset or Waimea Bay.

On the other hand, wiping-out is something that everyone should be proficient in—hotties included! If your limitations are exceeded, then at least you won't break your neck.

In brief, it's best to bail off butt first (with the legs slightly flexed and pointing to the side) and trying for the lower one-third of the wave face. Basically this technique prevents you being slammed straight onto the ocean floor. About 70% of the time you just pop out the back of the wave and nothing happens. If a trip over the falls does result, at least plenty of water has gone over before you, covering the bottom with more water. Finally, if you do hit, it's ankle and bum instead of neck and wheelchair.

MANAGEMENT

A spinal cord injury should always be suspected when someone collides hard with the bottom. Symptoms may start off with only some localized pain; alternatively complete paraplegia or quadriplegia may be obvious right away.

So you've just hit bottom at Uluwatu, Pipeline, Shark Island or Little Avalon and you've hit hard. A spinal injury is suspected. What do your mates do?

The basic principle is not to make the injury worse. This means making sure the injured person lies flat on their back and does not move from side to side. An ambulance should be contacted immediately. If movement of the person is essential (e.g., to escape pounding waves) or if there are no ambulances, the use of a surfboard for carrying could be considered if there were enough people.

Never let anyone manipulate the back until proper diagnosis has been made. X-rays are usually necessary.

Spinal injuries with spinal cord damage should be managed in a proper spinal injury center. Most Australian capital cities have such units. These units have the expertise to manage the spinal injury, prevent or minimize complications and begin early rehabilitation. If high-dose intravenous steroids are used within the first few hours, the outcome may be significantly better.

Medical care is aimed at getting the fractures healed without deformity, treating any correctable cause of spinal cord injury and making sure the spinal cord is not damaged any further. Major operations are rarely performed these days.

In Craig's particular case, skull traction was necessary to reduce the dislocated vertebrae and keep them in correct alignment while the various fractures healed. Careful treatment at this stage allowed the bones to heal without causing any severe pressure on the spinal cord.

Nursing skills in caring for the skin, bowel and bladder are very important—especially when the person has to be kept in bed. As the bladder is no longer able to contract, a catheter must be inserted via the penis. At a later stage, bladder training may help to train persons so they can pass urine "automatically." Bowel function is taken care of with correct diet and the use of special medication.

Rehabilitation care is aimed at:

● *Providing physical therapy (for pain relief, prevention of joints stiffening up, prevention of muscle spasms, and in some cases, keeping the muscles in shape for the time they begin working again).*

● *Helping a person to become physically independent (by providing and showing how to use a wheelchair and other devices), even though he may have permanently lost the use of his legs (and arms).*

● *Helping a person confined to a wheelchair emotionally adjust to a radically different lifestyle. Such adjustment or acceptance usually comes about when the person is convinced that he or she can still lead a satisfying life within the limits of disability.*

For example: Most paraplegics and a significant percentage of quadriplegics are able to drive a car, dress, feed and toilet themselves and in some cases, return to work. Most are able to start up a sport or hobby which is satisfying. An enlightened spinal injuries unit will include sexual techniques in its rehabilitation program. A percentage of spinal injured males are able to make babies! I know one paraplegic person who goes surfing using a specially designed (by him) surfboard which allows him to sit in the board.

There are no second chances once a spinal cord injury has occurred. Prevention is the real key. Remember, it can happen to you and the ocean bottom doesn't know, or care, who you are!

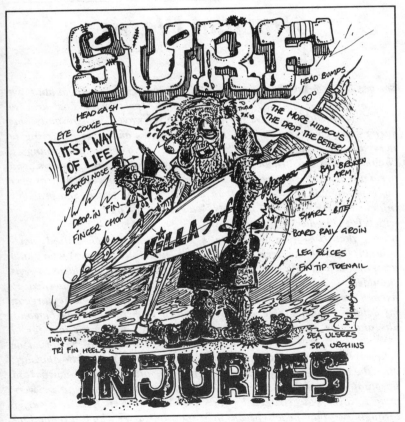

Cartoon drawn by Jim Davidson. This originally appeared in *Australia's Surfing Life*.

Disability: Arm Nerve Injury

Brachial Plexus

Dear SURF DOCS,

I'm 27-years-old, and have been a surfer since I was ten. In 1987, the nerve bundles to my right arm and shoulder were crushed in a rugby accident, leaving that part of my body paralyzed. It was called an injury to my brachial plexus, which is the name for the group of nerves that run from the spinal column, through the neck, into the armpit, and out into the arm and shoulder. I lost my C5 and C6 nerves, meaning that I lost use of my deltoid, rhomboid, biceps, radialis, and some triceps muscle.

Severely bummed, three days after the injury (one day out of the hospital), I borrowed my roommate's log and struggled out through two-foot beach break in front of my house. Though I could fight my way out, I couldn't get enough speed with one arm to catch a wave. So, instantly, my roommates and I started trying to rig me with rubber bands, bungies, pulleys, ropes-through-tubes...you name it. But none of the ideas ever made it to the water; and probably a good thing, too!

I started a search to find someone (hopefully a surfer) who could develop some of my ideas. I was getting desperate and needed to surf badly. My orthopedic surgeon agreed to help me find someone, and wrote a prescription for a device—if one could be found or made—to help me paddle and surf. Finally, after chasing down lead after lead, we found who we were looking for: Ken Kozole, a surfer and windsurfer who is a rehabilitation engineer, and George Mad-

146

Disability: Arm Nerve Injury

den, a windsurfer who is a certified prosthetist orthotist. They greeted me with open arms and showed compassion and stoke to get me back in the waves.

After many long hours and tortuous waiting periods, and fittings and re-fittings, and re-re-fittings, we finally got to a working model. We took it down and tested it, and although there were a few bugs in it, IT WORKED! Just a few minor adjustments were needed . . .

Then the insurance companies and the lawyers jumped in, told Ken and George they'd better stop right there if they hoped to stay in business, all the time yabbering about liability and malpractice potential—thinking I was going to go out with the device and drown, not realizing that even with one arm I was completely safe in the ocean (reflecting the general public's sheer ignorance of surfing!). Ken and George were frustrated; I was destroyed. All that time, energy, love, work, and hope down the drain.

We gotta get lawyers and insurance people on our side. We gotta find those that surf, and ask them to work with us!

Anyway, about this time, a kneeboarder relative from the Lost Coast in Northern California hears about me through the family grapevine, calls, and says "ever think about pulling on some fins and trying kneeboarding?" And he bought me an air ticket to Nor Cal, and picked me up in his plane, and off we went to his spot for me to try kneeboarding.

Since then I've been as stoked as ever. I went down to the swap-meet and had the little Chinese lady make me a custom-fit wetsuit to match my shriveled right arm. Malcolm Campbell carved me an awesome kneeboard with extra flotation, and Sam and the boys at Breakers Surf Shop/Club have been very supportive in and out of the water. I'm even starting to get some use back in my right arm, but I've got a long way to go.

DAVE DONHOFF
La Jolla, California

∎∎∎∎∎∥∥∥∥

Dear Dave,

There's a lot for us all to learn from your experience. First, compared to surfing, practically every other sport is more risky—particularly contact sports like rugby or football. And those kind of injuries can really set back your surfing.

Second, if a physician or other health professional keys into an injured surfer's drive to surf, an immense motivation and healing energy can be harnessed.

Third, we have a long way to go in educating the non-surfing world about the fact that surfing is not the life-threatening activity that they imagine it to be. The Surfer's Medical Association has a number of lawyer members, and any one of them would be happy to brainstorm with you on the dilemma that you and the rest of us face (societal psychosis manifested by a paranoia of being sued).

" . . . if a physician or other health professional keys into an injured surfer's drive to surf, an immense motivation and healing energy can be harnessed."

Fourth, that the fellowship and support of other surfers is essential for us all—in health and in sickness (especially in sickness).

And fifth, and what may be the most important lesson from your letter, that all forms of surfing are equal—from stand-up to kneeboarding, from boogieboarding to bodysurfing. No matter which method is chosen, the mere act of riding a wave is what makes a person a surfer. Prejudice among stand-up surfers towards kneeboarders and boogieboarders, and other non-standing surfers, has long been ingrained in our sport. The Surfer's Medical Association stands in vehement opposition to such bigotry. As you've discovered, Dave, you are no less a surfer if you are a kneeboarder.

Disability: Recovering

Surfing Despite Disability

Dear SURF DOCS,

At age two, I had polio, then became a victim of RA (rheumatoid arthritis). By age 15, I was living in Canada, and every winter would leave me badly crippled. By age 21, I was completely disabled—the arthritis destroyed my track career, and asthma and rhinitis/sinusitis stopped me from participating in even the simplest sports activities.

After researching the body's immune system, I found that all my illnesses were interrelated to immune system dysfunctions. I began experimenting with warm weather climates. I left Canada and went to Florida, Texas and California for winter stays. Finally, I came to Hawaii, and found the even weather patterns which allowed my arthritis to go into remission. It was a thrill to return to an almost normal lifestyle after years of living as a cripple.

I spent three years lifting weights and running before I started swimming. After about four months of swimming, I started surfing the south shore of Oahu. I ride a 6'2"thruster that's a little hot for me right now, but its narrowness and lightness make it easy to keep up with the boys. We usually surf 3-5' waves.

I'm 36-years old, and I waited a long time to fulfill my dream. Surfing is the most exciting sport in the world, and it's too precious to lose because of poor health.

My problem relates to the walking pneumonia I've had twice this year. I've found that my upper body strength has dropped considerably in the three months I've been sick. I would like your advice

*on how to get back into good
enough shape to surf the North
Shore waves.*

EDI
A lady surfer

■■■■IIIIIIIII

Dear Edi,

Judging by how well you took care of
your earlier medical problems, you flat-
ter us by asking for our advice on how
to build up your body after walking
pneumonia.

Walking pneumonia is usually due to
a virus, or something called *myco-
plasma* (which can be treated with
antibiotics like erythromycin or tetracycline). To regain your upper body
strength, you can do various exercises
or yoga (focus on the breathing technique), but most importantly, just surf a
lot.

Most important in recovery from
pneumonia are the simple things: Getting enough sleep (8 hours a night for
most people), and a balanced, healthy
diet.

Dizziness

Head Spins

Dear Dr. GEOFF,

I hope you can help me. I'm 18 and surf regularly. I've noticed though in the past few months I suffer severe dizziness and head-aches after a session.

Usually it goes away after a few hours but lately it lasts all day. The last time it happened I felt like spewing and even woke up the next day feeling dizzy.

It's really bad. I can't even walk down the passage without bouncing off the walls. Panadols don't seem to help (not even an over-dose). What's wrong?

P.S. I don't eat breakfast most mornings, but I really pig out later.

P.P.S. I don't want to give up surfing !!!!!

JAMES
Western Australia

Dear James,

One possibility is that your blood sugar is a bit low. Surfing sessions first thing of a morning in cold weather and with-out food inside can be pretty extreme. Try some light breakfast at least one-half hour before and then hit it.

Another possibility is that you're suf-fering from some type of overdose (booze, bongs, or whatever) from the night before.

Other possibilities include serious medical disorders which would ***need*** to be investigated by your doc. Persistent symptoms such as headaches, dizziness and vomiting in an 18-year-old need to be checked out properly. If your vision has changed in any way of late see your doc *straight away* to check you for a tumor.

Drug Use and Surfing

A Bad Idea Whose Time Has Gone

Dear SURF DOCS,

It seems to me that the people who do drugs surf better. For example, I heard that [names of two high-ranked PSAA surfers] go off. And there are lots of other people who do drugs and are good surfers. Some of the surfers around my area get stoned for breakfast, lunch, and dinner, and they are the best surfers around. Does pot have effects on surfing? Does it help some people surf better?

ZEB
Leucadia, California

▮▮▮▮▮▮║║║║

Dear Zeb,

The answer to your questions are easy: yes, pot does affect how one surfs—you'll surf worse. We apologize if that sounds like the opening act for Nancy Reagan's "JUST SAY NO" campaign, but that is what all available medical evidence tells us. To begin with, smoking anything—marijuana, tobacco, or clove cigarettes—is damaging to your lungs. And good lungs are essential to good surfing. Additionally, marijuana interferes with coordination and fine muscle movements, as well as mental concentration, which, again, will make you surf worse.

So, how do those guys do it, the ones who get loaded and surf so well? If you're friends with them (i.e., you know their habits), compare how they surf when they're stoned to when they're not stoned. What you'll see is that they surf better—and longer—when they're not stoned. The contest surfers you refer to, and the hottie-stoners in your area, are

Drug Use and Surfing

such good surfers that even when they're stoned they still surf better than practically everyone else.

Another ingredient to the puzzle is that some of these guys who are so good will—as part of the cavalier style of being ultra-hot—deliberately do things to make themselves seem even more impressive: surf on a beatup old board, paddle out at the hardest places, take off on seeming closeouts, and surf while loaded.

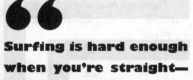

Surfing is hard enough when you're straight— being loaded just makes it harder.

Then there are some surfers whose emotional state is so frazzled when they're straight that being stoned is the only way they've found to get along in the world. They're the ones out in the lineup who—when not stoned—are always yelling at everyone, acting irrational, picking fights deliberately. But, when stoned, they seem mellower, and easier to get along with. It should be obvious, though, that drugs won't solve their basic problem; that will only come from digging in at a deeper level.

Hope that helps, Zeb. Surfing is hard enough when you're straight—being loaded just makes it harder.

Ears:
Surfer's Ear

Getting Drilled

Dear SURF DOCS,

I have surfer's ear. My doctor has told me that I have 95-100% closure of the ear canal. In the recent past I have had to stay out of the water to prevent further infections. I am reluctant to be drilled since seeing a friend go through so much pain and discomfort from the operation. He had to have his ear partially cut off and folded forward to access his ear canal. Ech!!

Lately I have seen so many new techniques involving laser technology that I'm hoping to wait until the operation can be made less painful and less intrusive. Am I whistling in the wind? Should I act as soon as possible? Will my hearing suffer further damage if I wait? I'm living in New Hampshire for two years—could this period of time out of the water improve the situation? For exam-
ple, I noticed that when I quit knee paddling, my surf knots eventually improved.

CHRIS
New England

Dear Chris,

Surfer's ear is still the number one topic of letters to the Surf Docs. Your letter gave us a chance to do an update, so we polled our Surfer's Medical Association ear specialists for the latest word on surfer's ear.

WHAT IS SURFER'S EAR?

Surfer's ear is when lumps of bone *(bony exostoses)* form under the skin of the ear canal. As the lumps get bigger, they can trap water, ear wax, sand, and dead skin next to the ear drum.

154

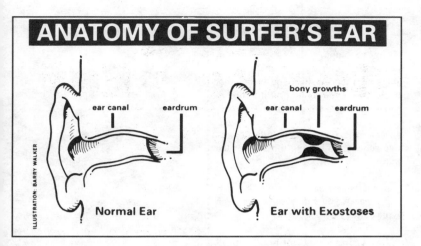

ANATOMY OF SURFER'S EAR

ILLUSTRATION: BARRY WALKER

Normal Ear — ear canal, eardrum

Ear with Exostoses — bony growths, ear canal, eardrum

What Causes It?

The bony exostoses are thought to be caused by repeated irritation of the ear canal by a combination of water, wind, and perhaps wave agitation. The skin of the ear canal is paper-thin: it's the only place on the body where the bone lies under the skin without an insulating layer of fat or muscle. Probably for this reason, surfer's ear develops more quickly in cold conditions. There also seem to be hereditary factors: in the same conditions, some surfers rapidly develop bony exostoses, while others go years with little or no growth.

What are the Symptoms?

Early symptoms (50-80% closure) are stuffed-up ears and ear infections; later (80-100%), there can be hearing loss and ringing of the ears *(tinnitus)*. Surfer's ear does not have any permanent effect on hearing or balance,

because it does not affect the delicate structures of the middle or inner ear behind the eardrum.

Can It Be Prevented?

For most surfers, using earplugs—along with a neoprene hood in colder waters—will prevent surfer's ear. Doc's Pro-plug's® are still the best for most surfers. Regular (one to two a year) ear exams are a good idea to see how your efforts at prevention are working.

Is It Reversible?

Surf knots, for instance on the knees, are essentially big callouses; leave them alone and they'll go away. Surfer's ear is bone and most ear specialists say that bony exostoses don't go away. Your ears will seem better if you move inland for a couple of years, but as soon as you start surfing again, you'll be back to the doctor.

Can Treatment Be Put Off?

If you've stopped the progression of surfer's ear, either by effective use of plugs and hood or by (God forbid) not surfing, then you can put off the surgery without doing any harm. If, on the other hand, you wait while your ears are getting worse, you may need more extensive surgery, with more time out of the water.

If your surfer's ear is stable (not getting bigger), you can postpone or even avoid surgery by:

1. **Using alcohol/boric acid drops to evaporate water from the canal.**

2. **Gently drying the canal after a surf with a blow dryer.**

3. **Getting your ears cleaned regularly by a doctor, especially before surf trips to the tropics.**

Are There New Treatments?

The surgery for surfer's ear is safe and effective; perhaps it's for that reason that there isn't much experimentation with treatments going on. We haven't heard much in the way of natural or holistic methods of treating surfer's ear, and there isn't much in the way of new technology either. Some orthopedists (bone docs) have been working with lasers to remove bone, but the lasers generate a lot of heat and tend to ricochet, both of which could be disastrous in the tiny spaces of the ear canal.

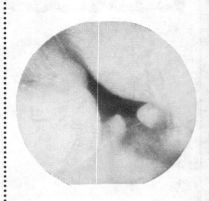

Be sure to check out the surfer's ear illustration on the inside back cover.

It looks as though for now we're stuck with surgery as the only effective treatment for advanced surfer's ear.

SURFER'S EAR SURGERY

Here is the current lowdown on surfer's ear surgery from our SMA ear specialists.

Technique

The skin of the ear canal is cut with a scalpel and peeled back. Bony growths are then removed using fine drills and burrs, and the skin is sewn back in place. Some surgeons prefer to get into the canal from behind, cutting the back of the outer ear and folding it forward to give better access. This approach can allow for more complete removal of bone and quicker healing time because of better skin repair. The ear is easily sewn back in place, but is more painful for the first couple of days than with the straight-in technique.

Cost

Covered by most medical insurance, the surgery costs $3500 to $5000 per ear in the U.S. Of that, $1200-2000 is the surgeon's fees, $1000-1500 is for anesthesia, and $500-1500 covers operating room/hospital charges. (We heard of a surfer from Oregon who went to Chile and had an excellent job done on his ears for one-third the cost in the United States.)

Time

The surgery takes from one to two hours, depending on the surgeon and how advanced the bony exostoses are.

Pain

Roughly comparable to having your wisdom teeth out.

Anesthesia

General anesthesia (totally out) is almost always used, but it's possible to do it with local anesthesia and sedating drugs.

Time Out of the Surf

You have to wait until the skin heals over or risk a major infection; the usual minimum is three to four weeks, although some lucky souls have been back in the line-up within two weeks.

One Ear at a Time vs. Both

Most surgeons like to do them one ear at a time, partly to ensure that you have one intact ear at all times and partly because it is demanding, tedious surgery. For the first week after surgery, your ear is packed with bandaging material and you are essentially deaf in that ear. If your surgeon is up for doing both ears at once and you're willing to be deaf for a week, then go for it.

Complications

With a good surgeon, this is a safe operation. As with any surgery, there is a risk of bleeding or infection, but our specialists report that both are unusual. There is an important nerve—the facial nerve—that runs in the bone of the canal and there have been cases where it was cut by mistake, leading to droopy facial muscles. However, it is now possible to use special monitors that are triggered if the nerve is touched, warning the surgeon to back off.

PREVENTING REGROWTH

For some reason, once operated on surfer's ear has a tendency to regrow unless you are diligent in using ear plugs and a hood. Even if you do everything right, it may still regrow. One SMA member, dear Rym Bone, has had to have his ears operated on 5 times! We now call him Ear Bone . . .

Ears: Swimmer's Ear

When Skin Goes Bad

Here's another surfer's ear question. I hate using ear plugs while surfing. Instead, I always put a few drops of rubbing alcohol into my ears after surfing to disinfect and help evaporate water. It does the trick, but I'm wondering if there can be any side effects. Also, would using hydrogen peroxide be safer or better? I previously used a product called Auro-dri (non-prescription): "Helps dry and relieve swimmer's ear." Then I read the label of contents: **Boric Acid 2.75% in Isopropyl Alcohol 97.25%.** *Now I just refill it with alcohol.*

Thanks for any advice.

PETE
Santa Barbara, California

▮▮▮▮▮▮▮▮▮▮▮

Dear Pete,

You've confused *swimmer's* ear with *surfer's* ear. While they can be related, they are not the same. Here's the scoop.

Swimmer's ear (or what doctors call *otitis externa*) is an infection of the skin in the ear canal. It happens when protective ear wax is washed away and/or water and sand get trapped in the canal. Wet, irritated skin forms a great place for bacteria to grow.

Surfer's ear is a bony growth under the skin in the ear canal that, if it gets bad enough, can block off the canal and cause hearing loss. It is caused by the irritating effects of water—especially cold water—and wind. Surfer's ear can lead to swimmer's ear because the lumps in the ear canal trap water, keeping the skin wet and irritated.

Both conditions can and should be prevented. Even though you hate ear plugs, they are still the best way to prevent surfer's ear.

But, if the plugs don't work out, it may be that a neoprene hood—by keeping your ears warm and shielding them from the wind—can do as much to prevent surfer's ear. We know plugs help prevent surfer's ear, and it looks like hoods do, too. The optimal solution is to wear both.

As for ear drops, they can help prevent swimmer's ear, but do nothing for surfer's ear. Alcohol evaporates the water from your ears and has no side effects as long as you don't drink it. Boric acid (which is gentle enough to use as an eye rinse) adds an extra kick: it makes the skin's surface more acidic,

by lowering the pH and making the ear canal inhospitable to bacteria.

Hydrogen peroxide is a lousy solution. It evaporates as slowly as water, further damages irritated skin, and dissolves protective ear wax. There is only one good use for hydrogen peroxide in the ears, and that is to clear wax build-up blocking the ear canal.

So, to prevent swimmer's ear, your drops are great. They won't do diddly to prevent surfer's ear, though. To do that, you'll have to keep wind and water out of your ears, using ear plugs and a hood.

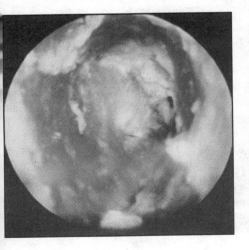

Swimmer's ear, not surfer's ear (bony closure), but the buildup of sand, dead skin, and wax (both natural and surfboard, how it got in this surfer's ear isn't known). All that junk stays wet and gets infected easily. *Photo courtesy of Dan Sooy, MD.*

Ears: Wax Build-Up

Whacking Your Wax

Dear SURF DOCS,

I am a 39-year-old surfer (24 years in the water). Lately I've been having a problem with excessive wax build-up in my ears. My chiropractor has been treating this problem with "ear candles," which have been somewhat successful, but he feels the problem is too much for this type of treatment and I should seek alternatives.

Thank you.

DENNY
Southern California

▮▮▮▮▮▮▮▏▏▏

Dear Denny,

Surfers are besieged by many kinds of ear problems, including so-called swimmer's ear or *otitis externa* (doctor talk, meaning inflammation of the external ear canal), impaction (jam-ups of wax and sand), surfer's ear (bony growths in the external ear canal), ear drum rupture and perforation, and middle-ear infections and blockage. Each of these problems can feel the same: pain, pressure, and trouble hearing.

What we are saying is that although you may very well have wax build-up, there can be other explanations for your problem. For instance, if your chiropractor has looked in your ears (something most chiropractors don't regularly do), he may have mistaken bony growths (surfer's ear) for ear wax. We see surfers all the time who tell desperate stories of trying to get help for surfer's ear, and being told by physicians that they only have wax in their ears (most physicians have never heard of surfer's ear, much less seen it).

The other thing that is important to point out is that ear wax is good. It waterproofs our ear canals and protects them from infections—that's why our bodies make it. Unfortunately, many people treat ear wax like boogers, and pick at their ears every chance they get with their finger, toothpick, or whatever pointed object they can fit in there. This usually pushes the wax farther into the canal, rather than out, and results in a wax ball that can be hard to get out. If you're an ear picker, that may be what started your "wax build-up."

" . . . many people treat ear wax like boogers, and pick at their ears every chance they get . . . "

Ear pickers also get more frequent infections by disturbing the delicate, one-cell-layer-thick skin of the ear canal, and that's all most bacteria or fungi need to get a foothold and *really* cause problems (itching, pain, swelling, discharge).

If you need to disimpact your ear (remove a jam-up of wax and other debris), try inserting three or four drops of olive oil (or any other vegetable oil) into each ear canal twice daily for up to a week. On the third or fourth day, begin flushing your ear canals with jets of warm water from a turkey baster or other bulb syringe (sold in drug stores). Don't stick it in farther than your thumb will go.

This will usually do the trick, and works as well or better than commercial ear wax removal products. Don't blast it too hard, you just want the water to gently dislodge the wax.

Ears: Ringing (Tinnitus)

Kill Your Stereo

Dear SURF DOCS,

Hi! Thanks for the great service. Most of us can't afford to get clinical advice.

My problem is this: At 26, with 10 years of surfing experience, I've developed (and been diagnosed as having) surfer's ear. I know that's pretty common. However, both ears ring constantly, and I've had some hearing loss. This has been going on for a couple of years, but has gotten worse over the past six months. I therefore have two questions:

1. Are my ears ringing due to surfer's ear? (I also listen to somewhat loud music.)

2. I won't have any sort of health plan for about another year. What risks do I run by waiting to have my problem cared for?

STEVE
Long Beach, California

▮▮▮▮▮▮▮|||||

Dear Steve,

Ringing in the ear (*tinnitus*, in medical lingo), can be indirectly caused by severe surfer's ear, when the ear canal becomes blocked—either by the bony growths themselves or a build-up of wax, sand and dead skin, especially if it's jammed up against the ear drum. Tinnitus can also occur in otherwise normal ears, often for no apparent reason. For more on tinnitus, write or call the American Tinnitus Association, P.O. Box 5, Portland, OR 92707, 503/248-9985. They hold international conferences on the subject of ringing ears.

Turning the volume too high on your stereo may have contributed to the ringing in your ears, and can cause permanent damage. The guys with the earth-shaking tape decks of today may be the

Ears: Ringing

hearing-aid wearers of tomorrow. Listening to very loud music is a habit, and after turning the volume down for a few months, you'll find your former noise levels almost painful.

If you're not having problems with ear pain or water being trapped in your ears, you can wait for treatment. You've got to start wearing ear plugs (such as Doc's Proplugs®) when you surf. Wearing a hood would be a good idea, too. Keeping your ears warm and dry will stop or at least slow the bony growths from forming in your ears.

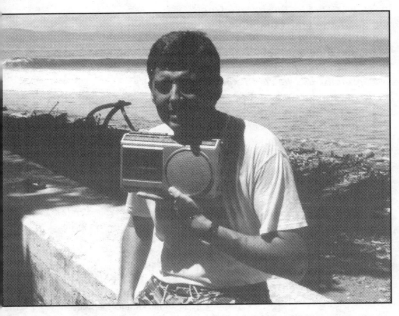

Boom-boxing your ears, or perfect endless lefts; take your pick. SMA Costa Rica Conference. *Beach Photos.*

Ears: Broken Ear Drum

Get the Zig-Zags!

Dear SURF DOCS,

*I am a 16-year-old surfer from Folly Beach, South Carolina. I have been surfing for 3 years. One day I got sick and went to the doctor, and when he checked my ears there was a pinhole opening in my middle ear. I have since gone to an ear specialist and he said I needed surgery, which I've just had (they cut in just above my ear and patched the hole—I think they called it a **tympanoplasty**). I'm told I should not surf for 4 to 5 months, that it will take that long for the patch to become positively secure. And they say if it gets wet it could hurt the healing.*

I was wondering if it would be at all possible to make something to keep water completely out of if my ear or if there is anything at all I could do to get in the water faster. The contest season is starting soon here, and I want to be in it!

JOHN
Charleston, South Carolina

▌▌▌▌▌▐▐▐▌▌

Dear John,

The eardrum is called the *tympanic membrane* ("tympanic" as in the tympany drum, those big copper kettle drums in orchestras). If you had a tympanoplasty, it means that a hole (a "perforation") in your eardrum was surgically sealed. The usual way of sealing small holes like yours is to plaster *(plasty)* it over with glue and a small bit of paper (some surgeons use Zig-Zag rolling paper—no joke!), or plug it with a piece of fat or similar body tissue. The idea is that if you can just cover the hole, it will then have a chance to heal.

If paper was used, you can see why you wouldn't want to get your ear wet too soon. Eventually the paper falls off, but by then, usually at about one month, the hole should be sealed over by the natural growth of the tympanic membrane. At that time, you probably could

164

safely get your ear wet, but it wouldn't be safe to surf yet. It takes a good six to eight weeks for most closed-over perforations to develop enough strong, fibrous tissue to endure a sudden pressure change (such as diving under a wave, or smacking the side of your head on the water during a wipeout).

For that reason, you should wait a full two months after having a tympanoplasty (for a pinhole sized eardrum perforation, and longer if the hole was bigger). Ear plugs, like Doc's Pro-plugs®, will do a pretty good job of keeping water out, but shouldn't be relied upon to protect your ear in the first weeks after surgery. Once you have healed, however, we would recommend you use earplugs to prevent other perforations or re-perforating the same spot because they do divert some of the force of a blow to the ear. Wearing a hood, helmet (i.e., Gath® or Radhat®), or swim cap also would lessen the chance of a perforation.

As to what caused your perforation in the first place, it sounds like you had an infection in the middle ear that caused a buildup of pressure and blew-out a weak spot (as when a tire is filled too high with air). Next time you have a cold, consider using decongestants containing pseudoephedrine to keep open your ear passageways.

Staying out of the water for four to five months sounds excessive to us. You should be healed far sooner than that; put in for your competition jersey now—you'll be wearing it soon.

The idea is that if you can just cover the hole, it will then have a chance to heal.

Elbow Pain (Tendinitis)

Self-Abuse Has Many Forms

Dear Dr. GEOFF,

I've just returned from my longest session (surf) for quite a while which aggravated an injury which has been with me on and off for over two years.

It consists of a pain on the inner side of my left elbow (neither caused or affected by drinking or self-abuse) which appears midway through each stroke when paddling hard. A couple of sharp twinges are usually felt once I am out of the water caused by nothing more than normal movements, then the problem disappears until the next lengthy surf. I have used an elastic elbow support with limited success and I expect the injury is something akin to tennis elbow, although I don't play tennis.

In addition to hoping you'll favor me with some words from your colleague, Dr. Frank Zappa, I am interested in your diagnosis and advice for treatment (if any) as I am sick of being creamed by clean-up sets due to my inability to scratch for the horizon with any great vigor.

> **CLEANED UP**
> *West Coast, Victoria*
> *Australia*

■■■■■■IIIIIII

Dear Cleaned Up,

There are a couple of possibilities. The most likely one consists of overstrain of the flexor capri ulnaris (FCU) muscle. This essentially comes about by continued forceful movement of this muscle while paddling, holding the wrist in position to get enough propulsion. However, there are other possibilities such as gradual irritation of the ulnar nerve. This would cause little electric shocks of pain going down the inner part of the forearm and sometimes into the little finger.

Elbow Pain

You don't say whether you're left- or right-handed and you also don't say whether you actually suffered an injury two years ago or not. Other important things to consider include what other activities you do other than surf.

The principles of management, however are:

● *Not to surf to the stage of getting pain. So stop when discomfort rather than pain first occurs.*

● *Avoid any other activities that also give rise to pain.*

● *Strengthen weaker shoulder, arm, and wrist muscles.*

● *Stretch tight muscles and ligaments; especially those that cross the elbow joint.*

● *Maintain equal range of elbow movement on both sides.*

● *If pain persists after activity, use ice and rest.*

Tennis elbow involves the outer part of the bone of the elbow *(lateral epicondyle)* and a tennis elbow splint would obviously be useless to a surfer.

The problem you describe is more common on the outside of the elbow and I would suggest that a trip to the doc be undertaken just to make sure that we are talking about the same elbow area.

Sometimes injections are necessary into the painful muscular attachment area. Great care is needed if it's on the medial side because of the presence of the ulnar nerve.

P.S. The esteemed Dr. Z. says: "In the fight between you and the world, back the world." I'm afraid that even with my overt optimism I would have to agree.

167

Epilepsy and Surfing

Grand Mal De Mer

Dear SURF DOCS,

I am 28-years-old and have been an avid surfer of the California and Latin America coasts for the past 15 years. While in graduate business school, I still found time to surf 145 times. I'm dedicated to the sport—it's in my blood.

Four years ago I developed partial-complex epilepsy, which means I'm prone to having seizures once in a while, without warning. My body goes into convulsions, my muscles tighten up, and my breathing becomes erratic.

The seizures have typically come while I'm sleeping. No problem. However, last September, I had my first one while awake. It came just as I was paddling into perfect 5-foot surf. Luckily, I was with three friends who understood my condition, and spotted it right away. They were able to get to me in time, keep my head up, and drag me back through the sets and onto the beach. Except for a little water in my lungs, I was okay—but it was a close call.

My neurologist has told me to stay out of the water, "Until we can completely control the seizures, and you have a seizure-free year, you shouldn't even consider surfing." I stayed out of the water for a week. Then, perfect waves and my love for the sport drew me out again. Since September I've surfed on a regular basis. I've had two more seizures—both on land.

I'm trying to find the right medication and dosage to control the seizures. I'm still surfing, and I'm concerned about my safety. What can I do to best protect myself while surfing. I can't give up my favorite thing on the Earth.

PAUL
Northern California

▉▊▋▍▎▏║║║

168

Epilepsy and Surfing

Dear Paul,

The safest thing would be to stay out of the water until you're sure the seizures are under control. But, since you've already made the choice to keep surfing—something we can well understand—here are some ideas to make it as safe as possible:

● *Don't surf alone! Surf with friends who will keep an eye on you. Make sure they know CPR and water-rescue techniques. Also, your neurologist may be willing to sit down with you and your friends to discuss the best way to deal with a seizure in the water.*

● *Consider wearing an inflatable neck collar, at least until your seizures are under control with medication. Called buoyancy compensators (BCs), these collars are sold in dive shops. When inflated, a BC will keep you from sinking or ending up face down if you should pass out from a seizure. If you have the kind of seizures that are preceded by a warning sensation (called an* aura*), you may have time to self-inflate the BC. Otherwise, instruct your friends that they should inflate it when they reach you during a seizure.*

● *Avoid surfing spots with long paddle-outs or difficult water entries and exits. Make sure there*

are adequate emergency services available wherever you surf.

> **Don't surf alone! Surf with friends who will keep an eye on you. Make sure they know CPR and water-rescue techniques.**

● *Tell your neurologist of your plans to keep surfing, and tell him or her to step it up on finding the right medication for you (it shouldn't take so long). And, remember, it's important not to miss any doses of seizure medication.*

It's easy to get pissed off and fed up while you're waiting to get your medications sorted out and are feeling the side effects, but stick with it. Seizing in the line-up is way too radical a maneuver for any surfer.

Exercise

Who Says Surfing Isn't Exercise?!

Dear SURF DOCS,

In an effort to justify surfing, I've been telling non-surfers for years that surfing is great exercise but I've never been able to back up my claim with hard facts.

Perhaps you could supply me with information on the cardiovascular effects of surfing, as well as how much exercise the body derives from it. Is surfing really such good exercise, or have I been fooling my parents, friends, girlfriends and myself all these years?

HANGIN' HOWIE
Encinitas, California

▌▌▌▌▌▌▏▏▏

Dear Hangin',

Our Research Kahuna, Brian J. Lowdon, of Deakin University, in Victoria, Australia is the foremost authority in the world on surfing physiology and he has provided us with the necessary facts.

Surfing is a whole-body exercise, utilizing most of the body's 600 or so muscles, particularly the heart. A recent study by Rudi Meir, of Byron Bay, Australia, involved monitoring the heart rates of surfers.

During an average go-out at a beachbreak, 44% of the time was spent paddling, 35% waiting for waves, and 5% riding waves (they averaged 21 waves per hour; the number would be less in big surf). While riding waves, peak heart rate was 171 beats per minute (bpm). While paddling, it was 143 bpm. The average for the entire go-out was 135 bpm.

Meir then calculated the energy expenditures required to sustain those heart rates, and came up with a figure of

Exercise

Calories Burned for Various Exercise

Sport	Calories used per hour
Running (10 mph)	1,285
Running (6 mph)	750
Cycling	660
Squash/handball	600
Surfing	**496**
Walking (level road, 4 mph)	420
Swimming (25-50 yards per min.)	360-750

496 calories (kilocalories) per hour of surfing—an impressive figure, in comparison to other sports.

Bear in mind that all surfers are not equally active in the water. You'd be burning a lot less calories if you weren't catching many waves, because of crowds, conditions, or being overly picky. Also, these numbers may not apply to cold-water surfing, which—depending on water and air temperatures and type of wetsuit worn—could be significantly higher.

The American College of Sports Medicine suggests the requirements of cardiovascular training to be:

F = Frequency: 3-5 sessions per week

I = Intensity: 70-80% of maximum heart rate

T = Time: 20-30 minutes per session

Surfing meets or exceeds each of the FIT requirements, so you're not fooling yourself or anyone else—keep surfing for fitness, health and fun.

Eyes: Trauma

Eye Scream . . .

Dear Dr. GEOFF,

About a month ago I had the unfortunate luck of being hit in the eye by the nose of my new surfboard.

I was fortunate in that I had the nose of the board rounded off and there was only bruising and slight bleeding in and around the eye. The bruising and bleeding took two weeks to clear.

I was wondering what steps should be taken if damage is done to the eye, e.g., the eye being popped out of the socket or being cut. If alone, what would you do? If with other surfers, what could they do to help?

Any information would be appreciated as I consider my eyesight too valuable to lose.

BIFOCAL

Dear Bifocal,

If the eye complex—be it eyelid, eye itself or bony socket (*orbit* is the medical term)—is cut (or broken) in any way, you must get to a major hospital as quickly as possible.

First-aid consists of placing a vaseline-impregnated large gauze pad over the eye and keeping it gently in place. This keeps the area clean and helps to stop bleeding.

If the eye is penetrated and the object is still in the eye, it's best to leave the object where it is. Tape a cup over the eye and the penetrating object to prevent its being bumped and doing more damage. It's a good idea to cover *both* eyes to minimize eye movement. It's unlikely that a surfboard would stay in the eye!

"Blunt" injuries (e.g., surfboard noses) literally burst the eye like a grape and that's the end of the eye. Very sharp objects (e.g., surfboard fins) are associated with slightly less force on the eye and it might be possible to save the eye using modern eye surgery techniques. A lot depends on what contents of the eye have been injured and how much of the contents have been lost.

> **" . . . prevention is the key and sensible surfboard design is the only way to stop these injuries from occurring. "**

It's very unlikely that an eyeball would be "popped out of the socket." It might look like it sometimes but it's unlikely in the usual type of surfboard accident.

Again, use of the vaseline-impregnated eye pad is the first-aid method of choice. In isolated areas, ring the emergency number and ask for the ambulance service. Tell them what's happened and they'll direct you to the nearest treatment center.

Recently, I was told of a horrendous accident in which a surfboard fin was embedded into a surfer's eye/orbit complex. The surfer literally pulled the fin out of his own eye, swam in, wrapped a towel around his head and went to the nearest hospital. Naturally enough, he lost his eye. Psychologically, it took him about eight months or so before he could face going back to surfing. It took him another six months before he'd regained full confidence and worked out techniques for surfing blind side. Take-offs and backhand surfing (his blind side) were the most difficult aspects to master.

Undoubtedly, prevention is the key and sensible surfboard design is the only way to stop these horrifying injuries from occurring. Blunting the nose (there are now standards for surfboard manufacturers in Australia) does not make any difference whatsoever on the performance of your surfboard. Therefore, insist on this and do not buy secondhand boards with "needle" noses.

Using a siliconized rubber tip (various brands commercially available, such as *Nose Guard*) is a good idea. They're cheap in the U.S. but expensive over here in Australia (mainly because of government charges).

They are recommended, however, as being a step in the right direction. I'm not saying that you won't lose your eye if you're hit by the protected nose of the board. However, the amount of force will certainly be far less. A few surfers have reported that *Nose Guard* has saved their eye or the eye of a person hit by their board.

Eyes: Glasses, Contacts and Surfing

Mr. Magoo Goes Surfing

Dear SURF DOCS,

I'm only 25-years-old, but I've been surfing for almost 15 years. I'm writing to you in the hope that you can help me with my eye problems.

First off, I've always had bad vision. I wear glasses, which let me see normally, but in the water, without my glasses on, I'm pretty hopeless. It's the one advantage to surfing with a crowd: when everyone starts paddling outside, I know there's a set coming. Surfing by myself is unthinkable, which really bums me out.

I tried various ways of rigging my glasses for surfing, but it just didn't work out. They'd fog up, mash into my face, or get torn off (there's probably a big tuna wearing them now!). I tried getting contacts a few years back, but they couldn't be fitted to me because they told me I had an "astigmatism." Plus, when I said I wanted contact lenses for surfing, I was told it was a bad idea because I'd lose them, and maybe get infections!

My other problem is that my eyes are really sensitive. After surfing, my eyes sometimes sting, especially if it was really sunny and I hung out on the beach. I've tried clip-on sunglasses (which all look pretty stupid), and have thought about trying to get prescription sunglasses, but they're awfully expensive, and I don't know what kind of sunglasses are best to get.

I went to one eye doctor who said, "Hang it up, kid," as far as

Eyes: Glasses, Contacts and Surfing

surfing goes, but I figure that must be crap (at least I'm hoping it is!). What are your thoughts?

MR. MAGOO
Pacific Beach, California

■■▮▮▮▯▯▯

Dear Mr. Magoo,

Given the fantastic optical technologies of today, there is no reason for you to continue surfing blind. If your vision can be fully corrected on land, it can almost certainly be fully corrected in the water. Here's how to see clear of this mess you are in.

First off, you need to find a eye doctor who is knowledgeable about vision correction for water sports. In coastal areas there are a surprising number of surfing eye doctors—ask around!

Contact lenses are probably your best bet. You'd be amazed how many surfers wear contacts. In a study of contact lens-wearing surfers, totaling over fifty thousand hours of surfing, there were no eye infections or eye damage, and about one lens was lost for every five hundred hours of surfing (about once a year for the average surfer). But there was a huge variation in the lens loss rate: some surfers would lose a lens practically every month, while others had never lost one. The difference was probably in how well their lenses were fit to their eyes, and their ability to keep their

eyes squinty or closed during intense situations (tube-riding, wiping out, diving under, etc.).

Contact lenses are generally "hard" or "soft," referring to the type of plastic used. When contact lenses first became popular a few years back, only the hard lenses were available, and many people (perhaps you) tried them on, hated how they felt, and refused to wear them. Then along came soft lenses, which most people found far more comfortable. Plus, soft lenses could be made to cover more of the eye, and they stayed on better during athletic activities, including water sports (they are called "sport lenses"). More recently, advances in plastic technology have led to highly gas permeable plastics, which can be made into both hard or soft lenses, including the "extended wear" and disposable-type lens. These high-tech lenses allow the cornea to receive more oxygen, which translates into greater comfort. The cost of contact lenses these days is significantly less than the old days. Plus, you can insure them against loss.

While there has yet to be a report of bacterial or parasitic eye infection relating to contact lens use and surfing in polluted water, the chance is minimized by routine and proper cleaning and disinfection of your lens every day, particularly on days you surf.

You mentioned you have an astigmatism, which is a common vision problem resulting from irregular eye curvatures that throws your vision off. These can usually be corrected with contact lenses.

You also described having sun-sensitive eyes. Again, this is not an uncommon problem, particularly if the cornea has been sunburned. Contact lenses—as do glasses—come in various tints, which may offer some relief. One product you might want to check out is a remarkable pigmented, sunglasses-like contact lens named Suntacts®. They were developed by an optometrist member of the Surfer's Medical Association, William Petersen, OD, in Dana Point, California.

If, for whatever reason, you decide that contact lenses aren't for you, some type of in-water goggle or glasses set-up is the next best option. Spex® is a unique water sports goggle which has a soft frame (it won't mash your face), floats (plus comes with a leash), and can be ordered with various types of lenses, including a prescription lens as well as varying darknesses of polycarbonate polaroid lens. Along with protecting your eyes from traumatic injuries, they also protect from ultraviolet. If your eye doctor hasn't heard of them, ask your local surf shop for help.

To make up your own pair of surf glasses, unscrew the side pieces (the arms that go from the eyeglass frame to the ears) from an old pair of your regular glasses, and attach an eyeglass sport band (from any drug store) to the eyeglass frame with snap swivels (from a fishing supply store) that fit through the screw holes. Add a tether that attaches to your wetsuit or to go around your neck so you don't lose them, and you're set.

As for the problem of glasses or goggles fogging up in the water, there are various antifog products, but a dab of liquid Downey® Fabric Softener lightly applied and then rubbed off both sides of the lenses will work just as well.

You definitely need a pair of sunglasses—every surfer does. These days practically all brands of sunglasses are excellent, including the real cheapos. Virtually all sunglasses offer 100% ultraviolet protection. As for all the bells and whistles (photochromic, polarized, gradient lens; color balance and absorption curves; lens coatings, etc.), it's a matter of taste more than anything. Just get a pair you like and wear them. One word of practical advice, though, for hard-core beach goers: glass lenses hold up better over plastic lenses when it comes to sand grit.

While every surfer has chuckled over watching the in-water antics of a poor looker like you, Mr. Magoo, you are in fact a disaster waiting to happen, whether it be running someone over to greeting a shark as a fellow surfer. Magoo, your goal should be to see so well in the water that we'll all feel more comfortable having you around, and ideally, for you, so that you'll feel comfortable venturing out into less crowded waters. Good luck!

Eyes: Retinal Detachment

Too Long in Drydock

Dear SURF DOCS,

I'm 21-years-old, and have been surfing hardcore for five years. In January of this year, my left eye was operated on for a detached retina. Later the same month, a procedure was performed on my right eye's retina to seal a tear. Usually, these conditions occur because of an injury to the eye, a blow to the head, or old age. The only cause I can think of for my problem is surfing—constantly receiving blows to the head, such as duck-diving, lips in the head, and wiping out.

Since the operations, everything is coming along fine, except for my surfing. The doctor said I shouldn't surf for six months (arrrrrgh!). Well, so far, I've been a good little homeboy, and followed doctor's orders. Even though he's a retina specialist, he doesn't surf—I want to get the lowdown from a doctor who does. Is six months appropriate for a young, healthy surfer who is healing well? I want to get back in the water as soon as possible because my life feels really empty. It sucks, being drydocked.

RALPH
Florida

■■■■IIIIIII

Dear Ralph,

Retinal detachment—when the layers at the back of the eye become separated—is a very serious condition that can lead to blindness. Fortunately, it's unusual in surfers, but you're right about the causes. It can happen any time there is a severe blow to the head. The first symptoms may not occur until days later, with a visual darkening (partial or complete), as though someone had pulled a shade down.

... remember that the waves will be there once your eyes have fully healed—you shouldn't take any chances with your eyes.

It's not clear why yours occurred. It may be an hereditary weakness. Also, nearsighted (myopic) people are more prone to retinal detachment. It is unlikely that the stresses of ordinary surfing would cause a detachment in both eyes.

Six months is longer than the usual recommended out-of-action recovery time—three-to-four months is more typical. Maybe your surgeon is concerned that whatever made you more prone to tears/detachments in the first place, may make increased healing time necessary. Also, doctors have an unfortunate habit of giving patients longer times (to take a medicine, to rest, etc.), because they think the patient will always cut it shorter (i.e., three months instead of six). We'd suggest you discuss it with your eye doctor. Maybe work out an arrangement whereby you'll start surfing again at three months and come in for weekly check-ups for a while.

Whatever you do, remember that the waves will be there once your eyes have fully healed—you shouldn't take any chances with your eyes.

Eyes: Floaters

Good Floaters and Bad Floaters

Dear SURF DOCS,

I've noticed black spots that float around in my left eye. They look like sperm under a microscope, a little ball with a tail. They move when my eye moves, and I most notice them when looking at a white wall or when I'm sitting in the line-up watching for waves.

I've seen an eye doctor and he said it was pieces of my cornea that break off when duck-diving or hitting the water at full speed, that I might need reading glasses in a few years, and not too worry or give up surfing—and that will be $80, thank you, cash or credit card.

A year ago I had a shoulder injury that the doctors up here said was nothing serious, but then it turned out I needed surgery. Can this be the case with what the eye doc told me, that it really may be a serious problem, or am I being overly cautious? I haven't the money to see other eye docs and haven't been able to get feedback from other surfers about this kind of problem.

> *Very worried,*
> **RANDALL**
> *Humboldt, California*

∎∎∎∎∎∎∥∥∥∥

Dear Randall,

We ran your letter by two of our eye doctors, who both agreed that you almost certainly have "floaters," a common and almost always harmless condition. Properly called *vitreous floaters*, they develop in about 60% of people by age 60, are more frequent and occur at younger ages in near-sighted people (as early as childhood), are usually lifelong

179

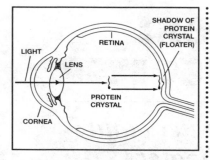

once they occur, and rarely require treatment.

The vitreous is a normally clear, jelly-like substance that fills the eyeball, acting as a shock-absorbing gel for the eyes' vital structures and giving the eye its ball-like shape. As the vitreous ages, protein, cellular, or pigment deposits may develop and remain permanently suspended in the vitreous. When light enters the eye, these free-floating deposits cast shadows on the back of the eye (the retina) and your brain perceives them as actual objects ("sperm," as you saw, or depending upon the shape of the deposits, "spots," "spiders," "worms," or whatever else you've got on your mind).

Apart from being annoying, and, for many, being the first reminder of getting old, vitreous floaters are completely harmless (unlike *real* floaters, from which we're anticipating an increase in surfers' ankle and knee problems). Unfortunately there isn't a medicine or a simple operation to remove them.

Most people's brain eventually gives up "seeing" them, and you'll rarely be aware that they're there.

However, all people who first develop floaters should be carefully examined by an eye doctor. On occasion, floaters can signal a separating or detached retina (often following a blow to the head or face, immediate surgery may be required), an infection inside the eyeball, or more general health problems such as diabetes or high blood pressure.

We hope your $80 eye doctor did a better job examining your eyes than in communicating with you: the cornea (the delicate, outer lining of the eye) has nothing to do with vitreous floaters. At some point, you might want to have an examination by a second eye doctor (either an optometrist or an ophthalmologist).

Eyes: Pterygium and Pinguecula

How Can I Get the Red Out?

Dear SURF DOCS,

I'm 32-years-old, and have been surfing for over 20 years. I constantly have red eyes (they ought to call it "surfer's eye"). I put drops into both eyes each morning, and sometimes prior to going out for the evening. I've been using the drops daily, for at least six years. Some days, after surfing all afternoon, no amount of eye drops will clear up my eyes. I've been drug-free for over eight years, but looking at me, you might doubt it.

My ophthalmologist diagnosed me as having pinguecula in both eyes. I was told I also have pterygiums. I would like to know about surgical procedures, costs, success rate, complications, and how soon these conditions could recur. One doc told me they could recur within a year, and that I shouldn't have the operation unless I was having a problem with my sight.

My employer won't pay to have my eyes scraped, because my eyesight is still 20/15, and all I have is a "cosmetic" problem. The growths seem to cause irritation and, therefore, redness—I can't win.

I am a pilot, and my eyes are my occupation. I have to be extremely careful about any operations. Should I have one done, or just settle for being red-eyed for life?

DON
Texas

Sick Surfers ASK THE SURF DOCS & Dr. GEOFF

Dear Don,

We, too, have probably left people wondering about substance abuse, when we show up for work after surfing with bloodshot, irritated eyes. Add to that the unusual sniffing, runny nose, and we must all appear to be drug-heavies. Just about everything out there in the surf irritates the eye: sun, salt, wind and spray.

Pinguecula and *pterygium* are varying degrees of the same condition. (See inside back cover.) They are those yellow bumps on the whites of the eyes, fibrous growths, caused mostly by UV radiation from the sun, but also worsened by wind, dust and spray. They are called *pinguecula* when they first begin, and *pterygium* when they start to cover the part of the eye we see through (the cornea).

Pinguecula/pterygium are not just cosmetic problems—they become easily inflamed, and can eventually interfere with vision. They can be removed by an eye surgeon. The usual method is to scrape them off with a special knife, or to use a form of radiation to treat the area. The surgery is generally highly successful, and costs between $400-800 in the U.S. Complications—including infection and scarring—are unusual, but as many as 5% of patients have slightly worsened vision. The growths do tend to come back, but with good care only about 10% will come back as severe as they were before the surgery.

The operation is a good option, but you should first do everything you can to stop the growths, perhaps avoiding surgery altogether. Follow the tips on avoiding red eyes, and be "obsessive" about wearing UV-blocking sunglasses during the day. You can cut down further on reflected UV by riding boards with cool colors and no gloss coat.

While on a recent trip to Tavarua, we used baseball caps with neck straps, and found they reduced sun and glare irritation a lot—especially if we used dark zinc oxide under our eyes. Another idea is to tuck an eyedropper full of clean, fresh water into your wetsuit sleeve, and periodically flush out your eyes (and when you get out of the water). Some eye doctors believe the formation of salt crystals plays a role in surf-related eye irritation.

Using lubricating eye drops (Artifical Tears® or contact lens rewetting solution) after surfing will reduce the gritty feeling and may prevent irritation. Placing sliced cucumber or used, cold teabags over your eyes will often help if you have eye irritation.

A word on eye drops that "get the red out." These drops use an adrenaline-like substance (nafazolin or tetrahydrazolin), which causes the blood vessels in the surface of the eye to clamp down and fade from view. That's fine, but the problem is that with constant use, the eyes develop a tolerance to them, and they won't work anymore—in fact, your eyes can end up more red than when you started! It's best not to use these drops more than two or three times a week.

Family Values

How Quickly We Forget . . .

Dear SURF DOCS,

I am 13-years-old and have been surfing for almost seven years. I have a steady girlfriend, and parents who are overprotective. They say I'm too young to single-date, and Tiffany (my girlfriend) and I completely disagree.

Both my parents are 42, and I've told them over and over they have no idea of what it's like to be a teenager these days. My Mom only replies with the typical, "Honey, I really do, but. . . ." And whenever it's my turn to talk, my Dad gets pissed and walks off. My parents even went so far as to send us to a counselor (a shrink)!

Now, don't get me wrong, I love both my parents very much. I don't take drugs, and the only time I tried cigarettes I threw up. But my family's suggestions suck: "Try a group activity. Have a costume party and bob for apples," they say.

If Tiffany and I ever decide to . . . ahhh . . . well, you know . . . we promise to take all precautions. But neither myself nor Tiffany are ready for that. Until then, we should at least be able to single-date.

I believe you can help, because my Dad reads **Surfer,** and he's three-quarters of the problem. Please reply—I will be grateful if you even print my letter.

DAMON
Del Mar, California

▪▪▪▪▪||||||

Dear Damon,

We surf docs are on your side—that you should be allowed to single-date—but before you fling that in your father's face, we want you to consider some things that may not have occurred to you. Based on how clearly you present your situation, it is obvious that you are a really together kid, and, for that reason, your parents feel they have a lot to protect. But neither you nor your parents seem able to solve the problem. Going to a "shrink" was a reasonable idea, but, really, it should have been you **and** your parents going.

Communication between you and your parents seems to be the main issue here—not Tiffany and single-dating. At thirteen, it's completely normal to want more independence from your parents—and most parents have a hard time dealing with that. You and Tiffany could easily sneak around behind your parents' backs, as most teenagers end up doing, but you want to be honest with them. So, what to do?

Have you talked to your father about what he was like when he was your age? Try getting him to open up to you, to trust you with what he really felt like. Our guess is that he was probably a lot like you—a surfer, passionate, wanting to be alone with a girl, yet also wanting his parents' approval. He may not have done so well with that dilemma, and he may still be searching for a solution.

The fact that your father is a surfer, and raised you as one, may be one way out. Does Tiffany surf? Does she want to try learning how? If so, would she be willing to spend a day going on a surf-trip with you and your family? That would be far better than "bobbing for apples." It would be a chance for your parents to get to know Tiffany, and see that you and Tiffany are comfortable and mature with each other. It would go a long way towards helping you gain their trust.

For older readers of *Surfer*, your letter raises some interesting issues. If they are still surfing by the time they have children, they will undoubtedly turn their kids on to it (as your father did). But surfing is more than just a sport; it's a way of life—and that's where the dilemma begins.

In our minds, growing up as surfers in southern California, we were all hell-raisers—scoring chicks right and left, cutting school, standing up to our parents, raging on surf trips to Mexico, drinking, getting stoned. But, now, as parents, most of us would worry if our kids did the same. The way out is to be honest in your remembrances; to free yourself from the media popularization of that time. How much of that stuff did we really do—particularly at age thirteen? Face it gang, we weren't as radical as we like to think.

Our guess is that you'll work things out with your parents, Damon. It may take longer than you think is reasonable, and, in frustration, you'll probably contemplate various rebellious acts. The irony of your situation is that one of those acts would be to give up surfing. Don't. Surfing, as we've explained, may be your best way out. Lastly, when the day comes that you "go all the way," we back you completely in recognizing that precautions against pregnancy should be taken. Unwanted teenage pregnancy is a total wipeout.

Fatigue

Surfing: The Cure,
Not the Problem

Dear SURF DOCS,

I'm a 33-year-old from New Jersey, who's been surfing for 20 years. I am not a hardcore winter surfer. However, December 20, 1986, I went out on a 4' glassy swell, stayed out too long, and got chilled to the bone. Or, as the article on hypothermia (Surfer, Vol. 29, No. 2) said, I was in stage one: sluggish thinking, slight confusion, etc. I've felt this way before, but usually snapped out of it after a warm shower and some hot food. This time I felt funny for days, and thought I'd caught a cold or the flu. To make a long story short, it's been almost a year, and I still have the same symptoms which the five doctors I've seen have been unable to treat, cure, or even diagnose:

1. Constant fatigue, listlessness, lack of energy.

2. Head and body feel hot, but there's no actual fever. Frequent night sweats.

3. Sore/tired eyes, and sensitivity to bright light or glare.

4. Frequent headaches right behind the eyes.

5. Constant ringing in the ears.

6. A lack of concentration, and that "dopey" feeling you get when you stay in the cold water too long.

The doctors have taken blood tests for mononucleosis, Epstein-Barr virus, parasites, thyroid functions, white blood cells, etc. I have also had a chest x-ray and given stool samples. All tests have come back negative, and proclaim that I'm in good health. The only diagnosis offered is that I have a "chronic viral syndrome," but I feel that some of the symptoms immediately followed my surfing experience in December '86.

I'm at a loss—if you have any thoughts or theories on my condi-

tion, I would greatly appreciate the information.

SCOTT
New Jersey

▮▮▮▮▮▮▮▯▯▯

Dear Scott,

We don't think your present problem is related to cold-water surfing (hypothermia). It appears that you have a chronic fatigue syndrome—it's hard to be more specific than that. It's unlikely that you have a potentially fatal disease, such as cancer or AIDS. It also seems unlikely that the exact cause of your fatigue will be discovered by the medical testing you've had so far. However, specific tests of immune function may point you in the right direction. Most labs call it an "immune competency" panel, which will include testing of vital immunological components, such as T-cells and natural killer cells.

The symptoms you describe are also consistent with something called *environmental illness,* and there are health practitioners who specialize in treating such problems: holistic physicians, homeopaths, clinical ecologists, and others.

You didn't mention if you've kept surfing this past year, but it doesn't sound like it. All your symptoms at this point could be caused by plain and simple depression, which usually accompanies physical illness, and often outlasts it. You may have initially had a viral ill-

> "**A**ll your symptoms could be caused by plain and simple depression . . . the treatment may be to go surfing. Give it a try."

ness, gotten depressed because you were sick for so long, eventually kicked the virus (studies show that very few people have chronic viral syndromes longer than three months), but still feel depressed. All the symptoms you have at present are commonly seen with depression. The treatment, in your case, may be to go surfing. Give it a try.

Feet: Painful Toe

Toe Jam

I am 38-years-old and after a 10-year layoff, I took up surfing again four years ago. I am 6'2" tall, weigh 180 lbs., and ride a 6'10" pin-tail. Surfing is as much fun as ever, and I'm in the water 3-5 times a week.

My problem is this: for two years now, I've been painfully jamming the big toe of my back foot into my surfboard when I stand up on it. Booties compound the problem, because they don't allow me to fully straighten the toe, so I sometimes end up standing on the first toe joint. The problem is worse in small, mushy waves. The pain of the jammed toe is quite debilitating, and is worst the first couple of times I stand up. After a couple of hours of surfing, both joints on my big toe are stiff, swollen, and painful to touch. Frequently they will "lock up." I wiggle the toe

until it cracks, and it feels better until it locks up again. If I don't surf for a few days, the pain and swelling gradually disappear.

I am concerned that this continual abuse of my big toe will cause me crippling problems later in life. Do you have any suggestions? Would wrapping the toe help? Thanks for any advice you can give.

DAVID
Southern California

∎∎∎∎||||||

Dear David,

When you jam your toe into the board, you're flexing it far beyond normal limits. This strains the toe joints, leading to injury and pain. Eventually, arthritis may develop.

You've got to work on your take-off. You're probably not getting your feet high enough as you hop up. Check it out on a surf video; you really have to suck your knees up to your chest. Practice hopping up in your living room first—it's hard to make fundamental changes in your style while out in the water. Doing sit-ups and burpees will help develop strength to really snap you to your feet.

Strengthening your toe muscles may also help. Find or make an elastic loop (use a big rubber band or bicycle inner tube). Hook one end around a table leg and the other around your big toe, then move your toe up and down against the elastic.

It is possible that you are dragging your back foot because of a problem with the nerves going to your leg and foot muscles. You can rule this one out yourself. Stand barefoot on the edge of a step, and "hang 10"—all your toes over the edge. Then have a friend press down on your toes while you try to bend them up. If both sets of toes seem equally strong, you're okay; if not, see a doctor.

To relieve your pain, take aspirin before and after you surf, or use over-the-counter pain medications such as ibuprofen (you may have to use big doses—ask a pharmacist how much is safe). Applying hot towels, warm water, and/or ice water can help, too—experiment.

Wrapping the toe probably won't help. Even a big wad of duct tape

> **You've got to work on your take-off. You're probably not getting your feet high enough as you hop up.**

wouldn't hold your toe in place, and would interfere with your surfing.

Consider seeing a podiatrist (foot doctor). He or she may take x-rays of your toe to check for degeneration of the joint or a hairline fracture, recommend prescription medications or an injection of steroids into the joint, manipulate the joint, refer you to a physical therapist, or advise you to have an operation. There are many options—you needn't worry about being crippled for life.

Feet: Bumps and Bunions

Same Shoes, Different Feet

Dear SURF DOCS,

I'm 15-years-old and have been surfing for two years. I go out a lot: almost every day in the summer, and on weekends and after school in the winter. I'm almost always in the water longer than my friends. Anyway, I've developed a large, hardish bump where my big toe joins my foot. Normally, it doesn't hurt, but is numb instead. I think it's due to surfing, because often when I kick out or come down off a floater it hurts a little. I went to the hospital, and they said it was my tennis shoes. I don't believe them at all, because my friends wear the same shoes, but don't have the bump.

I'm worried that because of the amount I surf the bump may turn into cancer, or something. I looked through some surf mags and found that many pros often tilt their back feet on the joints where the bump is.

Could my problem be caused by surfing? If so, is it going to hurt me in the future? Please help!

CONCERNED
Southern California

■■■■■IIIII

Dear Concerned,

That bump is probably a bunion, a hard lump on the bone at the base of the big toe (the first metatarsal bone). A bunion develops as a result of a first metatarsal bone being out of alignment, or from abnormal pressure on the side of the foot. Once a bunion starts to form it tends to get worse, unless you correct what's causing it. Bunions don't turn into cancer, but they can twist your foot out of shape and cause a lot of pain.

In your case the bunion is probably from dragging your back foot on take-off, or tilting it as you ride the wave. Adding to the problem could be the way you walk, the way your shoes fit, or the way your foot bones line up. Remember, your friends may have the same shoes, but not the same feet.

Go see a foot doctor (podiatrist). They're good at sorting out what causes the bunion, and will suggest ways to keep it from getting worse. For example, a podiatrist might make a custom shoe insert (called an *orthotic*) to hold your foot in the right position, or give you a flexible shield to keep pressure off the bone. While bunions can require

surgery, the answer could be as simple as better-fitting shoes.

As for surfing, we suggest you wear booties to minimize wear-and-tear on your feet. Also, check out your take-off and stance on the board—maybe even get a friend to videotape a few of your go-outs, so you can analyze the way you take off and position your feet when you ride.

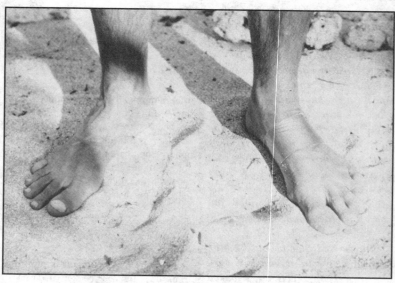

For a surfer, if it can't be fixed with duct tape, it probably can't be fixed. *Beach Photos.*

Feet: Rash and Itch

Athlete's Foot

Dear SURF DOCS,

I've been a surfer for 23 years, and have lived on Maui for two. For over 10 years, I've had minor bouts of athlete's foot on both feet, from time to time. Over-the-counter medications seemed to clear it up. About 6 months ago, it started flaring up again on my right foot. I used Tinactin® (tolnaftin), and it pretty much went away. Three weeks later, it got bad again, and Tinactin® didn't help. At that time, I was going barefoot, or in slaps everyday. I went through every over-the-counter medication there was, and it kept getting worse. After a month of this, my foot looked really bad—open, raw skin, moist and weeping.

I went to see a dermatologist, who prescribed griseofulvin tablets, a strong anti-fungus drug. He also told me to stay out of the water, which I did. After three weeks without improvement, he prescribed an antibiotic for staph infection. Meanwhile, he's still got me out of the water, and Honolua Bay was firing day after day.

A month later, I went to see another doctor—a podiatrist, this time. He decided I had a different type of infection, a bacteria, not a fungus. He took me off griseofulvin, and changed to Loprox® (ciclopirox olamine). My infection really started to clear up.

The podiatrist finally said I could go back in the water—my foot looked great. I surfed for three days without problems, then the infection came back, red and itchy, with little blisters, like poison oak. Back to the podiatrist.

Since then, I've been switched back and forth between various antibiotics, creams and soaks to no avail.

You guys, I'm beside myself. I've spent over $700 on this! I'm living in paradise, and I can't be in the ocean. What now?

TONY
Maui, Hawaii

∎∎∎∎IIIIII

Dear Tony,

The only way to truly get rid of your problem is to recognize the enemy, and fight fire with fire. Your previous treatments were in line, but dealing with a skin problem of your severity requires aggro care. Along with your fungal infection, you are also getting bacterial infections.

Our SMA foot specialist says no Maui surfer should have to miss one single day at Honolua. He recommends the full-court press:

1. **When you have a totally raw, weepy infection, start by soaking with a Burrow's (aluminum acetate) solution, which can be found in most U.S. pharmacies over-the-counter, under the names Dombro®, Bluboro® or Pediboro®. They come in packets or tablets, which you add to one pint of water. Soaking 2-3 times daily for 10-15 minutes should be enough. Don't overdo it—these solutions can dry out the skin, and cause cracking and bleeding.**

2. **When your skin has improved to the point where it is only red and itchy, begin using an anti-fungal cream along with a steroid cream. These will help with the itching. Use 0.5% hydrocortisone cream, which is non-prescription. Loprox® and Lotrimin® (clotrimazole) are good over-the-counter anti-fungal creams. There are also combination creams such as Lotrisone, which contains both anti-fungal medications and steroids. Don't use the steroid cream for more than two weeks, as it can cause skin damage itself. For most infections, continue the anti-fungal cream for four weeks.**

3. **Erythromycin pills (an antibiotic) are probably a good idea for a full-blown infection, but you'll need a doctor to write you a prescription.**

That's how to treat your problem, but even more important are preventive measures to avoid recurrences.

Heat and perspiration are the big predisposing factors here. Proper shoes and all-cotton socks are a big plus. Avoid rubber-soled running shoes—look for ones that breathe. Consider leather sandals instead of rubber slaps. A custom-designed pair of leather sandals may help keep toes separated, and avoid chafing.

> **The only way to truly get rid of your problem is to recognize the enemy, and fight fire with fire.**

Continue using anti-fungal cream for three weeks after the infection disappears, and keep using anti-fungal powder on a daily basis. If you really want to go all-out, get rid of all foot wear that has come in contact with your plague-ridden feet—it may be worth it, in the long run.

Staying on the beach doesn't seem to have done you much good, and there is no obvious reason why you can't surf—just take good care of your feet. Be sure to dry them carefully after you come out of the water (that would also be a good time for the Burrow's treatment, mentioned earlier).

The last idea would be to move to a less warm, less humid part of the island—maybe up on Haleakala.

Fish Poisoning

Ciguatera Will Smoke You!

Dr. Geoff saith:

Ciguatera poisoning is not the same as that encountered after eating at your local seafood restaurant, with just some vomiting and diarrhea.

Rather, it is a severe, sometimes fatal, neurological poisoning due to eating various species of local island fish which become toxic (for reasons not entirely known) hence its medico term: *ichthyosarcotoxism*. More than 400 species of fish have been found to be affected, with the greatest number in the Caribbean and Indo-Pacific. More than 75% of cases have been associated with eating barracuda, snapper, jack, or grouper. Plus, parrot-beaked bottom feeders in Hawaiian winters.

Ciguatera poisoning has been known since at least 2700 B.C. and is a world-wide phenomena. Various explorers, including the greatest chronicler of Pacific surf spots, James Cook, recorded cases in their ships' logs. In 1748, a British naval campaign against Mauritius was lost after 1,500 men died from this delightful poisoning.

To make things interesting, the poisonous quality of fish is variable and unpredictable. Sometimes it is localized to a species of fish on one side of the island; the same species on the other side being totally unaffected.

No one really understands the exact way in which poisoning originates. One theory implicates some change in reef algae, which are then eaten by small plant-eating fish and in turn pass along the food chain (similar to how DDT and mercury pass up the food chain, finally becoming concentrated in large fish which are eaten by man).

The fish itself appears to be unaffected but when man finally eats it, watch out!

Symptoms first appear about four hours after the meal and include numbness of fingers and toes, muscle tightness later followed by weakness and uncoordination.

Fish Poisoning

Death occurs from respiratory paralysis—this usually takes place within 48 hours. Death rates vary from 50% to 0.001%.

Apart from first aid care of the unconscious patient (lying on the side with the head down and to the side, mouth open and clear) there is nothing that can be done—apart from getting the victim to the hospital quickly.

Even local natives are occasionally affected, as I personally found out a few years ago while surfing Arcanum Island. Fortunately, none of us were particularly sick. However, it was scary as there was no way to get help—no radio, copra boat once every two weeks or so. Just local remedies (raau taero ia).

Whether it worked or not, I don't know. For those believers (or those desperate enough), we essentially ate small pieces of green papaya cooked in water.

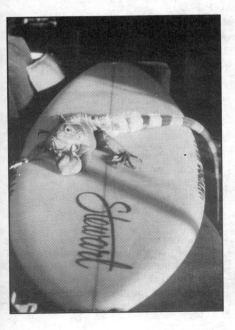

Surfing—everyone's doing it! Fluffy the Iguana. *Beach Photos.*

Fitness

Where There is No Surf

Dear Dr. GEOFF,

Around 4 months ago I moved out into the suburbs. Before this I had spent the previous 6 months surfing between 2 and 10 hours a day. Now I find that after about 5 waves my body feels like it's going to fall apart. I was pondering what to do about this and I figured I'd ask you to give me a simple exercise program aimed at the muscles used in surfing and paddling, and for cardiovascular endurance.

Running is out because my knee's playing up after being jarred, and there's nowhere to swim around here without being covered in wogs.

Thanks a lot,

MUSH

▮▮▮▮▮▮▏▏

Dear Mush,

Mate, your body sounds like it really is falling apart!

My suggestions are:

● *Move back to the Coast!*

● *Work on your cardio-respiratory endurance.*

● *Strengthen surfing muscles.*

CARDIO-RESPIRATORY ENDURANCE

Either an exercise or push-bike (i.e. pedal bike) is probably the go. A stationary exercise bike is the best, as you can monitor your own cardio-respiratory fitness and watch its improvement.

You need to figure out your maximal heart rate (as fast as your heart can be expected to beat if maximally exerted) and then to figure out your sub-maximal heart rate (the safer, sustainable, fitness-making heart rate). The objective is to

196

maintain sub-maximal heart rate for more than 15-20 minutes per session. This should be repeated 4 to 5 times a week.

You don't state your age, but assuming it's around 18 or so, a heart rate to aim for is between 150 and 160 beats per minute. Work it out yourself as follows the formulas exercise physiologists use:

Max Heart Rate = 220 - Age (in years)

Sub-Max Heart Rate = Max Heart Rate x .75

This probably is best organized in a gym where they have good quality exercise bikes and other little gadgets to measure heart rate. Once you start to get tuned into the feeling of your body working under load you will be able to monitor your own progress.

STRENGTHEN SURFING MUSCLES

The major groups involve the shoulders, neck and trunk (both front and back).

Again, at your friendly local gym they may well have the latest goodies which include a "swimming machine." This is a gadget which allows you to lie prone (face down) and pull weights in a swimming-like action.

However, it must be emphasized that these machines are not really able to accurately reproduce the forces involved in paddling. This is because paddling (or with swimming) is really a constant resistance action rather than suddenly moving a heavy load as you do when you lift weights.

Sophisticated machines working on an isokinetic (resistance of machine held constant through a full range of movement) principle are available, but nonetheless they're still only second best to the real thing (going surfing).

The muscles used for paddling are neck extensors (back of neck), pectorals (chest), deltoid (top of shoulder), triceps (back of arm), the various muscles attached to the rotator cuff (shoulder), levator scapula (neck), thomboids (by shoulder blade), subscapularis (below shoulder), trapezius (down back of neck), latissimus dorsi (down side of chest, around to the back) and the lower back extensors (lower back).

As well as all this, you must have a good range of movement (including flexibility), lightning reflexes and excellent balance, timing and experience. There is no substitute for surfing.

Flatulence!

The Science of Fartology

Dear Dr. GEOFF,

Can you help me? I suffer from flatulence. I can't seem to stop farting, no matter how many times I go to the can.

It's uncomfortable, annoying and embarrassing having to repress farts or waiting for opportune moments all day and night.

It's especially bad when I'm in my wetsuit. It keeps it all in, like a balloon. Then it suddenly releases around my neck or down a sleeve.

I'm a reasonably healthy male with a pretty good diet and lifestyle, so maybe you can help me with causes and remedies.

LE PETOMANE
*Sydney, New South Wales
Australia*

■■■■■IIIIlll

Dear Le Petomane,

Your interesting letter brings to the surface an ill-discussed, almost taboo subject, but nonetheless suffered by both sexes. A gentleman by the name of Joseph Pujol (not Pujab) packed out that famous nineteenth century French playhouse, the Moulin Rouge. His farting abilities were such that he was able to actually play tunes via the passage of rectal gas. His stage name was Le Petomane. Nylons, eat your hearts out!

Now let's explore the fascinating science of fartology.

First off, farting is normal, the sign of a normal, functioning bowel.

Flatus (fart gas) contains nitrogen, carbon dioxide, hydrogen, methane and oxygen. It differs from air in containing relatively little oxygen but greater concentrations of carbon dioxide, hydrogen and methane.

Odor arises from small amounts of chemicals of the indole, skatoles, mercaptans and hydrogen sulphide groups.

Flatulence!

Flatus is formed by:

● *Swallowing air*

● *Production of gas in the bowel*

The scientific method of "breath testing" (orally, not rectally), allows measurement of various chemicals (nitrogen, oxygen, carbon dioxide, methane, etc.). It gives a guide as to where the gas is mainly being formed within the length and breadth of the gastrointestinal tract. This in turn can give some idea as to why a person might be producing excessive flatus.

It has been estimated that most young adult males normally pass flatus 10 to 18 times per day, producing a daily volume of between 400 and 2000 mls (about 1-2 quarts) of gas.

Increased flatus can be defined as farting more than 25 times a day or passing more than 2500 mls of flatus per day.

The medical approach to excessive flatulence is to do a "breath test" and work out which gas or gases are present and decide whether they are in excessive quantities.

If the "breath test" shows high concentrations of nitrogen then excessive air swallowing is probably the cause.

Excessive carbon dioxide and hydrogen found using this same test means that various bowel/dietray factors are at

work. Hydrogen comes from bacteria breaking down fermentable substances; carbon dioxide comes from bacteria acting on non-absorbable carbohydrate. Pork and beans is a time honored method of producing excessive flatus with lots of carbon dioxide and hydrogen.

> " . . . most young adult males normally pass flatus 10 to 18 times per day, producing a daily volume of between 400 and 2000 mls (about 1-2 quarts) of gas."

Raisins, bananas and various juices (grape, prune and apple) will raise hydrogen levels in flatus as well. Antibiotics supress hydrogen-consuming gas bacteria, but not hydrogen-producing bacterial. Therefore antibiotics are not an answer.

Methane is produced by certain bacteria in the large bowel. Some people have these bacteria, others do not. You've got more chance of having these bacteria if your parents produce methane "smelly pardons." Statistics show that the chances are 90% if both parents are methane producers; 50% if one parent is a methane producer; and just 5% if neither are methane producers. If the breath test shows excessive methane then blame your parents—but in turn they can blame their parents and so on.

In a practical sense, unless you wish to emulate Le Pentomane's climb to fame in nineteenth century Paris, the best way to reduce flatus is:

● *Be aware of, and minimize, excessive air swallowing.*

● *Don't eat pork and beans, or similar food with high amounts of non-absorbable carbohydrates.*

● *Reduce the amounts of raisins, bananas and juices mentioned above. Grapes are a potent cause of flatus but I'm sure your inquiring mind has already grasped the obvious seasonal association between grapes and farting.*

● *If your parents are farters of the methane type, leave home.*

Although excessive flatus is rarely associated with serious medical diseases, if for any reason you are still concerned or there are other symptoms such as weight loss, diarrhea, vomiting, blood in the bowel or foul smelling feces, seek medical attention. It's easy enough to be referred to a bowel doc (gastroenterologist) who with a few quick tests can usually discover the cause of the problem.

Hand and Wrist Problems

Carpal Tunnel Syndrome

Dear SURF DOCS,

I've been diagnosed as having carpal tunnel syndrome in both hands, and was told I'd probably need surgery. Could you please give me more information on this condition, and also the chance of it recurring after surgery?

KIRK
Hawaii

■■■■||||||

Dear Kirk,

Carpal tunnel syndrome—while it sounds like something that afflicts commuters stuck in the subway—is actually a condition of numbness, pain, and weakness of the hands, due to a pinched nerve in the wrist. It's pretty common in surfers, a result of the way we use our wrists.

The carpal tunnel is an opening formed by the bones and ligaments of the wrist; through it runs one of the major nerves of the hand (the median nerve), along with all of the tendons that lead to muscles which flex the fingers. It's a tight fit through the tunnel, then the slightest swelling inside of it can compress and pinch the median nerve.

In an otherwise healthy person, the most common cause of carpal tunnel syndrome is swelling of the tendons (tendinitis), due to overuse. Any kind of repetitive motion that bends or twists the wrist can do it. For example, grocery checkers develop carpal tunnel syndrome from sweeping item after item over the automatic price scanner. Surfers can develop the syndrome from the motion of pushing up with bent wrists on take-off, from vigorous paddling with a lot of wrist action and even from the motion of waxing their boards (as well as shaping and sanding boards).

Also, if the kind of work you do involves repetitive wrist motion, going surfing might compound the problem and push it into the realm of carpal tunnel syndrome. If that's the case, quitting

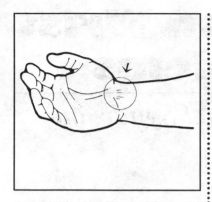

Area of the carpal tunnel. *Photo courtesy of the American Physical Therapy Association*

your job or finding a different way of working is often the quickest cure. Surfers who shape and/or sand boards for a living have a real problem!

A blow to the wrist (getting banged by your board) or an activity that puts a lot of pressure on the base of the palm (carrying a board) can also cause swelling in the canal. People who are very overweight or who retain fluid (such as in pregnancy) can get carpal tunnel syndrome. Some people develop the syndrome without any apparent cause, perhaps because their tunnel is narrower than usual.

Self-care of carpal tunnel syndrome is aimed at preventing or getting rid of the swelling in the tunnel. What often works is to fashion or purchase a splint that holds the wrist motionless in a slightly bent-upward position. The splint is worn mostly at night and while resting. Over-the-counter anti-inflammatory medicines like aspirin and ibuprofen can be useful. Given by an experienced doctor, steroid injections around the median nerve can provide relief. Weight loss, a low-salt diet, and diuretics (pills, herbs or teas that make you urinate a lot) may help.

Stretching before surfing or other wrist-tweaking activity can help. Wrist strengthening exercises, done gradually and carefully, can help prevent carpal tunnel syndrome.

If these things don't work, or if the problem keeps coming back, then you need surgery. The surgeon simply cuts through the ligament that forms the top of the tunnel, releasing the pressure on the nerve. Once the tunnel is opened there is nothing to compress the nerve, and 95% of the people who have the operation experience no further trouble with carpal tunnel syndrome. It's really important to have the surgery done by someone who's performed this specific operation many times.

While the results are often successful, there is a drawback—several of the muscles that flex the thumb are anchored to the ligament cut by the surgeon, and some grip strength—about 10%—is lost. This shouldn't affect your surfing, but may affect your work.

If you have surgery, recovery time is about 6-8 weeks, although you may be able to get back in the water sooner.

Head Injuries

Squash on the Rocks

¡Ola! SURF DOCS,

Six of us were on a three day bachelor party trip, camping at Punta San Jose, Baja California Norte on Labor Day weekend of '88. After an incredibly fine thunderstorm afternoon, several surf sessions, flash floods, many stories, and a huge spaghetti dinner, a neighbor wandered over to our camp to say "Hey, Howdy," and promptly walked off a sixty-foot cliff! "OUCH! Hey, I'm BOUNCING!..." Head meets rock.

Well, the six of us put down dinner and said "Where's the flashlight? First aid kits? Ah, Heck, we gotta save this dude and we never even met him!" The first crew sprints down the quarter-mile trail with duct tape and first aid kits. Phubba and I ready his new Vanagon Westfalia for ambulance duty.

The guy is semi-conscious, both jaws broken, possible internal, spine, and head injuries. We immobilize him as best we can on an 8'4" board. The guy weighs about 220 lbs.! We have to carry him 300 yards back to the car, trying not to drop him, and hey, did I mention that we had quaffed a few freshies ourselves that day?

OK! It takes 45 minutes to get to Santo Tomas over the wet Baja desert. Then on pavement, another hour to Ensenada. He's bleeding and throwing up all over Phubba's van. We had to stop twice on the way to the hospital to see about a pulse. So somehow, he lived. We definitely saved his life.

We had a heck of a time getting the blood and pellets out of our ambulance.

JOE BOB,
THE CLIFF DWELLER
Hermosa Beach, California

Sick *Surfers* ASK THE SURF DOCS & Dr. GEOFF

P.S. There are many more details to this story. Strong first aid knowledge and common sense of our crew was critical. In Baja and other remote areas, people should act less crazy, not more! And yes, I myself fell off a cliff of considerable height as a U.C. Santa Barbara freshman!

■■■■III|||

Dear Joe Bob,

It is a little recognized fact that cliffs and the hazards they pose play a big role in the life of the hard-core surfer. If the waves look good enough, surfers can be among the finest rock climbers in the world, and they do it in slaps, or booties, while carrying a board.

Every once in a while, someone takes the plunge. Luckily, you guys were there, and knew the right things to do. Using duct tape and a surfboard to immobilize and carry him out of the there was brilliant. We assume you used the tape to strap his head and neck in an immovable position, so that when you transported him there would be less chance of worsening a spinal cord injury (if present).

Quickly transporting him to the hospital, even if it was a long distance, and in Mexico, was also good-thinking. Some surfers might have been inclined to wait and see how he was before

deciding to hit the road. If a person has suffered a head injury and is only semi-conscious, or if internal or spinal injuries are suspected, waste no time. Get moving. Things can go from bad to worse in minutes. If you smell alcohol on their breath, your index of suspicion for a head injury should be higher—not lower—drunks fall down a lot.

We haven't heard of any good courses teaching common sense, but all surfers should be inspired by your example and be sure to have basic and preferably advanced first aid and CPR training. Emergency medical technician (EMT) training is worth considering—it only takes six weeks, and whether you go to work as an EMT, at some point later in your life, you will use what you learn to save someone else's life. To find out more about it, call your local Red Cross or ask at the nearest fire station.

Finally, your point about acting less crazy in remote places deserves underscoring. Especially dangerous is getting drunk. It sounds as if quaffing freshies was the major cause of this poor sot's fall.

As for your own fall in Santa Barbara, maybe we'll send you our special SMA t-shirt with a built in roll-bar!

Headache: Effort Migraine

It Only Hurts When I Surf

Dear SURF DOCS,

I've got a problem every time I go surfing (which is, unfortunately, very seldom): a strong headache occurs after about one hour. The pain decreases if I stay prone (lying down) instead of sitting up on my board. Also, I feel better if I hold my breath like when you compensate in deep water diving.

I don't know what it is. Maybe something related to the temperature of the water (but that doesn't seem to make a difference really), or to the high mental concentration I put into surfing since I'm a beginner? Have you ever heard of something like this?

ALEX
Biella, Italy

Dear Alex,

Yes, we have heard of this before. It sounds like a condition called "effort migraine," which follows just the pattern you describe.

An effort migraine typically occurs about an hour after exertion begins. Generally, it is felt as an ache throughout the head (rather than just one part of the head). It is most common in persons new to an activity (such as yourself, a beginner), and in persons who aren't in shape for what they're trying to do (again, this fits you perfectly, since you admit to not going surfing very often).

There are various prescription medications that can be successfully used to prevent and treat these kinds of headaches, for instance, ergotamine and propranolol, but the natural way would be far better: your headaches should go away if you get in better shape by surfing more. ◎

Heartburn

Surfer's Esophagitis

Dear SURF DOCS,

My problem is simple, but painful. Whenever I get up for a dawn patrol or early morning session, I don't eat any breakfast. I do this because if I paddle out minutes after I eat, I constantly belch and nearly vomit throughout the session. If I don't eat, I lack energy and then suffer from severe stomach cramps after I am out of the water and have eaten. It seems odd, but I get these cramps after I eat. Can you suggest an energy source before I surf that won't upset my stomach? I've considered one of those powdered drinks you see in health food stores, but I don't know if that's a solution. I don't suffer from any stomach disorders, and this only seems to occur after lengthy sessions.

TODD
New Jersey

Dear SURF DOCS,

Ever since I turned thirty, my surf go-outs invariably end in a severe and painful case of heartburn. What causes this condition? Is it strictly age-related? What can I do to prevent it from happening? All my friends have the same complaint and we're concerned.

TEAM ROLAIDS
Newport Beach

∎∎∎∎∎∎||||

Dear Todd and Team Rolaids,

Many surfers have had the sublime experience of barfing up doughnuts, granola, and the rest of their breakfast while struggling to get outside in the predawn light. The problems you're experiencing are all-too-common in surfers and have more to do with lying prone on a surfboard than with having any physical ailment. Paddling with back arched and abdominal muscles straining puts enormous pressure on the belly, often forcing stomach contents up where they don't belong. Some of the symptoms, such as belching and burping up food, are just annoying, but heartburn (also called *acid indigestion*) can lead to bleeding ulcers, and difficulty swallowing.

The problem lies in the way the stomach works. The stomach is a muscular bag connected on top to the esophagus (the tube between mouth and stomach) and on bottom to the small intestine. It holds your food for a while after you eat, grinding it with muscular contractions and releasing it bit by bit into the small intestine. The stomach also produces industrial-strength acid to help digest proteins: a special lining keeps it from burning holes in itself.

At the top of the stomach and the bottom of the esophagus is a ring of muscle called the *lower esophageal sphincter (LES)*. The LES relaxes when you swallow; the rest of the time it clamps down to keep stomach contents from going up the wrong way. High pressure in the stomach (lying on your board) or a weak LES can lead to food and acid sloshing back up into the esophagus.

If this happens when your stomach isn't producing a lot of acid, you just get belches and burps, perhaps a bit of breakfast recycling. If there is a lot of acid, the result is a painful chemical burn of the esophagus, a condition so common we've begun calling it *surfer's esophagitis* (*-itis* = inflammation). Repeated esophagitis can lead to bleeding

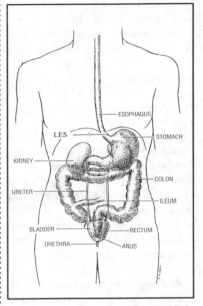

"From stem to stern."

ulcers and scarring of the esophagus, both of which are hard to fix. Esophagitis is more common as you get older. It's not clear just why. Hiatal hernia, where a part of the stomach balloons up into the esophagus, is a common condition that can cause a weak LES and is often the culprit in recurring esophagitis.

It is possible to surf without all the barfing and burning. You've got to eat before a go-out, so here are some tips to keep food and acid below the LES, where they belong:

● **Don't surf on a full stomach.** *Once food passes into the small* intestine, it can't come back up. It takes from one to three hours for your stomach to empty completely, so try to eat at least an hour—not "minutes"—before going out. Liquids pass through quickly, so powdered mixes might work. Use the carbohydrate-based ones like Carbo-Plex® or Carbo Fuel® and try mixing at half-strength since diluted liquids will pass through the stomach more quickly. Watch out for some of the glitz and pricey sports drinks that are little more than sugar water. One of our nutritionists recommends puffed-grain cereals with nonfat milk as a solid food that passes through quickly.

● **Keep a tight sphincter.** *Certain foods tend to relax the LES and should be avoided before a surf, including: coffee (caf and de-caf), caffeinated tea, carbonated drinks, citrus fruits (skip the OJ), some spices, chocolate (sorry), and fatty foods. Smoking (a bad idea anyway) also relaxes the LES, as does alcohol and various prescription drugs.*

● **Let gravity help.** *Just keeping things vertical will help keep food going in the right direction. Spend as much time as you can sitting on your board instead of lying on it. Don't lie down at home after eating.*

● **Minimize or neutralize the acid.** *Chances are, you're going to have some leakage through your LES when you surf. High-protein food stimulates the stomach to make acid, so stick with carbohydrates prior to surfing. Acid-neutralizing substances, like antacids (Rolaids®, Tums®, Maalox®, Mylanta®, etc.) can prevent symptoms: try taking a big dose (two tablespoons of liquid, five or six tablets) a half-hour before surfing. Waiting until you're in pain doesn't prevent damage to your esophagus.*

If you're still having trouble after doing all that we've suggested, it's time to see a doctor. You may have a hiatal hernia or a medical condition causing over-production of acid. Feel free to barf on any doctor who tells you the only way to solve the problem is to stop surfing. There are many prescription drugs (cimetidine, ranitidine, famotidine, omeprazole, etc.) that should work, so keep pushing until you find a solution.

Heel Tendon Injury

Achilles Heal

Dear SURF DOCS,

I am 20-years-old, and since age 12, surfing has been my life. I had previously hurt my heel, tearing the Achilles tendon in half, but my doctors said it was strong enough for me to resume surfing. I went back in the water, and tried, cautiously to tear up every wave I could. My leg felt very strong. Unfortunately, after only three weeks of surfing, I redamaged the tendon.

On an overhead day at a great La Jolla reef break, I took off much too late. I got hung up on a tubing, pitching lip, looking for a place to land, with both feet on my board. Upon impact with the bottom, my feet snapped up severely toward the knee. I felt a sharp pain in my right heel, and proned down on my board. I slid my hand back, and felt an inch-and-a-half break in my Achilles tendon.

After an hour-and-45-minutes of surgery, two days in the hospital, and a long-leg fiberglass cast, my questions are: Will I ever surf again, and if so, when?

ALEX
San Diego, California

∎∎∎∎∎∎∎∎∣∣∣∣

Dear Alex,

A completely ruptured Achilles tendon is a very serious injury. You will get back in the water, but it'll be a long road this time.

A big tendon like the Achilles heals slowly, and there's really nothing that can be done to speed things up. Give it lots of time. Experiments have shown that a completely torn tendon takes 18 months of healing to regain 90% of its original strength.

The doctor who repaired your tendon is the person who knows best when you can begin putting stress on it again (especially if he or she is a sports medicine specialist). Let the doctor know that you're serious about surfing again, and work together to figure out a schedule for your return to the water. A good physical therapist can help you stay in shape, and can monitor your progress until you're ready to get back in the water.

Keep in mind that striving to tear up every wave you can may tear *you* up, also.

As soon as your doctor says it's okay, start swimming to stay in shape. Our SMA consultant says you can probably begin bodysurfing with fins in nine months. Once you begin surfing again, work to develop a style that doesn't stress your tendon as much as before—watching surf videos will help you figure out what maneuvers to avoid. Keep in mind that striving to tear up every wave you can may tear *you* up, also.

Work toward a flowing, graceful style that goes with the wave, instead of tearing it up. In the beginning of your comeback, consider riding slightly longer boards that will get you into the wave earlier, helping avoid the kind of crunch that snapped your tendon.

Wearing a rubber bootie with a few extra layers of rubber glued onto the heel will put your foot in a position which puts less strain on the Achilles tendon.

Remember, the longer you let your tendon heal, the greater your chances are of surfing again without injury.

Helmets for Surfing

Head Jimmy

We *Surf Docs are often asked* what we think of the various surf helmets. Here's our review.

There are at present two major brands of surf helmets available: the Gath® Helmet and the Bradley RadHat®, both manufactured in Australia, but also sold in America. The Gath® helmet is the most common. Neither helmet has received the kind of rigorous, objective safety testing required by law of motorcycle, bicycle, football, or other sports helmets. Specifically, a helmet should be made to withstand trauma from sharp and blunt objects, and not buckle from side or top crushing forces.

Given that the safety and well-being of surfers isn't likely to become a governmental priority in the near future, at the Surfer's Medical Association 1990 annual conference at Tavarua, Fiji, we took it upon ourselves to subject the Gath Helmet and the Bradley RadHat to the most rigorous testing we could devise, in and out of the surf.*

NATURAL TESTING

Various members took turns wearing the helmets while surfing. The consensus was that both helmets were easy to put on, though the Gath Helmet plastic buckle-closure seemed superior to the RadHat's velcro-closure. Both helmets pushed through waves about equally, and didn't noticeably affect one's surfing.

---

* The Surfer's Medical Association does not make product endorsements, but will endorse health or safety concepts that form the basis of products. For instance, the SMA endorses the health concept behind surf helmets, but does not endorse a specific brand of surf helmet. This policy allows us to conduct objective, unbiased testing of surfing products which make health or safety claims.

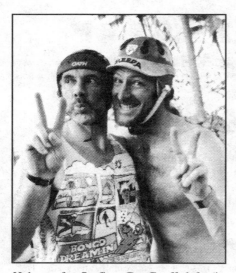

Helmets for Surfing. Dr. Geoff, left, (in Gath) and Dr. Renneker (in RadHat). Helmetology. *Photo by Sandy Campbell.*

There was no apparent risk to wearing either helmet; for instance, one's neck wasn't more likely to be wrenched in a wipe-out. Nor was peripheral vision significantly affected.

On appearances alone, everyone agreed that the Gath Helmet looked more stylish than the Rad-Hat. But, just in handling them, the RadHat was felt to be considerably more sturdy than the Gath Helmet, which was pliable, and easily distorted.

Both helmets did a good job of shielding the head from sun and wind exposure. The RadHat's neoprene visor shaded the face somewhat better than the Gath Helmet when it was without a face shield (as were the ones we were testing), but would be clearly inferior to the Gath Helmet models that come with adjustable, retractable visors, which are actually face-shields when fully extended. It would appear that the face-shields are easily scratched, and may need occasional replacing.

Eye protection from trauma would be superior with a Gath Helmet with a fully extended face-shield. Bradley has lately endorsed wearing a pair of blade-type sunglasses with unbreakable polychromate lens, which are held in place by the sides of the helmet and secured with small clips that come with the helmet.

The surfer's ear protection seemed about equal for both helmets, but neither provided as much insulation as a neoprene hood, which would still be necessary in extremely cold water. The Bradley helmet is adjustable, and could be made to fit over a hood. The Gath Helmets are not adjustable, so you might need to buy two of them, a smaller size for warm water, a larger one for cold water, to go over a hood.

Helmets for Surfing

MEET THE FLINTSTONES

How would these helmets stand up to the real test: a good head bash on the reef? Despite any number of foolhardy, behelmeted surf docs charging into unmakeable sections and flinging themselves head first onto Fijian reefs, there were no wipeouts so bad that the helmets' impact resistance could really be assessed. That testing would have to be simulated.

We set up the helmets on head-width tree stumps, as well as fitting them over head-sized coconuts, and used broken halves of surfboards to subject the helmets to successive forces that would equal surfing situations in which you might get hit in the head: a board loose in the surf, a board flying through the air, and someone riding their board straight into your head. We tried directing the boards nose-first, fin-first, and skeg-first.

The RadHat noticeably did better in terms of cosmetic damage, suffering only minor scratches, while the Gath Helmet sustained significant dents as well as scratches. But the RadHat failed miserably with the skeg test at even minimal forces. If a skeg happened to enter one of its eight vertical drainage slits, it would easily penetrate deep into your skull.

As for major trauma, for instance getting pitched on a huge wave and landing head first on a reef, we dropped an approximately 15 pound piece of coral from about ten feet in the air on to the Gath Helmet to see how it would stand up. It made a gruesome sound, but left the exterior of the helmet with only minor damage. However, the interior of the helmet showed some crush damage to the foam cells. In other words, the amount and/or thickness of the foam cells appeared insufficient to protect one's head (brain) from such a blow. At that point, one member scoffed: "You'd get about as much protection if you went surfing with a plastic bag wrapped around your head!"

Upon having a similar Flintstones-testing, the RadHat showed only minor exterior damage, and no internal damage.

ENTER THE AXE

A Fijian wielding an axe happened by as we were pondering the question of what would happen to a helmeted head if it was slammed into a sharp object, for instance the edge of a granite jetty rock. He happily obliged our wondering minds, and put the Gath Helmet to the ultimate challenge: the Fijian Axe Murderer Test.

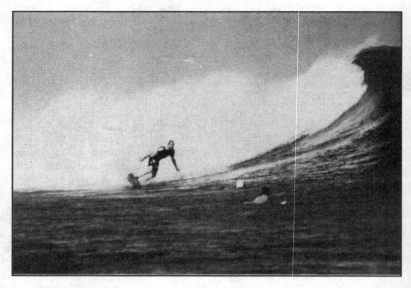

Geoff Booth taking aim at a Gath helmet, purely in the interests of concussion research. *Photo by Sandy Campbell.*

First we had him swing the blunt-end of the axe down onto the helmet, which caused a large crease and significant collapse of the underlying foam cells. Then we set him loose with the full axe blade. It was quite surprising how poorly the Gath Helmet stood up. The axe easily sliced through it, and would have spilled brains everywhere (if we had any).

Later, when the RadHat was hit with an axe, its outer shell cracked and buckled where it was struck. The buckled portion nearly impinged on the underlying plastic-ribbed head cradle; were the force greater or over a wider area, it too would have been distorted.

CONCLUSIONS

The Bradley RadHat and the Gath Helmet are about equal when it comes to ease and comfort in wearing them. The Gath Helmet looks better, and when used with the face-shield provides superior sun and eye protection. Both are about equal when it comes to surfer's ear protection. As for impact protection, our testing indicates that both helmets will protect you from minor scalp abrasions and lacerations, but

Helmets for Surfing

provide inadequate protection from major concussive head trauma, with the Gath Helmet faring worse than the RadHat.

Although it is evident that the Gath Helmet and Bradley RadHat both need to be improved, the Surfer's Medical Association strongly endorses the wearing of surf helmets. Even limited protection is better than no protection.

The Gath Helmets became commercially available in 1990 in Australia, and 1991 in the United States, and are distributed by Future Sports, P.O. Box 56, Margaret River, Western Australia 6285, (097) 572774, fax 61-97-572910. They retail for about $80, and come in four sizes. The Bradley RadHat is still largely a custom order item, direct from Jim Bradley, P.O. Box 131, Warilla, New South Wales, Australia 2528 (phone: 042 377297). They cost about $100 (including air freight).

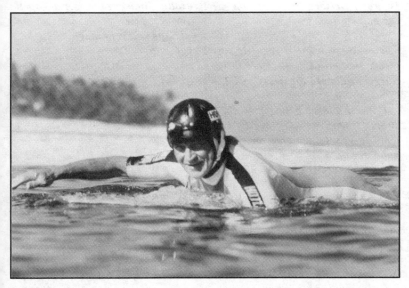

Helmets of different strokes. Dr. Robert Scott. *Photo by Sato.*

Hernias

Time Out for Healing

Dear SURF DOCS,

First of all, let me thank you in advance for offering your services to the masses via Surfer *magazine. I think what you doctors are doing is great. Besides, it keeps you off the golf course.*

Now the problem. I recently suffered a hernia while at work. Surgery followed the next day.

I was wondering just how long should I deprive myself of surfing? I'm 28-years-old, and in pretty good shape. I've been surfing for 14 years. This is the first major— major to me—surgery I've ever had. I have no idea how long it will take me to recuperate. I'll be asking the doctor, but he doesn't surf, so maybe he doesn't really know just what surfers go through.

I also golf and play soccer in a league. Could you please give me a timetable of recovery for these sports as well?

I'd like to get back in the water as soon as possible, but don't want to rush and cause another injury, resulting in a even longer dry spell.

Thank you very much.

DON
Oceanside, California

■■■■IIIIⅢ

Dear Don,

The most common type of hernia is when the contents of your lower belly begin to pouch out through a weak spot in the muscular wall of your abdomen. They are called *inguinal (groin) hernias*. Besides causing discomfort, hernias are potentially dangerous, because a loop of intestine may become trapped and twisted in the hole. This can cut off the intestinal loop's blood supply—a major league emergency.

216

Hernias

The operation to fix a hernia is pretty simple. The surgeon stuffs everything back in and sews the hole shut. But surgeons are like hairdressers—each has his own favorite technique of fixing hernias.

The most common method is to simply sew the muscle together layer by layer. If this is what was done to you, you'll need to be off your board for four to eight weeks. However, you can begin swimming 10 days after surgery to maintain shoulder and arm strength. Using a "pull buoy" between your thighs as you swim will take some of the strain off the operation site. Start as soon as you get home. Do a half-mile the first week, a mile the second week, and so on. Ask a swim coach at your local swimming pool for more specific instructions.

You shouldn't play soccer or golf until you're back in the surf—these sports are as hard on your stomach muscles as surfing.

> **Remember . . . healing is a process of exploring limits.**

If you're lucky, the surgeon did the "bionic man" type of hernia repair, where a piece of nylon mesh is put in to reinforce the muscles. With the mesh procedure, you could be back in the water within two weeks. Find out from your doctor which procedure he used.

Remember, whatever you do during your recovery time, do it gradually. Healing is a process of exploring limits. If it hurts, back off.

The most common cause of an inguinal hernia is genetics—you were born with a weak place in your muscle. But the surrounding muscle can be built up and strengthened, thereby possibly preventing future hernias. You have to be careful, though, to not strain yourelf in doing a workout and causing a hernia. Get with a trainer.

You said you got your hernia at work, so you may be entitled to worker's compensation. In case you were wondering, surfing isn't known for causing hernias—unless you're into tandem surfing and your partner weighs 250 pounds.

Hip Pain

Get Hip to Stretching

Dear SURF DOCS,

I am 35-years old and I've been surfing since I was 12. I'm 6' tall, and weigh 165 lbs.

About three years ago I was running eight-to-ten miles a week to stay in shape during the summer flat spells. I developed a dull ache in my left hip, but I continued running.

Within two weeks I experienced a sharp stabbing pain in the hip while running. I stopped running, but from then on the ache has been more or less constant. I still occasionally feel the pain in my hip when surfing, especially during the winter. It occurs particularly when I go from a sitting position to prone, in order to paddle for a wave.

I saw an orthopedic surgeon a year ago. After an x-ray and bone scan that ruled out a stress fracture, and a blood test that eliminated arthritis, my problem was diagnosed as bursitis. Anti-inflammatory pills had no effect. A cortisone shot gave me temporary relief, but the problem did not clear up totally, and returned to its former degree within six weeks. Application of a hot pad seems to make the problem worse.

Does this diagnosis seem reasonably certain, or would it be worth it to get a second opinion? If the diagnosis is correct, are there any other courses of treatment available? Finally, what is the probable long-term effect of winter surfing in New England on this problem?

Thank you. Your services are very much appreciated by thousands of surfers.

JOHN
Massachusetts

Hip Pain

Dear John,

Your doctor's diagnosis makes sense, but there may be more to it. Your *iliotibial band*—the fibrous band running over the muscles from the hip down the side of the leg to the knee—is probably too tight. This tight band snaps back and forth over your hipbone as you move, causing sharp pain. The snapping irritates the structures underneath the band, causing bursitis (inflammation). The resulting inflammation leads to constant, dull pain.

What to do? Stretch! A good program of stretching will lengthen the iliotibial band, letting the tension off the structures underneath it. Get a copy of Bob Anderson's book, *Stretching* (Shelter Publications, P.O. Box 279, Bolinas, CA 94924). There's a section on iliotibial stretches in it. Follow them religiously. Also, have a look at the stretches in the book for the front of the hip.

Beginning a yoga program would be an excellent idea. We'd recommend enrolling in a class. Look in the phone book, and if nothing under "yoga," then call a physical therapist (that will be listed in the phone book) for a referral.

Don't expect overnight improvement, but if things aren't better in three to six weeks, you may want to get a second opinion.

With a good wetsuit and pre-surfing stretches you needn't worry about the effects of cold water, even in New England's cold water.

> "**B**eginning a yoga program would be an excellent idea."

Healing should occur within two or three days, but if the pain is really bad, you'll need stronger medication from a doctor.

Once you've reduced the pain enough to keep surfing, don't start up running again. It would seem your running technique (muscle balance, foot movements, shoe type or too much distance) is probably what caused the problem in the first place.

Hip Replacement

Two Hip

I am a 46-year-old male who has been stand-up surfing for 29 years. About six years ago I was diagnosed as having a deteriorating left hip, perhaps due to a congenitally deformed joint (dysplasia) and osteoarthritis. About four years ago I was no longer able to catch waves because jamming my upper left leg to stand up caused too much pain. I began knee-boarding, which seems to minimize the getting-up problems and hip rotations and up-and-down movements are also minimized. I'm still stoked to be able to continue surfing four or five times a month. Kneeboarding's a gas and I'm getting more tube-time than ever before. However my pain has been steadily increasing, and I know it's time to consider surgery.

The main questions I have are these:

1. Can I realistically have a joint replacement which would allow me to continue surfing? Are there special custom-made types of replacements available for specific usages? I am more than happy kneeboarding, but wouldn't mind doing some stand-up riding, as well.

2. Where would I go to have the best possible consulting and surgical procedures to accomplish my goal?

3. How long and specialized is the rehabilitation period?

> **G. JOHM**
> *Port Angeles, Washington*

■■■■IIIIIII

Dear G. Johm,

Is it realistic for you to have a hip joint replacement? Our answer is yes and no.

220

Hip Replacement

You've heard of getting a second opinion? Well, we got a quadruple opinion for you. Four different surf doc orthopedists read your letter. Two said to go for it, two said no. Before we lay out their reasons, pro and con, here are some facts about hip replacements.

Joint replacement technology—whether for the shoulder, hip, knee or any other joint—has come a long way in the past few years, but is still not at the level most people imagine. It's not as if you can become a bionic man, replacing your worn-out joints with new ones whenever needed. There are the risks of an operation, infection, the joint not working, and when the replacement joint does work, there may be less range of movement; also, the joints sometimes wear out quickly. Most hip joint *prostheses* (the term for an artificial body-part replacement) only last about 8-10 years; less, if you engage in high-impact weight-bearing activities such as jumping and running. If you need a second hip replacement it can be quite difficult surgically, because there may be less of the natural bone contours to work with.

Hip replacement surgery is spoken of as "cemented" or "uncemented." The cemented technique has been around the longest, and involves simply cutting off the old hip bone and cementing a metal hip bone into place. The uncemented technique has only been around for about a decade, involves the use of a bone graft, and may prove to last longer than the cemented hips. One key fact is, cemented hips don't seem to bond as

well in young people (orthopedically, you're young if you're under 50).

The cost of making a custom hip prosthesis is usually from $2,000-$4,000 in the U.S., not including the cost of the operation. Recovery time will be about 10-14 days in the hospital, 2-3 weeks before you can swim and about 8-12 weeks before you can surf. The risk of dislocation (the bone popping out of its socket) is always there, especially in the first few weeks.

Why shouldn't you have your hip replaced? For one thing, you're still fairly young and able to surf. You may not be able to stand-up surf, but kneeboarding is every bit as legitimate. Also, courage willing, you're able to go out in all kinds of surf. With a hip replacement you may have to limit yourself to smaller, less radical waves.

Even though your bad hip causes you pain, you're probably still able to be more active than if you had a replacement hip.

● *Have you fully maximized your present hip care?*

● *Do you have a regular exercise and conditioning program to make your hip muscles as strong and flexible as possible, allowing your joint to be under the least strain?*

● *Have you tried applying heat to it before a go-out and icing it immediately afterward? You'll be amazed what a difference that will make.*

● *Does your hip feel better in warmer water?*

● *How good is your wetsuit?*

● *Have you tried padding the area with extra neoprene to keep it warmer?*

● *Have you fully utilized anit-inflammatory medication?*

On the flip-side, what would be the reasons for having a hip replacement now (using the uncemented technique)? For one thing, you could look forward to being pain-free. That is the most impressive benefit of the operation. In fact, you'll probably feel so good you'll charge out to make up for lost time, resuming all your previous activities and sports. Don't. Stick to surfing. You'll almost certainly be able to resume stand-up surfing, but you'll have to be careful. One free-fall late drop on a big wave and your hip replacement may be history.

An additional idea that may be feasible since it's usually only done for congenital hip conditions is to have an operation to slightly rotate your hip bone, to move the arthritic surface away from the chief weight-bearing part of the hip socket. It might decrease or eliminate the pain and the need for a hip replacement, at least for now. You'll

need to ask a surgeon if this is possible in your situation.

> **You've heard of getting a second opinion? Well, we got a quadruple opinion for you.**

There are excellent orthopedic surgeons in your area. Find out which ones take care of professional sports teams (i.e., sports medicine specialists) for instance in nearby Seattle. Find out who has done the most hip replacement surgery. Although there may be a technically better or more innovative surgeon somewhere else in the country, stay in Washington. Follow-up care is essential, you'll want the surgeon who did your hip to be nearby and who will make sure you get the best post-operative rehabilitation program.

Kidneys

Sucking Up Sea Water

Dear SURF DOCS,

I am 40-years-old, and surf two or three times a week. I find I unintentionally ingest a fair amount of sea water when I surf. At times I've taken in so much I've actually vomited. Up until last spring, that was the worst symptom I experienced.

Last March, after two weeks of four-hours-a-day surfing on the North Shore, my ankles and feet were swollen for three days. Even though that was my only experience with edema, I'm still concerned. Also, I passed a small kidney stone following last year's summer surf season.

Please tell me if sea salt could be the cause of these problems, and if surfers, in general, take in too much sodium from swallowing sea water.

LARRY
Virginia

Dear Larry,

Kidneys regulate the amount of salt (sodium) in the body. Too little salt in the blood and the kidneys hang on to it; too much and they dump it out in your urine. Sea water has the same proportion of salt as blood, and with healthy kidneys you could drink gallons of sea water without getting into trouble.

However, the swelling you describe may mean your kidneys aren't properly regulating salt and fluids. When your kidneys hang on to too much salt, your body retains fluid to maintain the proper balance—the swelling *(edema)* is the extra fluid. Some people who are on their feet all day often develop swollen ankles, simply due to gravity-induced fluid retention. Still, anyone who begins to have swelling like yours should be checked out by a doctor.

Having had a kidney stone in the past, you're more prone to kidney problems now. Again, go see your doctor—a few simple blood and urine tests should sort out what's going on. Most likely, your ankles became swollen and uncomfortable because you were over-taxing your body, not because you were sucking up too much sea water.

Knees: Sprained Ligaments

Putting Up Collateral

Dear SURF DOCS,

After a three- to five-foot session on a beautiful, sunny afternoon, I decided, as a photography hobbyist, to hike up the cliffs at Rincon and collect a few panoramics of the spot.

After the hike, I had a pain on the inner side of my left leg, at the knee. The pain traveled down my leg at first, and is now slowly lessening after a few weeks. Now I notice it mostly when I bend my knee to its maximum. Can this be the start of a more serious knee problem?

On my reluctant path to age 40, these little strains, pains and pulls sure put a damper on my surfing. I know I've neglected my legs, and that they could be stronger. What do you recommend for staying in shape? How about bicycle riding?

I've been surfing since around the age of 10—about the time of the first **Surfer** magazine, and movies like **Barefoot Adventure**—and would very much like to be able to look forward to future surfing adventures. Any help you can provide will be greatly appreciated.

BOB
Rincon
Santa Barbara

■■■■IIIIII

Dear Bob,

You're right, the pain in your knee is like a warning light on your car's dashboard, telling you it's time for some maintenance. The good news is, you've pulled to the side of the road in time.

Knees: Sprained Ligaments

Anatomy of the Knee Joint

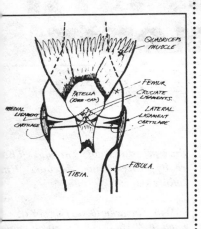

QUADRICEPS MUSCLE
FEMUR
PATELLA (KNEE-CAP)
CRUCIATE LIGAMENTS
MEDIAL LIGAMENT
CARTILAGE
LATERAL LIGAMENT
CARTILAGE
TIBIA
FIBULA

There is a lot you can do to minimize the strains, pulls and twists.

What probably happened is that you had a mild sprain of the ligament that runs along the inside of the knee (the *medial collateral ligament*). Were it simply a strained or pulled muscle it should have cleared up faster. This doesn't mean your knee is about to blow out, it simply means you've got to take care of it.

If the pain is going away on its own, that's great. It's time to start gentle stretches, avoiding anything that hurts. Check out Bob Anderson's book, *Stretching*, (Shelter Publications, P.O. Box 279, Bolinas, CA 94924) or talk with a sports trainer, physical therapist, or yoga teacher. Keep stretching daily, especially before any activity. Gradually begin working at strengthening your knee. A good way to start out is by swimming with fins in calm water. Bicycling is a good exercise, but stay in low enough gears to keep you pedaling at about 80 rpm. Using gears that are too high can damage your knee further. Nautilus-type gym equipment can be used to work on the specific muscle groups of your knee. Just remember to go gradually, and back off if it starts to hurt.

Once you get your knee back in shape, a few simple principles will help keep you in the water for another 30 years. Here are three keys to surfing longevity:

● **Proper warm-up and stretching.** *The sports experts now recommend gentle activity as a warm-up, then progressive stretching, then launching into full-on activity.*

● **Strengthening your muscles.** *Strong muscles protect the tendons and ligaments from strain and damage. This doesn't mean you have to bulk-out Schwarzenegger-style, just work at keeping your muscles strong and supple, especially the muscles around your knees, neck and shoulders.*

● **Avoid over-straining.** *Your activity should be regular, and you should avoid "weekend-warrior" spurts of heavy exertion followed by inactivity. This means you've got to surf regularly—doctor's orders!*

Knees: Torn Ligaments

Twist and Shout

Dear SURF DOCS,

I'm 19-years-old and have been surfing for nearly a year-and-a-half. About 26 days ago I was involved in a non-surfing accident in which I tore the inner ligaments of my left knee. At first I thought the injury was minor, because it didn't hurt much. I realized something was wrong when I discovered that I could bend my knee inward. Five days later I was operated on, and two ligaments were repaired. After the operation, my whole leg was put into a cast for three weeks. Next week the doctor will change the cast and put on a shorter one for another three weeks, with which I'll be able to walk.

Now, here is the problem: The doctor told me that I would be able to work my knee up to 99% of its full potential, with some exercise. Yet, several people have told me that my knee would not hold up to the pressures of surfing. This really worries me, because I'm totally stoked.

Will I be able to surf again like I used to? If so, how much time should I spend out of the water to ensure full recovery? What sort of exercises should I do in order to build up a strong knee? I would truly appreciate any piece of information you could give me.

DANIEL
Costa Rica

■■■■IIIIIIII

Dear Daniel,

Yes! You will be able to surf again, but it's going to take an incredible amount of patience and hard work. Healing yourself now will pay off in your being able to surf for years to come.

It sounds as if you completely tore your *medial collateral ligament*, which

226

Knees: Torn Ligaments

then let your knee buckle inward. Surfing puts a lot of stress on that ligament, particularly in low-crunching positions and when tube-riding. But, by far, the most common cause of surfers injuring their linear ligament is, as with you, a non-surfing accident. Watch out for those other "parallel" sports, such as skiing and snowboarding. They are real knee wreckers, compared to surfing.

Your injury points up the paradox that severe ligament injuries usually hurt less than minor ligament injuries (ligaments are fibrous straps that connect bone to bone; tendons hold muscle to bone). When a ligament is injured, pressure builds up because of inflammation. If the ligament is completely torn, the pressure is released and there is less pain.

An injury to a ligament generally is called a *sprain*; an injury to a muscle is generally called a *strain*.

Unfortunately, completely torn ligaments rarely grow back together—as do broken bones, for instance. That's when surgery may be needed, to patch the ligaments back together.

After ligament surgery, there are two simultaneous parts to the healing process. The ligament fibers must grow back together, and blood vessels must grow back to give a good blood supply. Your job is to avoid the stresses that will disrupt the delicate healing fibers, and to strengthen specific muscles that can make up for ligament weakness.

You need to work with a physical therapist to develop a training program to strengthen your knee. You're looking at 6-12 months of work before returning to full-on surfing (depending on exactly which ligaments you tore). Begin with exercises to strengthen quadriceps, hamstrings, calves and hips. Keep swimming to maintain endurance. A carefully planned yoga program could be invaluable.

Months later, you can begin running in a straight line, gradually progressing to curves and jumping. Your return to the surf should be gradual; don't try to rip your first time out.

Your doctor is probably right about the 99%. While your ligaments will never be 100% as strong as before your accident, muscle strengthening can return your knee to full strength. In fact, you may find yourself in better shape than before the accident. Find a good physical therapist to work with, and don't rush things—you'll be shredding again soon.

Knees: Cruciate Ligaments

Double-Crossed

Dear SURF DOCS,

I'm beached and bummed with a bad knee. Playing basketball a few months ago, a guy collided with me and I felt something snap in my knee. I could sort of walk afterward, but my knee felt wobbly. It still hurt after resting it a couple of days, so I went to the emergency room, where the doc said he thought I had a torn ligament. He wanted to send me to a specialist to be sure. That guy, an orthopedist, said I had torn the anterior cruciate ligament (he seemed pretty sure, although I couldn't afford to get the hideously expensive scan to prove it). He recommended surgery to repair the ligament, but I didn't have the bucks, so he helped me get set up in a strengthening program I could do myself.

Well, I've been doing the exercises and I know I'm getting stronger, but my knee still feels unstable. I want to surf full-on, but I'm afraid I'll wipe-out my knee and I remember the (non-surfer) orthopedist telling me that without the surgery I could have trouble with my knee down the line. As I try to save my pennies, I have one big question: do I need the surgery to be able to surf full-on? The hell with basketball, etc., I just want to surf.

STRANDED IN SAN DIEGO

■■■■IIIIII

Dear Stranded,

Most surfers with knee injuries didn't get that way from surfing. Knee injuries are uncommon in surfing, but when it's

228

flat, surfers find their way onto basketball courts, ski slopes, softball fields, and other knee-wrecking locales. Surfing is relatively easy on knees: your foot isn't locked onto the surfboard and water is much more forgiving on impact than some klutz in a basketball game.

The knee's ligaments and tendons are vulnerable to forces bending the knee in directions it wasn't designed to go. The anterior and posterior cruciate ligaments form a side-ways "X" inside the knee joint and keep the tibia (shin bone) from sliding forward or backward on the femur (thigh bone). The anterior cruciate ligament (ACL) is one of the most frequently injured parts of the knee—the ACL is injured thirty times more often than the posterior cruciate ligament. The ACL may tear if the knee is twisted on a planted foot, as in cleats or bindings, or in side-on collisions. The story with ACL tears is often like yours: a sound or sensation of something giving way, then a knee that will bear weight but feels weird and unstable.

Anterior cruciate tears are a drag, because the ACL doesn't heal by itself. You have to get it surgically repaired or do without it. With an unrepaired ACL tear, your knee is prone to re-injury and each injury leaves your knee more unstable. It's a vicious cycle, and can, in time, lead to a permanently stiff, arthritic knee.

Whether you can get by and still surf without the surgery depends on the stability of your knee, your age, and your style of surfing. If the rest of your knee is stable, you may be able to surf without problems. Most orthopedists say that younger athletes should get the ACL repaired, because they tend to have very good results and have years of strenuous activity ahead. Finally, if you're a soul surfer instead of a thrasher, your unrepaired ACL may not give you trouble.

In the hands of a good surgeon, ACL repair surgery usually turns out well and most people can go back to full activity. The surgeon takes a piece of tendon from the front of the knee, threads it back up where the ACL used to be, and puts in screws to hold it in place. The operation is done arthroscopically, using high-tech fiberoptic scopes and requires only a couple of small incisions through the skin. Usually you go home the same day.

The surgery is expensive: figure about $10,000 in the U.S., including surgeon's fees, anesthesia and hospital costs, and subsequent physical therapy. This is yet another case of why we recommend to all surfers to get health insurance.

Surgery also means four or five months of healing before the repair is strong enough to surf on, although you can start paddling after a couple of weeks.

For most young surfers who want to surf full-on, ACL repair is the way to go. But, since you don't have the bucks and you're not anxious to get back to basketball and other knee-nasty sports, here are some suggestions to get you back in the water:

1. Go back to your orthopedist or physical therapist and ask how stable your knee is after all the exercises you've been doing.

2. If they think your knee is relatively stable, surf gingerly on it. Give yourself weeks—not days—to gradually work back to your old style. If it hurts, back off. If your knee seems to be getting worse, go back to your doctor. Keep doing strengthening exercises.

3. You can try using a knee brace, but there is no reliable evidence that they help prevent re-injury in surfing or other sports. However, we know some surfers who swear by them. Some wetsuit companies, such as Body Glove, make neoprene knee braces.

4. Do everything you can to get health insurance. Beware, though, some plans won't cover you for pre-existing conditions. Also, don't think you can wait for national health insurance in the U.S.—it ain't here yet!

5. If your income is low enough, you may be able to get your surgery done for free at a public hospital.

6. Fear not, lots of surfers have had torn ACL's and returned to full-on surfing.

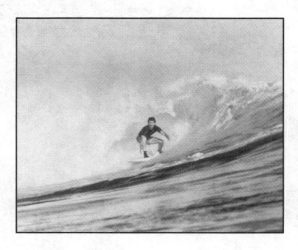

A knee specialist doing some field work. Tom Mc-Laughlin, physical therapist (Atascadero, California). Tavarua. *Photo by Sato.*

Knees: Water-on-the-Knee

Osgood-Schlatter's Disease

Dear SURF DOCS,

I'm a 14 year-old girl who is dying to learn how to surf. My mom is the one holding me back. She said that since I have water-on-the-knee, I could not surf. So, I went out and swam and worked out with my knee, and it started to get better. Then I went back to my mom to ask her again, and she said that I still couldn't because of my ankle (it snaps a lot).

So, I got an Ace bandage, started running on the beach (three miles each way) and got to the point where I could run without the bandage—even in loose sand! I went back to my mom and asked her again, and this time she said if I can get three doctors to say yes, then I can try to surf.

Well, I asked my father and he said that he would pay for one of them. I want to know if I should save up money to go to two more doctors. What do you think they will say? Do you think that I should just go with boogie boarding or wind surfing?

BEV
Ocean City, Maryland

■■■■II|||||

Dear Bev,

Start saving your money—not for doctors' fees, but to buy a surfboard. If your mother will accept the opinion of the Surfer's Medical Association, which has hundreds of physician members, then you don't need to go shopping for other doctors' opinions.

231

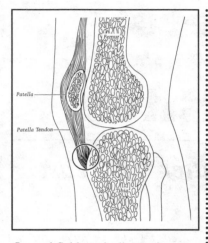

Osgood-Schlatter's disease is a tendinitis of the kneecap tendon. The
inflammation is at the junction of
the kneecap tendons and the tibia.
Reprinted by permission of The Putnam Publishing Group from *Sports Health* by William
Southmayd and Marshall Hoffman. Copyright
1981 by Quickfox.

We don't even need to examine you.
The "water-on-the-knee" condition you
had is a relatively common condition
known as *Osgood-Schlatter's Disease*.
It most often occurs between ten and
fifteen years of age, and has to do with
the growing end of the bone just below
the knee (called the *tibial tuberosity*)
being irritated by the muscle tendons
that attach there (the patellar tendon,
which includes the quadraceps muscles). It is quite different than surfer's
knee knobbies, which is due to external
irritation, for instance, from knee-paddling. But both are generally harmless

conditions. Osgood-Schlatter's usually
goes away within about two months if
forced knee extension activities are cur-
tailed. That means avoiding climbing,
running, and kicking. Once it goes
away, and as the bone fully matures, it
rarely comes back.

Based on the history you give, it is
almost certainly gone for good. And, if
it were to recur, surfing would not be
what brought it back. Surfing involves
practically no forced knee extension
movements. As for the snapping sounds
in your ankle, in the absence of pain or
swelling, 99% of the time such sounds
are completely innocent, only representing the normal movement of tendons
and ligaments, and the natural release of
pressure from joints.

It sounds to us as if the only real
problem here is your mother's attitude
about surfing: she's dead-set against it,
and will continue to find reasons to dis-
courage you from taking it up. You'll
have to help her realize what a healthy
activity it is, that many girls do it.
Maybe you could get her to go to a local
surf contest that has a girls' division,
and she could see for herself.

Knees

Kneecap Dislocated

Dear SURF DOCS,

About six months ago I went on a great trip to Punta Mita, Mexico. It was a killer 5' reef/point break. This was the best trip of my life, until we decided to frolic in the head-high shorebreak on the last day. When I ran out to dive under a wave, my foot got caught in a crevice. My kneecap became twisted over to the right side of my leg, and my ligaments were stretched and slightly torn.

When I finally got home, my doctor drained the blood out of my knee and told me I'd need open-knee surgery. Naturally, I got a second opinion from a more conservative doctor. He put a cast on my leg for a month, and I did three weeks of weight training after it came off. The problem was eliminated for four months. By July, my knee had become dislocated three more times. No ligaments tore

because they're so stretched out, but each time the knee dislocated I experienced severe stiffness and weakness for five days afterward. I really want to surf, but I don't feel confident with my knee the way it is.

What can I do to strengthen my knee? Will I need surgery? How long will I be out of the water? My doctor can't answer these questions—can you?

KEVIN
Northfield, New Jersey

∎∎∎∎∎∎IIIIII

Dear Kevin,

We consulted the SMA knee specialists, and came up with the information you need. It sounded to them as if you have a recurrently dislocating right patella (kneecap), or possibly (but less likely) a rupture of the right anterior cruciate ligament. It was hard to tell from the information you provided, which in itself may be one of the primary problems you're facing. Your doctor(s) haven't evaluated your knee properly, and/or they haven't done a good job of educating you about what's wrong with it.

Assuming the problem is with your patella (kneecap) and the ligaments that normally hold it centered over the top of your knee, this means that when you wrenched your right knee in the Punta Mita shorebreak, you stretched and weakened the medial patellar ligaments (on the inner side of your stance). This allowed the uninjured lateral patellar ligament (on the outside of your stance) to win the normally balanced tug-of-war over your kneecap, and yank it over to the right side (a dislocation). It's common to continue having dislocations until the weak side of the kneecap (ligaments and muscles) regains its strength, which is where exercises come in.

Despite the most vigorous exercise program, surgery is sometimes needed. This is usually done by arthroscopy, under general anesthesia. A thin tube is inserted into the knee, through which narrow cutting instruments are used to equally weaken the lateral ligaments. This may seem absurd—like fixing a twin-fin with a cracked fin by cracking the opposite fin—but there is some logic to it. At least then the originally injured medial ligaments will have an unstressed time to recover. The operation is successful about 90% of the time. The down side is the lengthy period it takes to recover. This isn't your "jump

off the table and play in the championship game the next day" type of sports medicine operation. It could easily take a full month to recuperate.

> **It's common to continue having dislocations until the weak side of the kneecap regains its strength . . .**

With or without the operation, you will be helped by quadriceps strengthening exercises. The quadriceps are a group of powerful muscles that run down the top of your upper legs, over the patella, and attach just below the knee (at the patellar tuberosity: the place where surfers get knots from knee-paddling). The quadriceps act to strengthen the knee. As you hop up to your feet on take-off, that's full-on quads. They are the chief stabilizing force of the knee, so strengthening and increasing your control over them is the first step in fixing your dislocation problem.

You can begin your program at home using simple materials. Start by sitting on the floor with your leg straightened out and the knee in a locked position. Put a 3-5 pound (1-2 kg) weight on your foot or ankle (i.e., get some sand, put it in a plastic bag and saddle it over your foot). Raise your leg to where your foot is about 12 inches (30 cm) off the ground and hold for five seconds, then lower it. Do this until your quads feel fatigued—10-15 repetitions is a decent number. Try to do this at least four times a day.

Gradually progress to fuller arcs (lifting your leg higher). Do it gracefully—you're seeking to regain control over your knee. Try doing it while sitting on the edge of a table. Do only comfortable arcs. Achieve fatigue (muscle tiredness), but avoid any motion that causes joint pain. As your quads strengthen, you may want to begin working out on a weight bench setup. Work on both legs. Progress to where you're lifting 50-60 pounds (22-27 kg) on single-leg extension. At this point, cautiously add curl-ups (straightening your leg from 90° bent position), and realize that the danger of the patella dislocating is behind you. Go as high as 30-40 pounds (13-18 kg) on the curl-ups. Also, begin strengthening your hamstrings (the muscles down the back of the upper leg that end in tight bands behind the knee) by lying face down and raising your straightened leg, adding weight for resistance as you progress.

When all your knee muscles are strong and moving gracefully—which will probably take about a month—you'll be ready to surf again. As for whether to wear a knee brace, this is a controversial area in the field of sports medicine. There have yet to be studies which show the braces to be effective, despite their widespread use. However, some injured-knee surfers swear by them. In your case, though, we'd look forward to a total recovery, and you're not even needing to consider using a brace.

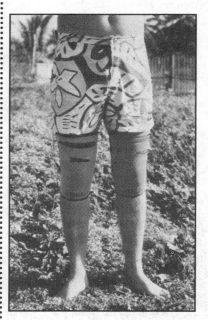

Knee braces—some surfers swear by them. *Beach Photos.*

Malaria in Surfers

They're Back . . .

*D*oes the average surfer need to worry about malaria, or is it just some exotic disease in darkest Africa? The Surf Docs suggest you carefully consider the following true story, by Surfer's Medical Association member, Mark Bracker, M.D.

It was early in the morning when I heard the car bouncing through the jungle towards our surf camp on a remote beach in Panama. Even before they got out, I recognized the all-too-familiar urgency in their faces. Our surf travel paths had crossed the week before and now they had come looking for me, knowing I was an American doctor. They told me about their friend, fourteen-year-old Jeff, who had suddenly developed a high fever and chills just two days before, and now was so weak he couldn't move.

After six hours over rutty jungle roads we reached their camp, and there I found Jeff. He had a 104°F temperature, was heavily sweating, wasn't able to answer questions, and was essentially unconscious. I had my suspicions about what might be wrong—including malaria—but, according to his father who was traveling with him, they had all been taking weekly chloroquine tablets to prevent malaria.

There wasn't much I could do for him there; I knew we had to get him to a hospital, fast. The nearest town was a good two hours away, the nearest airport at least a day's drive. We headed off right away, but shortly after leaving, Jeff had a major seizure and stopped breathing. Despite 45 minutes of CPR, I couldn't resuscitate him. Jeff, a fourteen-year-old surfer, was dead.

The autopsy, done back in the States, showed what had killed him: chloroquine-resistant falciparum malaria affecting his brain, which is called cerebral malaria.

Malaria is our world's worst disease, dwarfing AIDS or cancer. Over 3 million people die from it each year, 300 million people are infected with it, and the inci-

Malaria in Surfers

dence is increasing. What is malaria? It's a parasite, a protozoa, that lives in our blood cells and is transmitted by the female Anopheles mosquito. Once a mosquito bites you, it first spits under your skin, as a way of preparing for an easier blood feast. It's in that spit that you get the malaria, if the mosquito is carrying it.

The malaria belt extends worldwide across the equator, reaching to 40 degrees north latitude, 45 degrees south latitude, and up to 2,500 meters elevation.

The places surfers are most likely to get it include virtually every tropical place they regularly travel to, excluding Hawaii, Tahiti, and Fiji (which are all free of malaria). As for other dream spots—for example, Indonesia, the Philippines, Central America—we're talking about heavy risks of getting malaria.

Prevention is the key. All tropics-traveling surfers should carry a mosquito net, and use it. Dusk to dawn is when the mosquitos feed, so if you're not under your net at sunset, cover up and use DEET-containing insect spray.

Finally, take recommended medications as prophylaxis (prevention). Every country has its own recommendations, involving many different drugs. The recommendations change yearly, owing to the fact that malaria is a highly evolved parasite, able to develop resistance to virtually every chemical we have tried against it.

The present (1993) recommendations from the United States for preventing malaria are to take a drug named Lariam® (mefloquine), one tablet a week, starting one week before travel, weekly while in the malarial area, and continuing for four weeks after leaving. The drug is pricey, but worth it. Not all pharmacies stock it; call first. You do need a doctor's prescription.

Other drugs are recommended in other countries. The most common are proguanil and chloroquine. Chloroquine used to be the numero uno anti-malaria drug, but it was so widely used for so long that the mosquitos in most parts of the world developed immunity to it. However, there are still some places where it is effective.

It's best to find out which drug(s) are recommended for each of your destinations. Good sources of information for which drug is recommended for which country include travel medicine clinics (usually associated with major university medical centers), your local health department, and the voice-mail-like hotline of the Centers for Disease Control in Atlanta, Georgia, (404) 639-3311.

Don't necessarily rely on your physician to have the latest information on malaria prophylaxis; studies have shown that only 20 to 40% of physicians are able to give

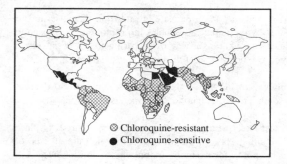

Malaria (falciparium) in the world, 1990.

⊗ Chloroquine-resistant
● Chloroquine-sensitive

accurate medical advice on malaria. The Surfer's Medical Association recommends that you take it upon yourself to answer two important questions:

1. **Is the area you are going to known to have malaria?**

2. **What are the presently recommended medications for preventing malaria in that place?**

Despite years of the best scientists in the world throwing everything they have at malaria, a successful vaccine against it has still not been found. But many will continue to be tested—the stakes are too high; more soldiers died of malaria in the South Pacific in World War II than were killed in combat. Malaria was a major killer during the U.S. Civil War before it was eliminated from this country by the use of DDT to kill the mosquitos.

The unfortunate truth is that all surfers may soon need to know even more about malaria. Chloroquine-resistant malaria is moving up the coast of Mexico, with a small number of cases have been reported in San Diego already. That led to studies of mosquitos living in the marshes around La Costa, in North San Diego county, and not only did they find that the right species of malaria-transmitting mosquito was living there (Anopheles), they even found some already carrying chloroquine-resistant malaria.

We are not suggesting that people in San Diego need to take such precautions as prophylactic medications, but we are saying that if malaria is again in our backyard here in California, think what it's like in the rest of the world.

If you are traveling, think malaria. If you're feeling invincible, and are maybe considering not taking anything, just wait . . . either you or one of your buddies eventually will be hit. And once you've seen firsthand the devastation of malaria, you'll be a believer in taking medications to prevent it.

Marijuana

Reef Madness

Dear Dr. GEOFF,

I am 17 and currently doing year 12 at school. Most Saturday nights I go out somewhere (party, etc.) and usually end up getting quite pissed. Very occasionally, I mix grass and booze. What I want to know is, will all this fuck my brains up? Does it affect memory at all? It may seem like a stupid question to you, but I don't want anything to affect my performance this year (every aggregate point counts).

PARA-NOID
Belmont, New South Wales Australia

Dear Dr. GEOFF,

Could you please tell me if smoking marijuana is bad by my health, and has any side effects. And what will happen if I continue smoking it, will I damage my lungs, etc.?

Yours faithfully,
SIMON
Silverstream, New Zealand

■■■■IIIIIIII

Dear Readers,

Marijuana usage has been raised by two of my faithful readers. I wouldn't have imagined any of my readers were drug users!

Marijuana usage is far more than a medical (health) issue. It has been politically tainted to such an extent that objective evidence in an ethically and scientifically valid form is hard to obtain. However, it is available if searched for.

At the moment, there is no medical evidence to show that the occasional user of marijuana (as such) has any major increases in health risks. "Occasional," meaning once or twice a month for about three or six months.

239

However, problems start to arise when:

● *Usage starts to increase above that considered usual for your social group (making the assumption, of course, that your's is a "normal" group)*

● *It is mixed with alcohol or other chemicals*

● *Social and personal relationships are* centered *around the use of marijuana (i.e., you feel you can't do anything without taking a toke)*

● *You either get busted or start to associate with the big boys (hard liners and crims)*

Under laboratory conditions, marijuana derivatives (essentially delta-9 tetrahydrocannabinol or THC) given to human subjects:

● *Leads to impaired decision-making involving complex psychological tests*

● *Impairs reaction times involving movement-oriented tasks*

● *Impairs short-term memory in* some *persons*

● *Impairs special types of sensation (e.g., vibration)*

● *Seems to potentiate the effects of alcohol*

● *Does damage the lungs; 1 (one) joint is equal in lung damage to a pack of 20 cigarettes*

Subjects reported decreased appreciation of time (being similar to the time distortion felt when inside a deep tube).

Recent articles in the medical press have incriminated marijuana in up to 15% of drivers involved in fatal car smashes.

Obviously, where you stand depends a lot on how much you read and also on your own principles.

My personal opinion is that marijuana is yet another example of exploitation by greedy egocentric individuals who cash in on the pressures of uncertainty, bewilderment, natural curiosity, and frailty of young people.

Whether it does or does not do harm is essentially irrelevant, although my personal view is that marijuana *is* harmful. It does, however, place yet another artificial (and profit-oriented) hurdle in the path of natural mental and physical training that could otherwise led kids to a greater awareness of themselves, and thus others.

Mono-Glandular Fever

The Kissing Bug

Dear Dr. GEOFF,

For the last 3½ months I have been home with a bad case of glandular fever. Well, after all this time resting I'm getting desperate to be fit and healthy again! I still get tired from little things like driving down to the beach. Another thing, my lymph glands in the neck and groin are still up. Some of my friends had it for four weeks, but my case seems eternal.

So whilst my friends are down the beach, I'm at home turning into the biggest vegetable. I had just bought a new kneeboard before I got this thing and I'm dying to give it a thorough thrashing. I've just turned 20 and used to be a fairly fit and active sort of guy, but now I'm just a total wreck. What should I do, Doc? My local

Doc reckons to just keep resting, but surely there must be something to get me active. I've been taking plenty of multi-vitamins but there's no improvement.

EL LETHARGO
*Ringwood, Victoria
Australia*

P.S. There must be more to life than Days of Our Lives.

Dear Dr. GEOFF,

My problem cropped up three months ago, firstly as a nagging fatigue. I took things quietly for a week or so and felt better so got back into it. After some heavy exertion I felt real bad.

The G.P. announced glandular fever after physical examination.

However the blood test came back clean. Nothing wrong.

I gave up all taxing activities like surfing, socializing but continued working as a tutor.

This went on without improvement for two months. Then I hit rock-bottom, feeling drained, and I've been in bed for three weeks.

My G.P. tells me to assume glandular fever and to "only do as much as you feel capable of, without tiring yourself."

I don't have ballooning glands. I do have a deep cough and chest congestion which is accentuated in a hot shower. Plus I get tired when I mill around too much.

Months of abstaining from life's pleasures are taking a toll on my good nature. My conceptions of the illness are that it is contracted by a punishment-oriented lifestyle. I had two years of living in a tent, traveling, surfing, squalor and general punishment of the body.

What does the illness do, how do you get it and how do you get rid of it for good? Would a sports medico be best equipped to deal with it? I would appreciate it if you could shed some light upon this hideous bug.

THANKS DOC
Blackburn, Victoria, Australia

■■■■II|IIII

Dear El Lethargo and Thanks Doc,

Your letters outline some of the problems and frustrations of the dreaded glandular fever ("mono").

There is no doubt that this disease, what medicos call *infectious mononucleosis* (or "mono" for short), is a most frustrating one.

As with all good things in life, it is due to a dreaded herpes-type virus (however, *not* the same one which plays havoc with lips and genitals). This one is called *Epstein-Barr virus*.

It requires intimate contact to spread, and is often called the "kissing virus." There are two major infection peaks: first at around age 5 years and later between 15 and 25 years. It is said that these peaks correspond to the age of "generous salivary exchange."

Mostly the disease is an acute one lasting a few weeks. Typically it produces a sore throat, a general feeling of being unwell, headache, loss of appetite, sensitivity to bright light, muscle aches and nausea. Swollen glands in the neck are commonly found but glands elsewhere also enlarged. These glands are the body's defense factories. Certain cells and chemicals (antibodies) are pushed into production by the stimulus of the virus being present.

Apart from the clinical presentation, a blood test (called the *monospot test*) can be done. However, it can sometimes be positive for other diseases. Also, it can rarely be negative even though the disease is obviously present.

A further test is available that measures certain antibodies produced by contact with this virus, and it can be used to confirm the diagnosis.

Sometimes the disease can stay around for a long time. It is also thought that the disease can come back. In some people, with other diseases and poor immune systems, glandular fever can lead to quite serious illnesses.

Certain complications can occur which can prolong the course of the illness and make it most unpleasant.

Hepatitis in a relatively mild form is very common. Mild inflammation of the outer layers of the heart and a form of pneumonitis (inflammation of the lungs) are other less common possibilities.

Epstein-Barr virus is also suspected of causing chronic fatigue syndrome, cancer of the nose and throat, and cancer of the lymph nodes.

Ongoing fatigue is unfortunately a common problem amongst the 15 to 20-year-old group. As you know, this age group is characterized by full-on physical behavior. Anything which slows down the normal daily rage is something to be dreaded.

At present, there is no treatment specifically available for this viral illness. Certain anti-viral drugs have been tried in life-threatening cases but without any apparent success. Vaccination against the human form of disease is a long way off (although a similar disease in chickens has been successfully prevented with the use of a vaccine).

Dietary supplements do not in general appear to help as long as a balanced diet is eaten. In the early course of the illness, especially if there is a fever and sore throat, fluid replacement becomes very important.

[In the chronic form of EB virus, nutritional, holistic, naturopathic approaches, and immunological therapies may prove helpful. In many U.S. cities there are offices of the Chronic Fatigue and Immune Dysfunctions Foundation, who can provide you information.]

Both letter writers have expressed their feelings of depression and frustration at being laid up for so long. However, sometimes it takes up to six to 12 months to feel "like your old self." In cases persisting longer than three months, a medical re-assessment is advisable and if neither of you have had this, I'd advise you to see your doc again.

If there is any doubt, ask for referral to a specialist physician.

Nutrition for Surfing

You Surf What You Eat

Dear SURF DOCS,

What's the best thing to eat before a surf session? I surf in the morning—half the time it seems like I barf up what I eat. I surf for a few hours most times, and get pretty rundown by the end of a session. Also, what about eating vegetarian? I'm trying to go veggie, and my buddy says I'll shrivel from not getting enough protein.

THE SALAD KING
San Luis Obispo, California

▪▪▪▪▪▏▏▏▏▏▏

Your Majesty,

Our SMA nutrition kahuna from Australia, Margaret Lowdon, PhD, helped us with this one. What you eat (and drink) before and after a surf session definitely affects your surfing performance.

The first question is whether to eat anything at all before surfing. Paddling can be difficult when you have a heavy, bloated feeling in your stomach. And a common complaint from some surfers is "paddle-out heartburn," from what docs call *reflux esophagitis,* and we call *surfer's esophagitis,* in which the food in the stomach comes back up (refluxes) into the esophagus (the connecting tube between mouth and stomach). Stomach acid burns the delicate lining of the esophagus. The pain can be like a heart attack.

Foods that increase reflux are the fatty ones (fried, greasy, meaty, creamy, buttery stuff) which take longer to digest and tend to sit in the stomach. Non-skim milk, alcohol, coffee, chocolate, and cigarettes also cause reflux, but other fluids (i.e., water) are fine.

If you must eat just before surfing, a small, light meal of starchy foods is best. Energy consumption during surfing is at a maximum during rapid paddling and riding, especially in big surf and heavy currents. During these peak

244

times, you need to burn energy efficiently. The fuel the body burns for energy is sugars. The sugars must be flowing through the bloodstream to be available for use as fuel.

Once you're revved-up from surfing for a while, eating high energy food between sessions—anything sweet or starchy—will keep you from getting rundown. Drinks with sugar can be the fastest way to get fuel into the bloodstream. Honey is a great source.

In general, fluid intake is more important to your sessions than food; you must replace the fluids lost to exertion to be able to function. Drinking just about anything will do. Water is fine, but avoid alcohol or caffeine drinks. Power down fluids before, but especially after surfing (and during a session, if you come into the beach). The much-touted "sport drinks" are mostly a waste of money. They offer no more energy than a soft drink or fruit juice and contain nutrients easily supplied by a food snack.

Surfing burns a tremendous number of calories, especially when done in cold water. Replacing this calorie loss is important if you want to keep shredding. This does not mean going overboard on proteins. All of your nutritional needs are easily met in a simple, well-balanced carbohydrate-based diet. Most Americans and Australians eat way too much protein.

Many people think that vegetarian diets can't supply enough protein. Don't

believe it. A vegetarian diet (no meat, as opposed to a vegan diet, which is no meat, dairy, or other animal products) can not only fulfill all your nutritional needs, but is better for you. Meat production (i.e., cattle) uses up a lot more land and resources than plant production (i.e., farms), so a vegetarian diet is good for the environment as well.

> **Surfing burns a tremendous number of calories, especially when done in cold**

Vegetarians do have to eat the right mix of foods. Hard-core surfers have higher requirements of calories and certain other nutrients which are present in smaller amounts in veggie diets. Nutrients for vegetarians and vegans to be aware of include:

● *Protein: Some vegetable proteins are short on essential amino acid components. By mixing the right sources of vegetable protein, it's easy to get the protein the body needs. Mixtures which supply good quality proteins are:*

"A vegetarian diet can not only fulfill all your nutritional needs, but is better for you."

＊ *Grains mixed with legumes (i.e., beans). Examples: rice with beans; whole-wheat bread with lentils.*

＊ *Grains mixed with non-meat animal protein. Examples: whole-grain cereal with milk; eggs in a corn tortilla.*

＊ *Soy beans are a complete protein themselves; tofu and tempeh are delicious and can be made to substitute for practically all "meat" dishes (i.e., "tofu" and tempeh burgers).*

● *Iron: Easy to get. Good sources are green vegetables, legumes (bean, lentils), dried fruit, whole grains, and potatoes. Iron is widely available in foods, but women, because of menstrual losses, need to consume plenty of iron-rich foods.*

● *Calories: Veggie diets are lower in fats (which is great, but fats are higher in calories), so make up calories by eating more complex carbohydrates.*

● *Vitamin B-12: You need only tiny amounts; there is plenty in milk and eggs. If you are strictly vegan (no milk or eggs), you will need to take a B-12 supplement or otherwise take special care to meet your requirements. A simple source of B-12 is fortified soy milk, but you must check the label to be sure you are getting 100% of the recommended daily allowance (some contain relatively little B-12). For a full discussion of potential B-12 sources, see* Realities of Nutrition, *Revised Edition, Bull Publishing Company, Palo Alto, California, (1993).*

To sum up as to surfing and nutrition: Surfers' energy needs are best met by complex carbohydrates: pasta, bread, cereal, grains, potatoes. For sweets, go for fruits and things with honey. Extra protein is not helpful and a vegetarian diet is great as long as it is well-rounded and balanced. Don't eat big or fatty meals before surfing and make sure you drink lots of fluids before and after a surf session.

Follow our advice, Salad King, and not only will you stop barfing (and you can trade in your yellow board), but you'll find yourself surfing stronger, longer, and better.

Nutrition: Building Muscles

Wouldn't You Rather Be Surfing?

Dear Dr. GEOFF,

Along with being a surfer, I have been a fanatic bodybuilder and weightlifter for the last four months. My question is about protein.

Firstly, I know that protein is essential for large muscles and is derived from meat, fish and dairy products. But these are usually high in carbohydrates and muscle with fat is not what I want.

Secondly, are protein supplements in the form of food drink (e.g., Paul Graham's food drink) a good way of deriving protein without carbs or is there even a way of getting protein and no carbohydrates?

Lastly, is there such a thing, which I have been told of, that is made purely of soybeans and contains protein but no carbs?

Best regards,

BRONX
Muswellbrook, New South Wales Australia

■■IIIIIIII

Dear Bronx,

I'm very pleased to see someone fired with enthusiasm for sport. Body building/weight lifting sure can be one ton of fun.

Diet plays an important part in all sports. But, it must be consistent with sound dietary and physiological principles and not crass commercial nonsense.

Various major categories of basic nutrients are needed by our bodies:

Fuel in the form of energy which is measured in kilojoules (calories) is derived from carbohydrate, fat and protein.

Vitamins are the "enzymes" essential for all cellular systems.

Carbohydrates in food are either complex carbohydrates (starches) or simple carbohydrates (sugars). Sugars are further divided into refined sugar (white, brown, honey and molasses) and naturally occurring sugar found in fruits, vegetables and milk.

Refined sugar only contains kilojoules; natural sugars (and starches) also contribute vitamins and minerals. Otherwise, there is no difference at all between these two types of simple carbohydrates.

Carbohydrate is the major source of energy fuel for our muscles. In anyone undertaking vigorous exercise, 50-65% of total kilojoules is required in the form of carbohydrate.

Carbohydrate is stored ready-for-use as glycogen. Excess carbohydrate is stored as fat.

Fat, although being an extremely concentrated source of dietary energy, requires about twice as much exercise to burn as an equivalent amount of carbohydrate or protein.

Dietary fat appears as vegetable and animal fat. Animal fat is rich in cholesterol. This substance, although essential in our bodies, if taken to excess leads to vascular disease which is manifest mainly in heart disease and poor circulation in the legs. Other organs such as brain and kidneys are also affected.

Dietary fat should be restricted to between 25-35% of total energy (kilojoule) requirements.

Protein products and the essential chemical building blocks (amino acids) for all parts of the body. Muscles, bones, heart, brain, etc., are amongst the more obvious and important body systems for the athlete.

Proteins are divided into:

● *Essential (i.e., they must be eaten as the body can't make them)*

● *Non-essential (the body can produce them)*

Sources of essential proteins include fish, poultry, meat, eggs, milk and cheese. Grains, seeds, nuts and legumes also contain *some* of the essential proteins.

Again, a *variety* of protein sources is necessary.

Protein is regarded as the magic elixir and is often taken in excess. However, only 10-15% of total body kilojoule intake should be eaten in the form of protein.

Protein can only be stored in limited quantities. Excessive protein not burned for energy will be stored as fat.

Nutrition: Building Muscles

A *balanced* diet contains all the vitamins and minerals necessary. Only persons with certain diseases or deficiency states need additional supplements. There is no definite evidence to suggest otherwise, despite many claims.

Because an exercising person sweats to maintain a constant body temperature, fluid replacement is essential. Hot, humid conditions require more fluid intake than cool, dry conditions.

A person undergoing active exercising needs to lower fat and simple carbohydrate intake. Energy requirements are best met by increasing complex carbohydrate in the form of fruits, vegetables and starches (breads, cereals and potatoes).

In weight lifting, the essential requirement is to have muscles which develop tension very quickly. This requires muscle strength. It also requires a very finely tuned neuro-muscular system.

Both of these can be influenced by training to large extent. However, to get to the top probably means that the individual was blessed with an optimal neurological and muscular system for that particular sport.

Muscle strength is directly related to cross-sectional area. The "larger" the muscle, the greater the strength. Each muscle is made up of 2 major fibers, the slow twitch (white) and fast twitch (red).

Weight lifters require muscles which develop tension very quickly. This is a property of fast twitch muscle fibers.

These muscle fibers actually enlarge with weight training. Training should be concentric (i.e., contracting against resistance such as in raising a weight) and eccentric (lengthening against resistance such as slowly lowering a very heavy object).

Muscle tension builds up muscle bulk (hypertrophy). Also, the slower the build-up of tension, the greater this hypertrophy. The principle is to gradually increase weights on a graded, graduated fashion with each set of lifts going to "exhaustion plus one more."

Each muscle probably has a set number of fast and slow twitch motor fibers. By specifically building up one fiber group (at the expense of the other) a cross-section of that muscle will therefore have relatively more bulk contributed to by the built-up group in comparison with the other.

"Timing, coordination and a full-on mental approach are the main requirements for suring."

A finely tuned neuro-muscular system essentially means having the ability to recruit as many motor units to fire at once as possible. Training at increasing levels of concentration can achieve this. Intensive concentration produces increased cortical "tone." This means that a larger number of brain cells are tuned up and ready to fire off a mass of coordinated electrical signals to various muscle groups. Therefore, many more muscle fibers are simultaneously recruited to do the same job.

So my dear Bronx, what all this means is that to achieve your ambition requires a balanced diet, avoiding excesses of any type of foodstuff. Stick to the 60% (carbohydrate), 25% (fat) and 15% (protein) type diet. This will provide you with requirements to allow muscle build-up in the correct way.

Avoid all types of fad diets of "health foods." They often don't work and may be potentially damaging.

If you find you can't get to the massive dimensions you wish or are striving for, it may reflect the fact that you weren't genetically endowed with the optimal number of red fibers in the first place.

It is interesting to note, that some surfers from time to time "bulk up" via weightlifting. Usually this is not helpful. Timing, coordination and a full-on mental approach are the main requirements for surfing. I tried three months of using the "Matrix Principle" (Ron Laura) and put on many inches of muscle bulk in arms, chest and thighs. It was truly amazing. However, it didn't help my surfing (paddling into waves, etc.) one bit. If anything, I felt slower. Other surfers who have tried to improve strength and muscle size have reported the same feelings.

Best of luck and remember the famous words of Little Lotta: "Let's eat again real soon."

Peeing in Your Wetsuit

Urine the Line-Up

Dear SURF DOCS,

I am concerned about wetsuit bathroom-users. Is there any harm in this? Is it bad for your suit or body? Can fungus develop?

Following my after-surf showers, my suit and legs reek. I always soap up thoroughly, and wash out my suit after each use with soap or shampoo. Would wetsuit shampoo help? A friend of mine suggested putting the suit in the washing machine. Any information you could give me would be great.

DUMBO
Santa Cruz, California

■■IIIIIIIII

Dear Dumbo,

To pee or not to pee, that is the question (assuming *that* is what you meant by "wetsuit bathroom users"). Peeing in your wetsuit has long been one of the less-publicized pleasures of cold water surfing. Whether it's a good idea is still a matter of debate. Believe it or not, the Surfer's Medical Association made it a subject of discussion at one of their recent conferences.

More than just the quest for warmth, there is a physiological basis for the strong need to pee when you are surfing. There are many factors: the kidneys actually begin to produce more urine when the body is simply immersed in water; a drop in body temperature (*hypothermia*) triggers the kidneys to put out more urine; the adrenaline rush of surfing stimulates the urge to pee; and, finally, lying on your board puts direct pressure on your bladder.

So, the odds are stacked that you will need to pee when you are out there. While urine is not something most people choose to bathe in, it's not exactly toxic, either. Healthy urine contains no germs, and its most prominent ingredient—urea—is commonly used in skin care products. Urine does contain

251

Sick *Surfers* ASK THE SURF DOCS & Dr. GEOFF

ammonia, and can burn the skin if in direct contact for long periods of time (as in a baby's diaper), but that shouldn't be a problem in the surf.

However, some of the Surfer's Medical Association's doctors think that peeing in your wetsuit can cause "wetsuit folliculitis," an acne-like skin reaction. Another problem is that fungi and bacteria grow well in urine, and grow like crazy in a pee-soaked wetsuit. This can lead to skin irritation, allergic reactions and possible infections of the skin.

According to manufacturers we called, urine won't harm your wetsuit as long as you rinse it out. Wetsuit shampoos contain chemicals that lubricate and preserve the neoprene in your suit, but they're probably no better at getting rid of the smell of urine than any other soap or mild detergent (such as a dish washing soap).

Never put your wetsuit in the washing machine—that's a good way to destroy it.

In the long run, peeing in your wetsuit is probably more risky socially than medically.

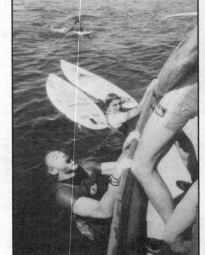

Why pee in your wetsuit when you can water your bro's. Dr. Geoff getting a mouthful from Rym Bone. SMA Photo.

Penis

Bent Pecker

Dear Dr. GEOFF,

I hope you can help me with my problem. If involves my pecker (cock). The problem is, although it is normal in size and function, the bloody thing bends. What caused this, since it's been like it since birth? I'm too embarrassed to flash it in front of a chick. What can be done and who should I see?

Yours thankfully,
ANGLE OF THE DANGLE
*Maroubra, New South Wales
Australia*

Dear Angle,

Penile bends are completely normal. Whether to the left or right, it doesn't matter. Provided the angle is less than 90 degrees, you've no worries!

In fact, you're probably at an advantage in having this most interesting biological variation.

How much more engaging in conversation to be able to say "Would you like to see my bent member" compared with "Want to see my Valiant Charger with mags?"

Pollution

Crap in the Water

Dear SURF DOCS,

During the summer of 1986, I went surfing in the South Bay (Manhattan Beach), and that same night I started experiencing sneezing, heavy nasal congestion (to the point of not being able to sleep at night), a tight head and a loss of taste. I felt like I had been hit by a truck. I had heard of the problems that were being associated with the polluted South Bay, and could see suspicious "crap." My next time out in the South Bay produced the same results. I then experimented by surfing away from the South Bay, at San Onofre, and experienced no problems. I experienced no problems at either place during the winter surf of 1986/87. My initial conclusion was that the warmer water in the summer, combined with the polluted South Bay, had set off some kind of allergic reaction in my head.

Yesterday, after surfing at San Onofre, I experienced the same problem. The water was warm and I did notice brown, foamy garbage of some kind floating in the white-water. The symptoms started five-to-six hours after getting out of the water. I experienced no taste sensation during dinner, and after being in bed for about two hours, I woke up and could not breath at all through my nose. In the morning, I took a couple of shots of Afrin® nasal spray, and that opened up the passages.

My guess is that I am definitely allergic to something in the ocean, and the polluted waters have caught up to me since the summer of 1986. Any advice?

MIKE
Southern California

■■■■IIIIIII

Pollution

Dear Mike,

Your guess is probably right—that you are suffering from an allergy, and have what is called *allergic rhinitis* (*rhin*: nose; *itis*: inflammation), or simply "runny nose." In an allergic reaction such as yours, the lining of the nose and sinuses become swollen and produce so much mucus you may feel like your head is going to explode. Your loss of taste is probably not from the effect of a neurological toxin or pollutant, but is from your nose being stopped up and interfering with your sense of smell (which normally stimulates taste). The severity of your allergic rhinitis suggests that you have a hypersensitivity to something in your environment. The question is, what?

Seasonal pollens can be carried through the air and into the water. Were there offshore winds, and did anyone with known hay fever or allergies also complain of symptoms? Ask other surfers.

Marine micro-organisms, particularly plankton—which is what makes up the "red tide" commonly seen in the warm summer months—can cause allergic reactions identical to yours. Also, red tide doesn't affect every beach at the same time, because of varying water temperatures, currents and swells.

Finally—and what you're obviously most worried about (and we are, too)—is whether sewage, toxins or chemical pollutants might be at fault. Brown, foamy "shit" in the water gives us all heebie-jeebies when we see it, but is usually the result of swells pushing the natural slime from kelp (called *surfactant*) into the wave zone, where it fluffs up like meringue. Untreated sewage supposedly isn't set loose in "civilized" countries like ours, but there are exceptions, and varying degrees of sewage treatment. It's possible you have a hypersensitivity to sewage treatment chemicals or their byproducts. We'd recommend you contact the Surfrider Foundation to see if there are any known peculiarities of the sewage outfall, industrial or shipping discharge in the beaches where you are affected.

The goal is obviously to find out what you're allergic to, and avoid it. If you determine that it's a problem with sewage or chemical pollution, do us a favor and be sure to report it. Offhand, though, it doesn't seem as if you're facing the toxic avenger in this case. If the surf looks too good to pass up on a day when you think you'd be affected, try preventing an attack by taking an antihistamine before going out (available over-the-counter—look for the chemical name *chlorpheniramine*).

Antihistamines should also work when you are suffering from an attack, and might be helped by *pseudoephedrine* (Sudafed®) and *triprolidine* (Actifed®), as you've discovered. A prescription nasal spray called *beclomethasone* (Vancenase® in the U.S.) also works well, especially if this becomes a chronic problem. Let us know how you make out.

Pollution

Diagnosing Ocean-Borne Diseases

Dear SURF DOCS,

I'm 25-years-old and have been surfing for eight years. I surf in Northern California, in the Pacifica area.

Last January, I began having abdominal cramps, diarrhea, loss of appetite, and weakness, which continued off-and-on for months, and which my doctor could not diagnose. One day, while surfing, I saw a large clump of what appeared to be sewage floating in the water. I went to my doctor and asked him if my disease could be related to surfing in sewage-contaminated water.

He did a special stool test which showed that I had yersinia enterocolitis—which he said is an unusual infection of the intestines. He then knew which antibiotic to treat me with—something called Septra® (trimethoprim-sulfamethoxazole) and it quickly cleared up.

My doctor thinks it's possible that I got the infection from surfing in polluted water. What do you think? Is there any way to prevent this from happening again?

RICK
San Bruno, California

■■■■III||||

Dear Rick,

Yersinia enterocolitis is, as you unfortunately now realize, a weirdo disease. The symptoms are as you describe, though sometimes there is also vomiting, fever, joint pain, and strange patches on the skin. The diagnosis is rarely made outright, it's so uncommon that most doctors don't think to test for yersinia (it requires special staining and culturing procedures of stool specimens). It is, as in your case, a diagnosis usually made weeks or months down the road, often by accident.

It's hard to say if you got it from shit in the water, but, for sure, you got it from shit somewhere—that's the only

256

way it's known to be passed on. It's what doctors call the "fecal-oral" route: exposure to food or water contaminated by the feces of an infected person or animal. With yersinia, man is thought to be an accidental "host" (victim). Yersinia is an animal lover—it takes to an animal's gut the way condo developers take to southern California. It prefers dogs, cats, pigs, and various wild animals.

If your symptoms had begun shortly after you saw the scum in the water, and if other surfers had come down with it about when you did, then you could make a strong case for having acquired it from the scum. It appears, though, that your symptoms began before you saw the scum, and, to your knowledge, other surfers weren't affected, which argues against the yersinia coming from ocean-borne contamination.

However, it is possible that there was a low-level of contamination all along, and that, for one reason or another, you were the only surfer infected (perhaps related to how often you surf or how often you wipe out, i.e., how much sea water you swallow). Another factor which makes it possible that the ocean water was contaminated with yersinia is that, unlike most other bacteria, it thrives in cold temperatures. Also, you got sick during rainy season, when more waste runs into the ocean.

Another ingredient to the puzzle is urban runoff—the water that runs off the streets. During storms, large amounts of urban runoff are discharged.

> *Yersinia enterocolitica* is a bacteria similar to the one that caused the Black Death in the Middle Ages.

At present, urban runoff receives no sewage treatment, isn't usually monitored, and would be a possible source of yersinia (and other infectious agents), considering the huge amounts of pet and animal feces on city streets and sidewalks.

Yersinia enterocolitica is a bacteria similar to the one that caused the Black Death in the Middle Ages (the Plague). Are we seeing the beginning of a Brown Death epidemic, from sewage being poured in the ocean (if not from yersinia, then from one of the many other known micro-organisms that can cause disease in man)? It sure seems so, but governmental agencies generally say "no," that current sewage treatment methods eliminate such organisms, and that sufficient monitoring is done to insure our health.

It's hard to believe such claims. It isn't as though they're lying, it's just that sewage monitoring doesn't tell you everything. Most sewage monitoring only involves "coliform counts," a crude measurement of a class of bacteria (*coliforms*) that are not generally a health problem. If the coliform count is high, it means that more shit is in the water than usual—but it doesn't tell you what's in the shit. A better sewage monitoring system is being introduced around the country (not yet in California), which theoretically will give a better indication as to whether human infection-causing bacteria are present in the ocean. It won't tell you anything about yersinia though.

Yersinia and other potentially disease-causing bacteria (of which there is a fairly long list) are never routinely tested for. It turns out that it is very difficult to do bacteria studies on seawater, due to its high salt content. Finding out whether a virus, such as hepatitis, is present in the ocean is even harder.

Definite proof of the presence of a disease-causing organism requires actually recovering it. As we have ex-

"**Short of mass epidemics, proof of sewage-dumping causing disease is very difficult.**"

plained, though, this is not easy to do for ocean-borne infections. We called various county and private laboratories to see if they would test sea-water samples. The San Francisco County Health Department (Environmental/Water Quality Office) will do coliform counts, but say they don't have the capability to test for yersinia, and certainly not for a virus such as hepatitis. Private medical labs will do routine bacteria cultures, if you have a physician order the test, for about $30-$40 per sample. Their testing system will not usually pick up yersinia or vibrio (another major class of ocean-borne bacteria associated with human infection), and it won't tell you anything about hepatitis.

In your case, Rick, you should take sea-water samples to the lab that diagnosed you, because they obviously are capable of detecting yersinia. Also, test the stools of any pets you have.

There is a unique lab in Newark, Delaware (Microbial I.D., Inc., 302-737-4297) that can do highly sophisticated, fatty-acid comparison studies on bacteria to link an infection in a person to an organism in the environment (about $50 per sample). It turns out that if something like this gets into court, it can be claimed there are so many different strains (types) of, for instance, yersinia, that finding it both in the ocean and a sick person is not sufficient proof (i.e., it's not enough to say that a blue 1975 Ford Fairlane was involved in a crash, you have to prove it was the same color blue by a paint analysis.)

Pollution

This is the kind of crap facing coastal-environmental groups who are trying to clean up the ocean. Short of mass epidemics, proof of sewage-dumping causing disease is very difficult. But in every situation where it appears to be the case, we surfers should do what we can. If you see what you think is untreated or undertreated sewage or pollution at your surf spot, call the county health department and ask for assistance. If nothing else, coliform counts can be done—which may tell you if you're on the right track. Then you can consider additional testing, for instance the Delaware lab mentioned above.

There is something of an upside to the downside of ocean waste dumping in Pacifica. Linda Mar, one of the most heavily surfed beaches in Pacifica, has a urban runoff storm drain alongside its main beach parking lot with a locals-favoring feature. A bell sounds before the gates open and the runoff is discharged onto the beach to run down into the ocean. Locals have learned not to leave their towels or beach stuff anywhere near the drain, and take fiendish pleasure in hearing the bell sound and watching non-locals' stuff get swamped.

Surfrider Foundation
122 S. El Camino Real, #67
San Clemente, CA 92672 USA
1-800-743-SURF

259

Pregnancy and Petting

Bases on Balls

Dear Dr. GEOFF,

Being 15 (nearly 16), I really enjoy a bit of petting with girls.

Well my latest love, who I found to be very friendly and lives next door, enjoys it too, and we made a terrible mistake of heavy petting. Desperately I need the answers to some questions:

1. **How long does sperm live for?**

2. **During heavy petting can a girl become a Mummy from a good hard finger (depending on how long sperm lives for on bed sheets and hands)?**

3. **What's the most fool-proof birth control?**

HELP ME!
Melbourne, Victoria, Australia

▮▮▮▮▮▯▮▯

Dear Help Me!

Here are the answers to your questions:

1. **48 hours**

2. **Yes**

3. **Abstinence**

Now before you go out and commit suicide, or worse still, tell your girlfriend's dad, let's put some perspective on these answers.

Girls only become Mummys when the boys' sperm fertilizes the girls' egg (ovum). Whereas boys make lots of little sperm cells (looking like tadpoles under a microscope) nearly all the time, girls only make one ovum per month. If your girlfriend has not yet started having periods (bleeding or menstruating) she's probably not producing an ovum. On the other hand, if she's menstruating regularly it's likely that she is producing an egg each month.

Pregnancy and Petting

An ovum only is ready for fertilization for a few days each month—usually between the 10th and 14th days, counting the first day of bleeding as day 1, and assuming a 26-day cycle. This is based on an ovum being released 14 days before the next period begins, and allowing 2 days for the sperm to remain alive. Before all you kids suddenly become interested in math, there are a few traps in this rule. Firstly, the rule only applies in retrospect—that is after the next period has begun. One can never be sure that the particular cycle actually occurring at the time of "heavy petting" will actually last 26 days. Secondly, if the cycles are irregular, then the dates above will obviously vary. Thirdly, it is best to add-on a few more days to be "safe." So in a 26-day cycle, truly safe days would occur between the 1st to 7th and 19th to 26th days respectively.

I'm not aware of any studies performed to establish the active life span of sperm on hands, sheets or other assorted devices. So the figure of 48 hours probably only applies to sperm survival inside the vagina.

About the only completely safe method of contraception is an aspirin-held very tightly by the girl between her knees.

The good news is that becoming pregnant from heavy petting (assuming there is no penis penetration) is a million-to-one chance.

Let me know next month whether you are a lucky Australian!

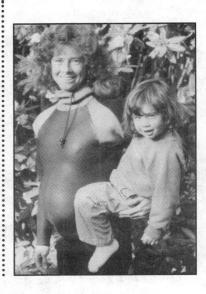

Surfing into her ninth month, Joan Emery. *Captain Trips Photos.*

Premature Ejaculation

Troubled Tube-Riding

Dear Dr. GEOFF,

I would like you to picture this. 12 foot, offshore Pipeline perfection, big spitting barrels, Simon Anderson turns and strokes late into the biggest set of the day. Imagine the amazement on his face as the big spit blasts past before he's even got to his feet, even before the lip has thrown out, eh! A Premature Blowout . . .

What am I driving at? Well, unfortunately for me, I have this problem. Not at Pipeline, but with my girl. I have this problem that occurs whenever I get, let's say stimulated. The lower appendage drops into overdrive well before I'm in the home stretch and I'm left with this damp feeling in my jocks. A premature blowout of the embarrassing kind. What is the problem? I can't go on having my girl troubled with sticky fingers. And my mum will soon become suspicious if I keep "spilling egg white" on my pants every time I visit my girl, eh!! (I mean no one eats that much egg white do they!!) Please help!!

MR. DAMAN DAMP

▮▮▮▮▮▮▮▯▯▯

Dear D.D.,

Premature ejaculation, "Prejac" (sounds like a new T.V. series) is a very common concern. Nearly all age groups mention this as a problem. Learning to manage it successfully when you are young makes life a lot easier. . . .

A number of reasons for this phenomenon are possible. Consider in your case some of the following:

● **Anxiety:** *Are you trying to get it off in the back seat of a Charade, parked in front of your girlfriend's parent's place, and she is due home in 5 minutes?*

Premature Ejaculation

● **Sexual technique:** *Many males do not spend enough time stimulating their female partner before intercourse, nor do they do so during intercourse. At the same time the male may in fact not be stimulated enough prior to intercourse. That means that on insertion there is a sudden overpowering mass of stimuli which trigger the male ejaculatory reflex.*

● **Conditioning:** *There might be an over-conditioned ejaculatory reflex. In other words all those early years of wanking have "primed" you to expect orgasm as soon as sexual play begins.*

Now with all these factors occurring it's a wonder that all males do not suffer Prejac.

Handling the problem is usually easy if you have an understanding, cooperative, and concerned female sexual partner.

Discussion between the two of you and an experienced sex therapist, aimed at explaining the above factors in more depth and allowing both partners to express their feelings/concerns will often lead to resolution of this problem.

Other simple remedies such as "distraction" techniques can be used. These involve concentrating on something outside your body (e.g., 12' Pipeline tubes) or another part of your body (e.g., biting your tongue).

For more complex measures, we owe thanks to Masters and Johnson, the loving American couple/researchers who spawned the sexual revolution.

Their techniques are given in a sequential program. The most "popular" technique utilizes the "squeeze technique." This involves instructing the partner to use a special squeezing (with the hand) technique of the penis to reduce the urge to ejaculate. It requires practice, firstly without intercourse to get the technique "down pat" so to speak. The technique is then tried during intercourse. Other methods are available if this fails.

The squeeze technique and other techniques are discussed in detail in various popular books (like *The Joy of Sex*). You can do a lot to treat yourself—but we'd recommend doing your homework before heading to bed.

If you (or others) have a genuine problem and are prepared to do something about it, make an appointment with a sex counselor. Ask you own doc for guidance or contact your local community health center for precise details.

Rescue Techniques for Surfers

*T*he *following material* was adapted (and somewhat modified) from the "Surf Survival" program of Australia, developed by Jim Bradley. Jim Bradley is an esteemed kahuna of both the Surfer's Medical Association and the founder of the School Surfing Association of Australia. He has been a pioneer in the field of surf safety.

You're paddling out after a nice ride, just as your buddy maneuvers into a set wave. You know it's going to be a late drop, and give him a hoot of encouragement. As you scratch over the shoulder, you hang back for a second to see if he made it. The last you see he's hanging under the lip, heading into the pit. After the wave passes by, you watch from behind, hoping to see him pull out at its end. But he doesn't. Figuring he didn't make it, you scan in over the jumbles of whitewater, but, again, you don't see him anywhere. Then, close to where you'd last seen him, you catch a glimpse. He's face down and motionless. What do you do?

GET TO HIM

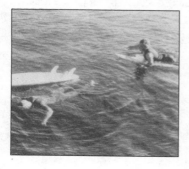

Your first task is to get to him as swiftly as possible. But give top priority to preserving your own safety. If he is, for instance, caught on rocks or wrapped in a lobster trap-line, proceed with utmost caution. To help him, you need to be cool-headed and safe.

As soon as you get to him, grab his hair or the neck of his wetsuit and lift his head out of the water. There may be another wave coming, so brace yourself. Don't let go.

Slide off (and abandon) your board, and move onto his board. Unleash your ankle strap; from now on his board will be your rescue station. If he gets loose from you and sinks when a wave washes over, you'll be able to pull him back to the surface by his leash. (If he was surfing without a leash, or if his leash broke, you'll need to use your board as the rescue vehicle, in which case, put your leash on him.)

GET HIM BREATHING—AT LEAST GET SOME AIR INTO HIM

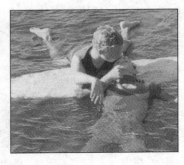

Lay on the board sideways (perpendicular), and, using it as a table, pull him onto it, with his face up. This is easiest done by reaching under his armpit, and securing a pistol grip on his chin; lift only his shoulders and head onto the board.

Assess whether he is breathing. If he was face down when you got to him, he'll need air. Can you see his chest rising and falling? Is he gasping for breath or coughing? If not, or if in doubt, GIVE HIM FIVE FULL BREATHS, ideally mouth-to-mouth if you can (while pinching his nose), or mouth-to-nose (while covering his mouth). You'll know if your breaths are getting in because you'll see his chest rise and fall.

(The idea of giving five breaths (vs. two) does not conform to standard cardiopulmonary resuscitation guidelines, but, not surprisingly, such guidelines do not cover surfing rescues, where it may be difficult to give breaths while balancing on a surfboard, and it may be quite some time before you can get a victim to shore.)

THE RESCUE ROLL: GETTING A VICTIM ONTO THE BOARD

The major concern now is to get him onto the board and paddle him to shore. This is the trickiest (and cleverest) part of a surfboard rescue operation. It is hard to get an unconscious victim onto a board (unless they are quite small and the board is large, in which case you can more easily manage lifting and pulling them onto the board). Here's how to do it with the average-sized surfer and the typical short board.

After you've given your life-saving breaths, pull the board out from under him, and turn him so he's face down. Turn the board upside down. Pull the arm closest to the board's tail across the deck and slide the board so the rail is into his armpit. This will be the fulcrum by which you'll be able to lever him onto the board.

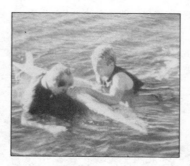

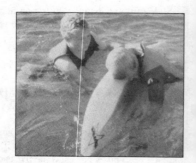

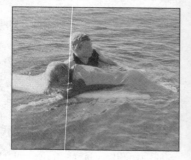

Keep rolling the board under him, until it is deck up and he is fully on it. Drape his arms and then legs over the rails of the board, getting him as balanced as possible. Position yourself between his legs, with your chest over his backside, as if you were paddling out for a tandem session. Try to keep the board's nose tipped up, which should help to keep his mouth out of the water, and will let you paddle it more easily.

PADDLE FOR SHORE

If you are still in the wave zone, and the surf isn't gigantic, you should try to ride the whitewater into shore. If the surf is huge, and each time it pushes you both off the board, angle toward calm water. Your goal, obviously, is to get in as quickly as possible. Use your discretion about giving more breaths, based on how long it is taking to get in. After four minutes of not breathing, brain death is likely to occur.

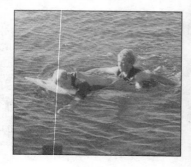

As you reach shore, if no one is waiting to help at the beach, having noticed what is going on, begin yelling for help. Paddle up onto the sand as far as you can (sacrifice the fins; it's his board anyway!). Now comes the hard-part, if he is still unconscious, and perhaps not breathing: getting him out of the shore pound up onto the beach.

Rescue Techniques for Surfers

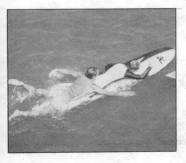 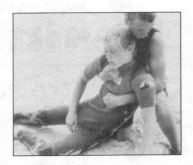

If someone is there to help, terrific. Ask if they have already called for emergency rescue. If not, send them off to do that. Very often people will stand around at the scene of a disaster completely paralyzed by fear; you'll have to be in charge and direct people until professional help arrives.

As you think through getting him up the beach, bear in mind there could be a spinal cord injury, so you'll want to take special care to not twist or pull on his neck. If you are alone, get behind him and bear hug him, with your arms under his armpits, and your hand(s) keeping his head steady. Moving backwards, drag him up onto the beach. If other people are there to help, coordinate their lifting him so that his head and neck remain in a neutral, untwisted position.

Once you get to a safe position on the beach, proceed with CPR. SEE *CPR FOR SURFERS* (page 101).

Resin Fumes

Styrene Dreams

Dear SURF DOCS,

I am 27-years-old and have been glassing surfboards for different factories for about five years. When I first started glassing, friends used to joke about my getting a cheap "high" from breathing in the resin fumes. At first it was funny, but now I'm kind of scared.

These days, I feel spacey after a heavy glassing session, and I think my memory is getting worse. Am I frying my brain, or what? Are there really risks of working with resin? Is there any chance of permanent damage? What can I do to reduce my risk? Any advice would be much appreciated.

Thanks,
RALPH THE RESIN MAN

▮▮▮▮▮▯▯▯

Dear Ralph,

Our resin fumes expert, Dr. Gary Groth-Marnat, from Curtin University in Perth, Australia, has researched your questions, and provides us with the following information.

Breathing fumes is no joke—they can be dangerous! And, yes, your symptoms exactly fit the picture of resin fumes intoxication. The good news, though, is that it's doubtful you're on your way to becoming a zombie. Here's what you and every other surfer needs to know about the health hazards of resin.

Resin is a conglomerate of many chemicals, most of which are pretty safe to be around (unless you're involved in the day-to-day manufacturing of resin). The bad stuff in resin, what causes you to feel cuckoo, is called *styrene*. Styrene is what makes the resin get strong ("cross-link") after a catalyst is added. It's what gives resin its characteristic smell. It makes up about half of the total volume of resin. Ten percent of the styrene evaporates as the resin hardens, which means that as you're glassing a board and waiting for it to dry, there's a lot of it in the air. That's the danger time.

Resin Fumes

U.S. worker's health standards are that 50 parts per million (ppm) of styrene in the air is considered to be a safe average level of inhalation exposure during an 8-hour work day for nearly all workers. One hundred ppm is the maximum acceptable level for a 15-minute interval. Most people can detect the odor of styrene when the concentration is between 0.5 and 1 ppm.

The styrene levels—and health hazards—in surfboard manufacturing have never been formally studied, but a pilot study was conducted by Greg Raymond, M.S., an industrial hygienist and a founding member of the Surfer's Medical Association. He did a limited amount of air sampling of styrene at a custom surfboard and sailboard manufacturing shop in the summer of 1986, at distances of 5-20 feet (1.5-6 meters) from the point of resin application, in rooms with varying degrees of ventilation.

His findings (styrene concentration):

● *Laminating/glassing area: 4-30 ppm*

● *Sanding/glossing area: 60-100 ppm*

● *Polishing area: up to 20 ppm*

The glossing area, where the highest levels were found, was where the ventilation was the worst (no open door to the outside, no forced ventilation).

These findings probably underestimate direct maximal exposures to workers, because they were taken at distances reflecting overall levels. If your glassing style is to keep your face close to the board during the laminating process, watching for missed areas, bubbles, and places needing squeegeeing, your styrene exposure will be considerably greater.

If you're really curious, it is possible to measure your blood levels of styrene. Contact ESA Laboratories in Bedford, Massachusetts.

Styrene exposure would be considerably lessened by:

1. **Improved ventilation (good air flow with open doors and windows, wall-mounted fans to remove room air).**

2. **Keeping the glassing room at a cool temperature.**

3. **Using a respirator containing organic vapor (charcoal) cartridges (paper face masks don't cut it).**

4. **Using protective clothing and gloves (PVA or polyethylene are best).**

Styrene causes a sense of irritation or burning if it gets on your skin and/or mucus membranes, so be extra careful to keep your skin, mouth, and eyes covered, particularly if you have open cuts and sores.

If your sense of smell is reasonably intact, the degree to which you can smell the resin fumes is a good measure of how protected you are. Fully decked out by the above precautions, you should barely be able to smell the resin (if at all), and it may take changing your respirator cartridges as often as every day to keep it that way.

If styrene is making its way into your brain, you'll begin to notice any number of problems, starting with worsening of short-term memory ("Did I remember to add the catalyst to the resin?"), trouble concentrating, slowed reactions and incoordination (explaining why some pinstriping looks so nutty); as well as irritability, tiredness and headache ("Why are all these surfers bugging me to get their boards done, I'm only a month late!")

Symptoms usually go away within a matter of hours or days, but in particularly susceptible people, can last longer and be more severe. In one case, a guy with only two years of styrene exposure became completely psychotic for an extended period of time, with persistent visual hallucinations, paranoid thoughts, insomnia, and depression.

Long-term exposure to styrene (i.e., 10 years or more), has been associated with permanent liver damage, numbness and weakness, and a slightly increased risk of cancer (lymphoma and leukemia).

Breathing resin fumes will make you "high," via depressing the central nervous system, with effects similar to sniffing glue. The difference, though, is that the toluidine in glue actually kills brain cells, whereas styrene usually doesn't. Exposure to another solvent, such as acetone (which many glassers use to get the resin off their hands) may make the styrene effects worse. Use acetone sparingly.

Real and unpredictable problems can occur when combining styrene with other central nervous system depressants, such as alcohol and various other drugs. Driving a car after a heavy glassing session, when you feel spacey, would not be a good idea; a beer or two after glassing and then driving a car would be a terrible idea.

For the average surfer doing backyard ding-repair jobs, the styrene exposure risks would obviously be far less than for a professional glasser, but the above safety precautions should still be considered.

As for your mental concerns, Ralph, we doubt that your brain has been turned to mush. Stick to the above recommendations and you should be fine.

Rib Pain

Stress Fracture

Dear SURF DOCS,

I am 25-years-old and have been surfing for three years. My physical condition is generally excellent. Two years ago, while surfing I suddenly developed a pain in my side, under the right armpit. The pain increased, making it difficult to lie on my board, or even to take a deep breath. I don't recall any impact or injury associated with where the pain is—nothing intense enough to break or crack a rib, I'm quite sure.

The pain kept me out of the water for two weeks, then I went back to surfing with no pain or problems. A few months later, the pain returned. I kept surfing as much as I could, but after even an hour in the water, it was quite painful.

After a few more months, I noticed a bump on my right rib, at the front of my chest (the first rib below the pectoralis major). The size of the bump was such that it was just barely noticeable. Any compression of the rib hurt. I dealt with the problem by holding my surfing to the threshold of pain (perhaps 10-15 hours a week).

After a year, I finally went to see an orthopedic surgeon. He felt the bump, took an x-ray, said it "don't look like any broken rib he'd ever seen," and referred me to a chest specialist. Next, I had a bone scan, which revealed intense deposition at the site of the bump. The chest specialist decided he wanted to do a biopsy-type surgery, to get a section of rib and have it analyzed for malignancy. The thought of bone cancer reared its ugly head. Both doctors put a lot of weight on the fact that I couldn't remember any impact sufficient to break a rib.

At the last second, I bailed on the surgery and fled to Seattle for more testing. I was seen there by a prominent oncologist (cancer specialist), who ordered more x-rays and a full bone scan. She also did *a complete physical examination (the first of all the doctors to do so!). The Seattle doctors came to the conclusion that I had cracked a rib, and that the constant irritation of surfing had kept it from healing. They recommended that I rest it.*

Of course, I haven't. It's been a year now and I've been surfing more than ever. I am still bothered by a dull pain, and if I drop suddenly onto my ribs, it's a sharp pain. When I'm surfing a lot, the pain is basically constant—it feels like a broken bone. I would appreciate any advice you may have for me.

MARK
San Diego, California

∎∎∎∎∎∎∎∎∎∎

Dear Mark,

What's really amazing is that you had to go to Seattle, a surfless city, to get a sensible diagnosis of your surfing injury, and to a cancer specialist, no less. What she told you makes sense for two reasons:

1. **Ribs can be fractured (cracked) without a significant preceding impact or injury (people have broken ribs from sneezing).**

2. **Fractured bones need rest to heal; rest that your ribs haven't had.**

You've probably got a stress fracture of your rib. Stress fractures aren't usually caused by getting lip-launched and bouncing off the bottom; that causes full-on fractures. Stress fractures are the result of long-term forces on a bone, usually in a direction the bone wasn't designed for. For example, when you paddle your board with your head held high, you exert enormous downward forces on your ribs. Eventually these forces may cause tiny cracks in the bone, cracks so small that normal x-rays will miss them.

> **"Stress fractures are the result of long-term forces on a bone ... "**

It's not clear why your rib suddenly became so painful, maybe you finally stressed it over the edge. The bone began to heal itself by laying down new layers of bone. Each time you subsequently surfed, you undid its progress. Trying to hold things together, the bone gets bigger and bigger, but doesn't accomplish much, because the forces that originally fractured the bone are still there.

Rib Pain

As all of us have done at one time or another, you ignored the advice to rest because it interfered with your surfing. Ignoring the orders of non-surfing doctors is a time-honored surfer tradition, but this time they were right. There's no way you'll surf pain-free again without giving your rib a break (so to speak). It's excruciating to sit on shore as clean fall and winter swells roll in, but putting it off may mean an even longer healing time when you finally do rest.

Ignoring the orders of non-surfing doctors is a time-honored surfer tradition . . .

You've got to let that thing heal. We hate to tell you this, but two weeks isn't enough. It's going to take 6-8 weeks off your surfboard.

But you don't have to stay out of the ocean. You can stay in shape by open-ocean swimming. Mellow bodysurfing may be okay after the first three weeks. Don't sleep on your stomach, and avoid rib-crunching sex.

If you don't get better with rest—which is unlikely—go back to the doc-tor in Seattle. There are other rare causes of rib pain, such as bone infections or tumors, that may need to be checked out.

Safety

How Safe is Surfing?

Dear SURF DOCS,

I'm 14-years-old and have been surfing for three years. For the first two years I just surfed small waves at Newport and Huntington Beach. This summer me and a friend, Candy, tried some pretty big waves at San Clemente and San Onofre.

At San Clemente, I suffered my worst wipeout ever, and it got me to thinking: is it common to be killed or seriously injured from surfing? And, is there anything I can do to prevent injury?

JEFF
Orange County, California

■■■■■Ill|||

Dear Jeff,

Have you ever noticed that most non-surfers think of surfing as an incredibly dangerous activity, on par with bull-fighting ("matadors of the sea") and mountain climbing ("riding moving mountains")? The general public thinks that a shark is certain to eat us every-time we paddle out. All mothers know that as fact.

The truth is that surfing is an extremely safe sport. In fact, the rate of injuries associated with surfing is equal to fishing! Members of the Surfer's Medical Association, in our respective beachside communities, have conducted a number of studies on the frequency of serious or fatal surfing injuries. We looked at injuries that led to out-of-water time (i.e., deep cuts, sprains, fractures, etc.) It works out to about 4 injuries per 1,000 days surfed (or 1 in 250). Big-wave surfing was not associated with the most injuries; surf under four-foot was. Colliding with your own board and the bottom were common mechanisms of injury; shark attacks, drownings, and deaths were extremely rare.

If you surfed every day, those statistics mean that you'd be benched at least once a year. But who surfs every day? The grim reality is that no matter where

"The truth is that surfing is an extremely safe sport. In fact, the rate of injuries associated with surfing is equal to fishing!"

you go in the world, the surf (and weather) is far from good every day. The average surfer surfs two days a week or less.

Get out your calculator and you'll see that most surfers can expect about one injury every two to three years. How does that rate of injury stack up to other sports? Compared to football and rugby, with close to ten times the rate of injury, surfing should be every parents' dream sport for their child.

According to the U.S. Consumer Products Safety Commission, in 1979, in the United States, there were 9,900 surfing injuries (3,900 requiring emergency room care) but football caused 1,370,900 injuries, and cheerleading 15,200!

All sports have risks and injuries, otherwise there wouldn't be a field of sports medicine, and there wouldn't be a need for an organization like the Surfer's Medical Association.

You will go a long way towards preventing injuries and being a healthier surfer if you religiously follow the SMA Ten Commandments.

THE SMA TEN COMMANDMENTS:

Thou shalt:

1. **Drive safely to the beach.**

2. **Know CPR.**

3. **Blunt your fins and nose.**

4. **Avoid sunburn.**

5. **Wear sunglasses.**

6. **Protect against surfer's ear.**

7. **Be a strong swimmer.**

8. **Know your limits.**

9. **Help other surfers.**

10. **Respect and protect the ocean.**

(Dr. Geoff recommends an eleventh commandment:

11. **Covet not thy fellow-surfers wave (unless he/she rides a sponge, mal, goat-boat, or jet-ski).**

School, Surfing and the SMA

Out of the Closet

Dear SURF DOCS,

I have been surfing since the age of 13. In high school, I surfed 4 or 5 times a week and maintained a 4.0 grade point average.

I am now 20-years-old and have just completed my junior year at UCLA. Striving for a bachelor of science degree in biology, I have taken several courses in chemistry, physics, math, and biology. In the last three years this heavy course load has greatly reduced my surfing time. I average about thirty hours each week of studying and sometimes don't surf for two weeks straight. I participate in clubs and sports at school (UCLA ice hockey team), but surfing is my primary source of relieving stress, and relaxing.

In two years I will be attending medical school. I know it will be a full-time commitment, but I am hoping that surfing will not be cut out of my life during my years at medical school. I want to know how the doctors who belong to the Surfer's Medical Association survived medical school and still had time to surf.

I am also interested in getting information about the Surfer's Medical Association. Is it possible to join if you are not yet a doctor?

SCOTT
Calabasas, California

███████║║║

Dear Scott,

It's time for an exorcism, care of the Surfer's Medical Association! You appear to be possessed by a devilish notion held by many in our society, that surfing is frivolous and incompatible with other more serious life pursuits, be it working hard in school, having a career (in medicine or any other field), or maintaining relationships and raising a family. Nothing could be further from the truth.

It's clear from your letter that surfing is dearly important to you, and you're now struggling with what you see as a process that is taking it away from you. But is it the time demands of school that are keeping you from surfing? It seems unlikely. No matter how busy you are, or how serious you are about school (or, for that matter, work or family), there is time to surf (if you live anywhere near the ocean). It's a question of priorities.

Since you didn't express sorrow in your letter that school was robbing you of time for ice hockey, then why are you spending time playing on the ice hockey team? This is just a guess, but it would seem that at present you'd be more likely to list on your medical school application that you played on the ice hockey team at UCLA, rather than emphasizing the surfer side of you. (Did you consider being on UCLA's surfing team?)

A lot of pre-professional students (pre-med, pre-law, etc.) try to mold themselves into what they think admissions committees are looking for, rather than realizing that those kind of charades usually backfire. The most successful people, regardless of what they're seeking to do, are those that are upfront and well-integrated within themselves.

" . . . the more you surf, the better your grades will be."

It's unlikely that surfing takes away from your studies. Who can study effectively when they're tense and anxious? Given that surfing makes you happy and relaxes you, it's far more likely that it will actually aid your studying—that the more you surf, the better your grades will be.

So, how to help you to continue being a surfer? You must first confess that, first and foremost, you are a surfer—and expect no absolution on that point. Be proud of being a surfer, don't be in the closet about it.

Joining the Surfer's Medical Association (SMA) may be just the ticket for you—and we would welcome your membership. Although the intention of the SMA isn't to provide a way of "coming out," it's a natural byproduct of joining, a legitimization of one's surfing side.

The Surfer's Medical Association began in 1986, when a group of surfers interested in the health aspects of surfing held a conference on Tavarua Island, in Fiji. Days were spent surfing, nights were for seminars. The surf was unreal, the exchange of ideas hot . . . the Surfer's Medical Association was born.

The Surfer's Medical Association (SMA) is an international organization of surfers committed to helping all surfers be healthier. The organization consists of surfing physicians and other health professionals, scientists, and "barefoot doctors" (surfers interested in the health and medical aspects of surfing). **Every surfer is welcome to join.**

There are presently over 600 dues-paying members, representing all ages, backgrounds, and parts of the world—along with Nobel prize winners from America are high-school surf rats from Australia. Everyone is equal in the SMA. About 25% of the members are non-doctors. Membership includes a decal, membership directory, twice yearly journal, and invitations to all SMA conferences. There is a membership category for every person. Here's a partial list (dues amounts are in U.S. dollars):

● **Barefoot Doctor Member:** *The Surfer's Membership—for surfers interested in learning how to take better care of themselves and others ($20)*

● **Health Professional Member:** *The Surf Doc Membership—for those who spent too much time going to school and now want to surf more ($50)*

● **Professional Member:** *For non-health professionals with real jobs ($50)*

● **Surf Parent Member:** *For those who want to see Johnny come home in one piece ($30)*

● **Surf Family Membership:** *The family that surfs together, stays together ($30; $60 if any family member puts a degree after their name)*

● **Surf Widow Member:** *For spousal equivalents of surfers—the SMA can help ($10)*

● **I'll Join Anything Member:** *For non-surfers who think it would be cool to join a surfing medical association ($19.95)*

The number one goal of the SMA is to educate surfers so they can spend minimal time hassling with doctors and maximal time surfing. Other goals include: to conduct and support research and educational activities on surfing and health; to represent the sport of surfing in the fields of medicine and science; to teach physicians about the unique health problems of surfers and how to better care for surfers; to create a network of barefoot doctors and surfing health professionals around the world; and to protect and preserve the surfer's natural environment—the waves, ocean, and beaches.

School, Surfing and the SMA

Annual SMA conferences are held in Tavarua, Fiji, but other conferences have been held at Pavones, Costa Rica ("Rainforests and Coastal Ecology"); the Bluff, Western Australia ("Diseases of Surfing"); Todos Santos, Baja California ("Marine Medicine"); Grajagan, Java ("Surf Camp Medicine"), and many other choice locales.

The SMA has a number of ongoing health-related projects, particularly the Nabila Health Project in Fiji, in which surfers have been working with villagers to achieve better health for all.

The Surf Docs' column in *Surfer* magazine is another example of an SMA project. There are many more.

Is there a lot of stoke in the SMA? Yes! Are we proud of being surfers? Absolutely.

For more information, and to join the SMA, write to: The Surfer's Medical Association, P.O. Box 1210, Aptos, California 95001-1210 USA.

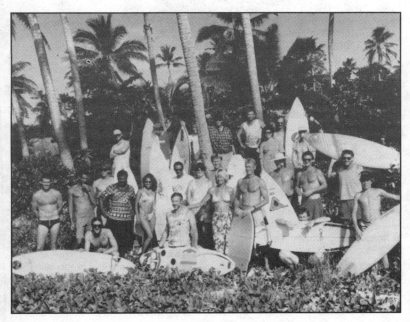

SMA members at one of their annual conferences in Tavarua, Figi. From doctors to students, stand-up surfers, body boarders, Americans to Australisans—everyone is welcome to join.

Sea Snakes
Drop-In Specialists

Dr. Geoff saith:

Most species of these beautiful serpents are found in the northern waters of Australia and adjacent Indonesian archipelago. However, apart from the Atlantic Ocean and Caribbean, sea snakes are found throughout the tropical and subtropical waters of the world.

Like some of their land counterparts, sea snakes have a venom gland. The venom produced is highly toxic. A few species have venom *many* more times potent than the most toxic land snakes.

Like surfers, some species are extremely tolerant (and therefore never bite) while others are very aggro (and quick to bite).

Hundreds (yes my little ones, *hundreds*) of fisherman are killed in south-east Asia each year by sea snakes. Most deaths are associated with shallow water net-fishing. However, I've heard of a surfer dying from the effects of a sea snake bite in Indonesia. With the sudden increase in surfers in such areas, more deaths can be expected.

Death from sea snake venom is unpleasant! Muscle breakdown occurs, resulting in paralysis. Excruciating muscle pain—even when the limb is passively moved—follows. Because of the effects of muscle breakdown chemicals, even if a person recovers, permanent damage to muscle, heart and kidneys can result.

Forget the crap you may have read in various pseudo-intellectual glossies. Sea snakes:

● *Aren't deterred by surf*

● *Can swim faster than you can paddle*

● *Can stay submerged for at least half an hour*

Sea Snakes

- *Can dive to a depth of 50 meters (164 feet) or more*

- *Do eat flesh*

- *Can easily bite you and inject their venom*

Whereas effective antivenemes are available, it's another thing obtaining them! Imagine getting bitten at G-land and getting to a large hospital in a hurry. Makes you laugh, doesn't it.

Okay, what if one of your mates is bitten? Research work by Dr. Straun Sutherland showed that by applying a firm (not tight) crepe bandage to the bitten area and full length of appropriate limb—as well as immobilizing that limb with a splint—venom movement into the general circulation is virtually stopped.

(Of historical interest are some of the old methods used for snake bite—amputation of the affected limb with an axe; heaping gun powder on the bite and igniting it; using a shotgun to blast off part of a bitten hand; giving massive quantities of alcohol and forcing the victim to walk up and down for hours.)

Once the bandages (strips of clothing can be used) are applied they should not be taken off until medical help is reached. Do not use a tourniquet or waste time trying to enlarge the wound and suck out the poison.

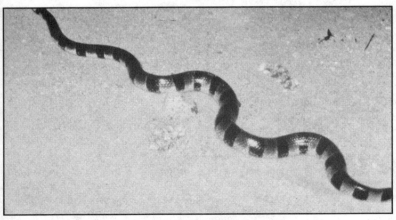

Tavarua sea snake. *Beach Photos.*

Sex, STDs and Pregnancy

On Being Horny

Dear SURF DOCS,

I'm 17 and all I can think about is sex and surfing. I'm worried about getting a disease or getting some girl pregnant, but I'm getting confusing information. Write back quick, man, I'm gonna explode!

HORNY AND WORRIED
Santa Cruz, California

▌▌▌▌▌▏▏▏

Dear Horny,

Sexually transmitted diseases, STDs (what used to be called "VD," venereal disease), and unplanned teenage pregnancies are on the increase in a big way. A "Just Say No" approach to teenage sex hasn't worked; neither has beating around the bush when it comes to sex education. We think young surfers can make intelligent and responsible decisions about sex. Like anyone else, they need the facts.

STDs are passed from person-to-person by sexual contact: penis to vagina, mouth to penis, mouth to vagina and all such permutations with the anus, if you're into that. It's almost impossible to spread STDs by kissing alone. Here are the major STDs you need to know about:

● **Herpes:** *Painful sores on penis and vagina that come and go, sometimes for life. Medication (acyclovir) may help, but there is no cure. Rarely serious enough to put anyone in the hospital, but active sores can make lying on your board a tricky experience.*

● **Gonorrhea:** *Nasty yellow goo from penis or vagina ("the drip"), burns when you pee. Curable with antibiotics. Rarely fatal, but can put you in the hospital if not treated promptly. Bad news for females, who can develop severe pelvic inflammatory disease.*

Sex, STDs and Pregnancy

● **Syphilis:** *More common than people think. Usually starts with a single painless sore on penis or vagina, can progress through all kinds of symptoms to insanity and death. Curable with antibiotics.*

" . . . one sure way to lose lots of surfing time is to become a teen mother or father."

● **Genital Warts:** *The number one STD on college campuses. Painless, small (⅛-¼ inch; 3-6 mm) broccoli-like growths on or near the penis and vagina. Associated with cancer years later. Easy to remove when small; getting out big ones can be a real downer.*

● **Chlamydia:** *The word no one can remember or spell. A mysto disease; sometimes there are no symptoms at all. Usually gonorrhea-like symptoms in men; often fever and belly pain in women. Can put you in the hospital; especially serious in women where it can make it impossible to ever have a baby. Cured by antibiotics.*

● **AIDS:** *AIDS kills. No cure.*

Now, before you sign up for life in a monastery, realize that there is such a thing as safe sex. Anything that prevents direct contact of the penis with the vagina prevents the spread of the germs that cause STDs.

Some, although not all, of the things that prevent pregnancy also help prevent STDs. Here's the lowdown on currently available birth control methods, looking at how well they work and how well they protect you from STDs:

● **Abstinence (not having intercourse):** *Requires both man and woman to participate. Foolproof birth control; foolproof STD protection. We've heard that there are surfers using this method; we just don't know any of them personally.*

● **Condoms and Foam:** *Men and women. Almost foolproof birth control; almost foolproof STD protection. Blocks direct contact with STD germs, kills anything that gets through.*

● **Condoms Alone:** *Risky. Condoms can tear, especially if longingly carried around in a back pocket for a long time.*

● **Foam Alone:** *Woman only. Lousy birth control; lousy STD protection. Better than nothing.*

● **The Pill:** *Woman only. Foolproof birth control;* **No STD pro-**

tection. *Has to be prescribed by a doctor; be sure to ask about safety and side effects.*

● **I.U.Ds:** *Woman only. Fool-proof birth control;* **No STD pro-tection.** *Must be inserted by a doctor; again, ask about safety and side effects.*

● **Diaphragms and Cervical Caps:** *Woman only. Almost fool-proof birth control; lousy STD pro-tection. Must be fitted by a doctor. Kind of a hassle, some people think teens are too immature or impulsive to use this method. We think that's nonsense.*

● **Injections and Implants:** *Woman only. Foolproof birth con-trol;* **No STD protection.** *Not widely available now, may be the wave of the future. Must get through a doctor; ask about safety and side effects.*

The main function of these methods is to prevent pregnancy: one sure way to lose lots of surfing time is to become a teen mother or father. Pick a method of birth control that really works; adding a condom if need be will provide good STD protection. If you're too young to find a reliable method of birth control, then you're too young to have sex.

No method of birth control works unless you use it right. If you don't have a doctor that you trust, the best place for

> **If you're too young to find a reliable method of birth control, then you're too young to have sex.**

teens to get birth control and informa-tion is at clinics like Planned Parent-hood. For college students, the best place is usually the student health ser-vice. These resources are inexpensive (or free) and care is confidential.

Whichever method you choose, do it right away—half of all pregnant teens get that way within six months of the first time they have sex. Getting an STD now could make your life miserable down the line. Until you find a good method of birth control, you should approach sex the same way you approach cold-water surfing: the wetsuit stays on until the excitement is over.

Shark Attacks

A Case of Shark Bait

During a small, clean swell in September 1974, Kirk, Ed and Charlie went down Highway 1 to a long, isolated beach known for its postcard-beauty, with a lighthouse capping the scenic promontory at the beach's end. A powerful beachbreak, it is only rarely surfed. The three paddled out into perfect three to four foot waves, with hard offshore conditions.

Kirk soon lost his custom Ono board (no leash), swam in, retrieved it, and paddled back out. Just after he went to sit back up on his board, he felt someone (something) push him forward. He thought it was a friend, Ed or Charlie, playing a joke, until it took him and his board deep underwater and violently shook him. He struck out with his hand, hit something hard—and was released. He surfaced in a panic,

saw mushrooms of blood around him, his board being blown further out to sea and a large white shark. He let out a primal scream as the shark started toward him again.

Luckily, a wave appeared, and Kirk backstroked into it and managed to bodysurf to the beach. He lay there bleeding. Ed and Charlie quickly came in, and were in a state of panic. Kirk told Ed to go to the nearby lighthouse for help. Ed ran a mile-and-a half to the lighthouse, unthinkingly carrying his board the whole way. Kirk could see he had severe wounds, mainly to the lower body. He told Charlie to tie a tourniquet. Charlie wrapped all of their beach towels tightly around Kirk's wounds and the bleeding slowed.

It took four hours to get Kirk to the hospital. He got 150 stitches and spent two-and-a-half weeks in the hospital. He spent three months

in rehabilitation and physical ther-
apy, and was back in the water 4
months later.

He now goes by the nickname
Shark Bait *and still surfs. His*
board was never found.

TOM
Salinas, California

■■■IIIIIII

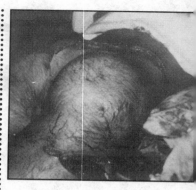

Shark Bait's shark bites.

Dear Tom,

If you surf major coastal promontories, where marine wildlife such as seals, sea lions, and sharks tend to congregate, be prepared for trouble. In this case, Kirk managed to save his own life by luckily getting to the beach, but he probably would have bled to death there on the beach if it hadn't been for his friends. Kirk's board may have been a factor in his survival: it had a super strong glass job and may have kept the shark from being able to fully close its jaws on him.

The size of the shark in this case was apparently enormous (fifteen-foot plus). But sharks of small size, under six-foot even, have been known to inflict fatal wounds. Still, it must be kept in per-spective how few shark attacks occur worldwide. According to John McCosker, director of the Steinhart Aquarium in San Francisco, there have been little more than 50 shark attacks in Northern California since 1926, and only about 10% resulted in death. Eleven of those attacks were on surfers—with ten (but

counting) since 1972. The rate of shark attacks, especially on surfers, is clearly on the in-crease. McCosker describes their attack pattern: They wait well underwater, down current, swim rapidly up at a 45-90° angle, take one big bite, then swim away and wait for the victim to die before returning to eat it. Rarely does the victim see the shark before the attack.

As horrible as it all sounds, keep in mind that shark attacks are extremely rare. Your risk of dying from a shark attack is insignificant compared to your risk of dying from a drive to the beach.

Sharks and Menstruation

Periodic Danger?

Dear SURF DOCS,

I am a healthy 25-year-old female. I live in the Caribbean, and have been surfing for ten years. I try to surf every day, even when I'm menstruating. Obviously I wear a tampon.

About three years ago (I had my period at that time), I saw a shark while surfing. An outside swell passed over it, and gave me a view of its entire back. It was pointed in my direction, and scared me pale. Luckily, I caught the next wave in.

I know we have many species of reef sharks—they like the same area we surfers do. Every single month now since September, I have seen sharks—and always when I have my period. I feel like the boy who cried wolf. I think I hold the record for shark sightings by a surfer. I know sharks can smell blood and urine a mile away, but can they also pick up my scent when I'm menstruating and wearing a tampon?

I know you're going to recommend that I stay out of the water during my period, but it lasts 5-6 days out of every 28—and always when we have a swell! Maybe with some scientific facts, I would consider it.

**SCARED OF SHARKS, BUT
HOPELESSLY ADDICTED
TO SURFING**

■■■■IIIIIII

Dear Scared,

It turns out that the "scientific facts" on sharks and menstruation are few and far between—it just hasn't been studied. The experts we consulted didn't think that you're in more danger of being

Sick *Surfers* ASK THE SURF DOCS & Dr. GEOFF

attacked during your periods. However, it does sound as if your shark sightings are related to your surfing during those times.

Staying out of the water would be the safest thing, but you sound like a hard-core surfer. Wearing a tampon is a good idea but small amounts of blood can seep through. Our SMA gynecologist consultant suggests wearing a contra-

ceptive diaphragm while surfing during your period. Also, consider wearing a full wetsuit (1-2 mm, for the tropics). Wearing a diaphragm, tampon and wetsuit should virtually eliminate blood seeping into the water, and may allow you to turn your shark-sighting record over to someone else.

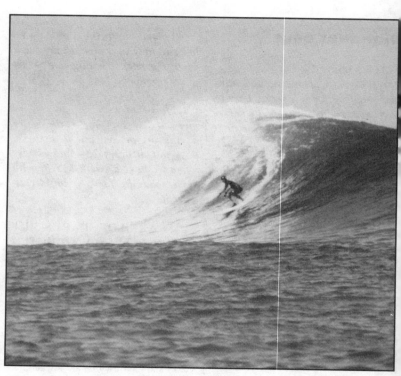

"I've never seen anyone capable of carving as severe a turn as Wombat."
—M.R. McTavish. Cloudbreak, Fiji. *Photo by Sedge Thomson.*

Sharks and Jellyfish

Double Whammy

Dear SURF DOCS,

I live in South Carolina, and am going to start surfing. Could you please give me some info on shark attacks and man-o-war jellyfish? How can I protect myself from them? Do they come out at high tide, low tide, day or night? Are they attracted to brightly-colored wetsuits and swimsuits? Thanks for your help.

TALI
South Carolina

■■■■II|IIII

Dear Tali,

First off, all surfers are at greater risk of getting in a car crash on the way to the beach than of anything that might happen to them once they get there. Many surfers have never even seen a shark, but just about everyone can tell you of a hair-raising brush with death in a car.

So, fasten your seatbelt and drive sanely. Meanwhile, here's what you need to know about sharks and man-o-war.

There are many different species of sharks, and only a few of them have been known to attack man. Why they attack when they do isn't known. In many cases it's thought to be mistaken identity. For example, off the coast of California and Oregon, attacks by Great White sharks are more common in areas heavily populated by seals, their favorite food. It may be that surfers—especially in their black wetsuits—are mistaken for seals. In these instances, brightly-colored wetsuits instead of black ones could · help prevent the attacks.

On the other hand, many attacks in Florida have been in murky water near rivermouths, and are more common at dusk. Tide seems to have little to do with the occurrence. It's not clear what effect bright colors have. Many experts believe they attract sharks.

"If you do spot a shark, paddle calmly and smoothly in to shore. *Don't panic and thrash . . .*"

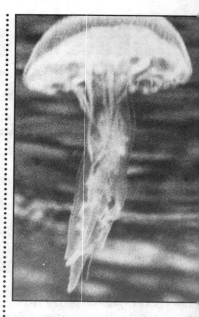

Your best weapon against a shark attack is common sense. Generally, sharks like to hang out where the pickings are easy, and they'll eat just about anything. The waters around harbormouths, rivermouths, prime fishing spots and marine mammal congregations are more likely to have sharks. Chances are if you talk to local fishermen and surfers you can find out what spots in your area have a bad reputation for sharks. Also, sharks aren't very daring, and prefer to attack lone victims, so it's a good idea not to surf alone.

If you do spot a shark, paddle calmly and smoothly in to shore. ***Don't panic and thrash***—it appears to attract and agitate sharks. If you are actually confronted by an aggressive shark, be aggressive yourself. Believe it or not, even Great Whites have been known to be chased off by a solid punch in the nose.

Once an attack has occurred, prevention of bleeding is the essential step. Get your mates to stuff towels, clothes, etc. into the wound and press firmly. Tourni-quets should not be used unless bleeding is not able to be stopped by the above method.

If you're in a developed country, do not move the victim. Instead notify the hospital and get them to send an ambulance. In Australia (particularly N.S.W.) the system is to contact the nearest surf club or police station. They in turn notify the ambulance, local hospital and blood bank. A specially prepared ambulance is sent to the victim and immediate resuscitation is begun.

Experience (mainly in South Africa) has shown that the victim's chances of survival are greatly increased if resuscitation is begun on site.

Sharks and Jellyfish

If you're in a remote area, you'll have no choice but to transport the victim. Use a surfboard as a stretcher and keep those towels pressed in tight. Basically, the odds of survival are related to degree of blood loss and how quickly the loss can be replaced.

As for man-o-war, they don't attack anybody, they just drift around stinging whatever they bump into. Man-o-war have trailing tentacles up to 1,000 feet (305 meters) long, with detachable stingers called *nematocysts*. They like warm water, and drift into the Florida area in summer, when the warm Gulf Stream shifts toward the coast.

When the man-o-war's tentacles come in contact with an object, the nematocysts are fired off, releasing venom. The long tentacles are transparent and hard to see in the water. If a man-o-war drifts into the surf, your only protection is to be covered, either with a wetsuit or a rash guard. It's been reported that having sunscreen on reduces the chance of being stung.

If you do get stung, either by a man-o-war or other jellyfish, immediately rinse off the area with saltwater. ***Don't use fresh water,*** it will stimulate the nematocysts to keep stinging. Apply something to inactivate the venom. Alcohol is best, including rubbing alcohol, strong liquor, or even perfumes containing alcohol. Other liquids that will work in a pinch are vinegar, urine (really!) or olive oil. Meat tenderizer also works. Experts disagree on the effectiveness of these remedies.

> **If you do get stung, by a man-o-war or jelly-fish, immediately rinse off the area with salt-water. *Don't use fresh water...***

Whatever you use, leave it on for at least 30 minutes without touching the affected area. Then carefully scrape away any nematocysts that are still on the skin (they can still sting). The best way to get them off is to apply shaving cream and shave the affected area, but you can also scrape them off using handfuls of wet sand.

Man-o-war stings can be incredibly painful, and can be fatal if a person has a severe reaction to the venom. If someone is stung and begins to swell, and/or has trouble breathing, get them medical attention as quickly as possible. As for treating the pain, soaking the area with cold packs or ice is surprisingly effective.

The Shoulder
Rotator Cuffed

*D*r. *Geoff saith* all surfers should have a working knowledge of the shoulder —it's that fundamental to surfing. And we're not talking about that place on a wave where barnies and hoppers dwell.

There are seven joints which make up the shoulder complex. However, only the gleno-humeral joint (the true "shoulder joint") will be discussed. It has the greatest mobility of any joint in the body.

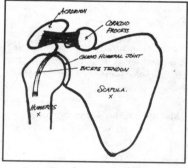

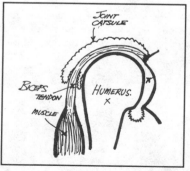

The humerus (upper arm bone) is joined to the scapula (wing bone or shoulder blade) by the gleno-humeral capsule. This capsule is weak and basically serves as a kind of lubricating sac. In front, the capsule is strengthened by ligaments and the whole structure is surrounded on top by a cuff of tendons formed from four major muscles, called the *rotator cuff*. The rotator cuff consists of the supra- and infra-spinatus, teres minor, and subscapularis muscles. Passing through the capsule is the biceps tendon.

Protection of the "roof" of the gleno-humeral joint is via the strong coraco-acromial ligament. A specialized joint space (called a *bursa*) is present between the cuff of muscle tendons on top of the humerus and acromion.

Blood supply and mechanical irritation are the critical areas in shoulder problems. All tendons have a relatively poor blood supply. The most critical area of the

The Shoulder

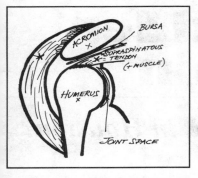

cuff, as far as shoulder problems are concerned, is found in the supra-spinatus tendon just below the coraco-acromial ligament. This area is subject to a lot of wear and tear. Movements associated with paddling and swimming make this wear and tear worse by bringing the head of the humerus up against the coraco-acromial "roof." Inflammation occurs as a result of both the blood supply being squeezed off and direct wear. The tendon swells up and pain occurs.

At first, pain is localized and is noticed only in part of the range of shoulder joint movement. If inflammation spreads to involve the gleno-humeral joint, all movements become painful.

Most shoulder injuries in surfing are the result of continual low-grade irritation. These are called *overuse* injuries. To a major extent most shoulder injuries of this type are preventable by using correct paddling techniques, pre-paddling warm-up exercises, and stretching exercises.

Warming up consists of at least 90 seconds of the following exercises:

1. **Arms outstretched by the sides in the horizontal position, then crossed in front. Alternating right over left and left over right. Palms down.**

2. **Arms straight at sides with palms in. Bring straightened arms up from side to meet above head, palms together.**

3. **Static stretches for about 30 seconds are performed by bringing right hand to reach upper back from above, left hand to upper back from below. Hook fingers of both hands. Repeat to alternate side.**

Correct paddling should be carried out to prevent the arm from being too outstretched to the sides. Ideally, the arm should glide deeply and directly beneath the rails of the surfboard.

Shoulder Pain

Overuse Injury, in Houston?

Dear SURF DOCS,

I'm a 19-year-old surfer and I've been surfing a little over half my life. After a session about a year ago I had a warm pain in my shoulder, right at the joint. I proceeded to rotate my arm and the pain rotated my body. Whenever I lift my arm up or back I feel the binding-like pain. It's bothered me ever since. It tends to hurt more after the longer sessions.

MATT
Houston, Texas

■■■■III|||

Dear Matt,

It probably won't surprise you to hear that we receive a lot of letters asking us about shoulders. It's not that surfers have genetically deficient shoulders, it's just that the most work in surfing is done by the shoulders. Paddling takes its toll. No one has ever counted the total number of paddle strokes in an average surf session, but it could easily top 1,000 if you're catching a lot of waves and the rides are long. At a place like Ocean Beach in San Francisco, where paddling out through rows of whitewater frequently takes upwards of thirty minutes, you can hit the 1,000 mark before you've even caught a wave.

To make matters worse, the strokes in catching a wave are triply intense in terms of strain on the shoulder, because you're paddling as hard as you possibly can, driving your arms and hands deep to get as much distance as possible. After a long surf session, your shoulders are fatigued. After a three or four day swell, they are ready to quit. They have been over-used.

That sounds like what you have, Matt: an overuse injury of the shoulder, which is the most common shoulder problem for surfers. Short of resting it (the more days the better; can you go a week?), here's what we recommend:

1. **Warm up at beachside before going out by slowly stretching your shoulders through their full range of motion (do it slowly and deliberately, as if you were doing Tai Chi).**

2. **Consider using a board that paddles easier (slightly thicker and/or longer).**

3. **Don't use paddle gloves (we're anticipating an increased number of shoulder problems as they become more popular).**

"**N**o one has ever counted the total number of paddle strokes in an average surf session, but it could easily top 1,000 . . . "

4. **If you aren't going to make a wave, don't dive off your board with your arms outstretched.**

5. **Come in early if it starts to ache.**

6. **After coming in, do cool-down stretches, focusing on counter-stretching the shoulder (putting it into the opposite motions from paddling, i.e., back-stroke kinds of movements).**

7. **Ice it for twenty minutes after doing the above.**

Your shoulder will slowly improve. Eventually, you'll forget that you ever had the problem. Just don't forget to keep doing your stretches. Finally, we'd like to know where there are good enough waves near Houston to have brought on this problem. We'd like to go there!

Sinus Problems

Pott's Puffy Tumor

Dear SURF DOCS,

I'm 16-years-old, and have surfed for about three years. I began having severe headaches in late April, which the doctors told me were a sinus infection, and would go away. However, in mid-May it got worse, and a trip to the hospital was necessary. CT-scans done on my head showed a build-up of infectious pus in my brain cavity, which evidently put pressure on my brain, causing the headaches. After hours of brain surgery, the pus was drained and my head felt normal again.

I returned to the doctor three weeks later, and got his unofficial diagnosis: sinus infection—as a result of surfing in seawater—that was forced into my brain by water going into my nose. The doctor wasn't positive about his theory. Result: no surfing for 6-12 months. It has been two months since then and after antibiotic treatments, more CT-scans show my brain free from infection.

Please answer some questions for me. If the infection is gone, why can't I surf? I feel 100%. What about noseplugs? They should stop water from entering my nose, which would reduce the chance of another infection (if it did, in fact, come from the water). Even if I got another sinus infection, I would know enough to stay out of the water until it was gone.

Please correct me if I'm wrong, and give me some suggestions to help get me back out in the water as soon as possible.

TOM
Aptos, California

■■■■II|||||

Dear Tom,

Our SMA brain surgeon consultant says you're lucky just to be alive. Based on the information you provided, it sounds as if you had a "Pott's puffy tumor." It's not really a tumor (for sure, not a cancer); just a silly-sounding name for an unusually fatal condition. Pott's puffy tumor has a 60-90% mortality rate.

What happens is this:

1. **An infection gets into the frontal sinuses, which are bone-encased hollows above your eyes that connect down to the nose.**

2. **An abscess (pus-pocket) forms.**

3. **The abscess eventually "puffs" (erodes) through the skull into the brain.**

Antibiotics alone can't get rid of these kinds of infections. It takes surgery. Either opening a small hole through the forehead into the frontal sinus, draining the pus out, and hoping the brain infections clears up—sometimes done by Ear, Nose and Throat docs for less severe infections. Or, for worse infections, the forehead part of the skull is taken off and the brain infection is scooped out. The eroded-away bone is replaced with a piece of plastic, a procedure only performed by brain surgeons.

If the lesser surgery is done, you can go back in the water in about 3 months, a lot sooner than the 6-12 months usually recommended for the more radical surgery, which sounds like what you had. We'd recommend shooting for the full 12 months. When it comes to these kinds of infections, you don't want to cut corners.

But, rest assured, Tom, you will be able to safely return to surfing. Here are our recommendations:

● *Use a helmet while surfing*

● *Forget about noseplugs; some studies show they **increase** the risk of infection*

● *Don't use any nasal drugs, legal or illegal*

● *Treat any allergies you may have with medications*

● *Avoid flying for a year*

Finally, keep in mind that surfers frequently have sinus problems. It appears to be because of the constant irritation from sea water, plus barotrauma (pressure from diving under waves). We'd suggest early treatment of the pressure-like facial pain of sinusitis. Start with heat: hot packs (a warm wash cloth) or a hot shower directed on your face. Next, try decongestants: oxymetazoline hydrochloride-containing nasal sprays (Afrin® in the U.S.) and/or pseudoephedrine-containing tablets (Sudafed® in the U.S.). If these don't open things up (less pressure and/or pain) within 24 hours, you may need antibiotics. As you learned the hard way, it can be dangerous to wait too long.

Skateboard Injuries

Father Knows Best

Dear SURF DOCS,

Although I am 15 years of age, my dad will not permit me to ride the skateboard I have bought. Being a doctor, he claims that skaters have a great potential to fall and crack their heads open or be hit by cars. The skateboard, being a traditional and necessary means of getting to the beach, cannot be too dangerous.

I was wondering if you might be able to find out the number of tragic injuries caused by skating compared to those caused by surfing. Please, this is vital to my surfing opportunity! Without this transportation, my surfing days are numbered.

BILL
San Diego, California

∎∎∎∎∎∎❚❙❙❙

Dear Bill,

Father knows best, sort of. Your doctor-dad may have picked up on some of the cautionary press in medical journals on skateboarding. To quote the *Physician and SportsMedicine*, August 1989 issue:

> *"Skateboarding injury numbers are climbing like a rider zooming up a stunt ramp, and the American Academy of Pediatrics (AAP) has become concerned enough to erect a big caution sign. The AAP has issued a report urging that skateboarders wear protective gear, that skateboards be banned from streets and highways, and that children under 5 years old not be allowed to ride them."*

Are those recommendations too extreme? Does this mean that they'll soon be issuing similar restrictions on surfing? Probably not. If you look at the injury and death numbers put out by the United States Consumer Product Safety Commission (1979), skateboarding comes

298

Skateboard Injuries

out looking extremely dangerous (137,900 injuries) compared to surfing (9,900 injuries), which weighs in as being less lethal than badminton (11,100 injuries).

Only a handful of surfing injuries result in death, but thirty to forty skateboarders die every year. However, that is a fraction of the number of deaths from jogging or bicycling. And keep in mind that simply driving a car tops the accidental death charts. Still, we think you should be allowed to ride a skateboard. The question is how to do it in the safest way possible.

" . . . surfing weighs in as being less lethal than badminton . . . "

About 17% of skateboarding injuries involve the head and neck (the worst kind of injuries), but in young children the percentage is much higher. As with surfing, injury rates are highest for beginners. Unlike surfing, where most injuries are caused by the surfboard itself, the problem with skateboarding is not the skateboard—it's the skateboarder.

But, even for the most reckless skateboarder, use of safety gear—elbow and knee pads, gloves, shoes, and, most importantly, a helmet—will go a long way towards preventing injury.

Where does that leave you? You're older and more mature than most skateboarders, and we're assuming you're not a beginner (that you've been practicing on the sly). We say go for the acid test: put on a skateboard demonstration for your dad, complete with safety gear, including a helmet (maybe buy one of the new helmets designed for surfing, and use it for both activities.)

Be responsible and safety conscious and your father will almost certainly give in and let you skateboard to the beach and everywhere else. If your father is an absolute holdout, don't forget that a bicycle is also a traditional surfer's way of getting to the beach.

Skin: Fungal Infections

Haole Rot

Dear SURF DOCS,

I am a 28-year-old surfer and beach goer. Over the years of surfing, I have noticed that when summer rolls along I develop what some people say are "sun spots," or some type of fungus. They appear as white blotchy spots over my upper back and chest. Don't get me wrong, I am not covered totally, but enough to make someone notice and mention something about them.

I tan real easily, and it seems as if the only place I do not is in the areas affected. They start off like small pimples without a head, then gradually start to grow into these spots. They can sometimes get irritated. My wife says it's from too much sun. My mom says it's because I sweat and am working outdoors all the time.

I've tried different shampoos, soaps, and lotions. Can you please tell me what is causing this? Do I have to take medication? And is this medication over-the-counter? Thanks for your help.

NATURE BOY
Corpus Christi, Texas

▌▊▊▌▌▐▏▏▎

Dear Nature Boy,

You've got what dermatologists call *tinea versicolor*, a mostly-harmless skin condition caused by a common fungus. Hawaiian natives, connecting their white spots with white tourists, gave it the much more interesting name of *haole rot*. Haole rot is the work of Pitysporum orbiculare, a fungus that is present on our skin all of the time, but which tends to get the upper hand in warm, moist climates—such as summer on the Gulf Coast or in Hawaii.

P. orbiculare makes chemicals known as phenols, which inhibit the pigment-making cells in human skin—hence the white spots. Haole rot tends to show up

Skin: Fungal Infections

on tanned summer skin, but can exist unnoticed on pale winter skin. Sometimes haole rot can block hair follicles on the skin, causing the pimples and irritation that you mention. Usually, though, haole rot is harmless and causes no symptoms other than skin spots. It will not lead to skin cancer or permanent skin changes.

. . . a mostly-harmless skin condition caused by a common fungus.

To treat haole rot, use a prescription-strength selenium sulfide shampoo (Selsun® or Exsel® with 2.5% selenium sulfide). Selenium sulfide is the active ingredient in over-the-counter shampoos like Selsun Blue®, which are often not concentrated enough to do the job on haole rot. To use selenium sulfide shampoo, lather up your scalp and the affected areas on your body. Do it last thing before going to bed and then don't rinse it off. Let it dry on your skin, then **leave it on all night** (don't worry, it won't stain the sheets). Rinse it off thoroughly in the morning, scrubbing vigorously to remove skin flakes around the spots. Repeat the process once more in a week. Be aware that the white spots can take as long as a few months to fade.

Leaving selenium sulfide on the skin overnight can be irritating. If so, try putting the shampoo on for ten minutes for three consecutive days. Don't use selenium sulfide on broken or already-irritated skin, or for more than three days in a row.

If your skin can't handle selenium sulfide, there are other treatments that work. Try anti-fungal creams like 1% clotrimazole applied to the area around "rot spots" twice daily for two weeks (clotrimazole is now available over-the-counter; ask the pharmacist). The problem with this treatment is that it can be very expensive to treat all the involved areas with anti-fungal cream. If you can't afford clotrimazole or a visit to a doctor for prescription-strength selenium sulfide, try the over-the-counter 1% selenium sulfide shampoos—they will work for some people.

To prevent haole rot from coming back:

1. **Keep your skin dry: wear cotton, change clothes frequently.**

2. **Rinse your wetsuit out well and allow it to dry briefly in the sun.**

If the selenium sulfide works for you, repeat the treatment every three months to keep the fungus at bay.

Oh, and Nature Boy, listen to your wife. You probably are getting too much sun.

Skin: Sunsuits and Wetsuit Allergy

Itching to Know

Dear SURF DOCS,

My problem concerns wetsuits, and came up while I was learning to scuba dive in 1978. When I'm exposed to the adhesive bonding used to adhere neoprene to nylon, I break out in an allergic reaction (I don't react to the cement used to put the seams together). This usually happens after about two weeks of wearing a wetsuit a couple of times a week. Bandage adhesives also cause the same reaction, but only when I've been exposed for long periods of time.

My answer to the problem was to buy a custom no-nylon, neoprene suit. However, it will not hold up that well for surfing, as the nylon helps strengthen the suit. Are there any other alternatives? Are suit makers still using adhesive-bonded neoprene suits, or have they found a new way to make them?

Luckily, I live in Hawaii, where I don't need to wear a wetsuit, but I do occasionally surf on the mainland where one is needed. Please let me know if any new products are presently available on the market. Thanks.

CAROLYN
Aiea, Hawaii

∎∎∎∎∎∎||||||

Dear Carolyn,

Your problem has our consultants scratching their heads. They tend to agree with you, and think it's likely that you're having a reaction to the adhesive bonding, not the nylon, which is one of the most inert, non-sensitizing and non-irritating of the polymer/plastic-types of chemicals. However, it's also possibe that you're reacting to coloring chemicals, cross-linking agents, UV-inhibitors, fungal inhibitors, or any of the many other chemical agents that go into the making of a wetsuit. So, what to do?

Consider trying out a polyester/lycra rash-guard garment that has been made into a vest, short john, long john or a full bodysuit. Although generally used as undergarments for wetsuits to avoid rash and provide insulation (allowing the use of a thinner wetsuit), they would also give your skin a protective barrier from the wetsuit's nylon adhesives. Dive shops carry them, and some surf shops.

A number of our SMA members don these Superman-like bodysuits at our Tavarua conferences, calling them "sunsuits," and were able to survive two weeks in the searing, midday equatorial sun without burning. Given the bane of Tavarua surfing—burned backs of the legs from the long paddle-backs—our sunsuits are life savers. (The backs of the legs are where sunscreens seem to wear off the fastest, generally ending up on your board's rails, making them woefully slick.)

One last thought, Carolyn, remember to rinse your wetsuit thoroughly after each use. We know of one other case like yours, involving a surfer now nicknamed Bobby Stinkbomb. It seems he was also allergic to his wetsuit, but Bobby was one of those in-the-water bathroom users. His rashes went away once he began washing out his suit.

> **. . . it's possibe that you're reacting to coloring chemicals, cross-linking agents, UV-inhibitors, fungal inhibitors, or any of the many other chemical agents . . .**

However, his friends still don't sit too close to him in the lineup.

Skin: Fun in the Sun

Sun Sanity

*D*r. *Geoff saith:*

Australians have the highest rate of skin cancer in the world. The Americans aren't far behind. Right now 125,000 Australians have skin cancer and don't know it.

The challenge to all surfers, male and female, in terms of reversing the ridiculously high incidence of skin cancer, is three-fold:

● *To read and understand what you find here*

● *To believe it can happen to you*

● *To actually "take the drop" in terms of positive behavioral change by lessening your sun exposure*

THE SUN

Where does the sun come into all of this? Quite simply, the sun—or should I say sunlight (and in particular the ultra-violet or UV wave band)—causes skin cancer. We don't know precisely how ultra-violet radiation (UVR) does this. Scientific evidence points towards a number of factors in this puzzle. Some of the known factors include:

● *Intermittent sunlight exposure*

● *Age at which exposure first occurs*

● *Length of time of exposure*

● *Genetic factors, including skin type and actual susceptibility for getting skin cancer*

Skin: Fun in the Sun

There are also a number of unknown factors. However, there seems to be good scientific evidence to show that the earlier kids expose themselves to hefty quantities of UVR, the higher the chances of later developing skin cancer. Regular use of a sunscreen for the first 18 years of life is estimated to decrease the lifetime incidence of skin cancer by 80%.

Sunlight is made up of a bewildering array of electro-magnetic (E-M) energy waves. While it is true that the earth's atmosphere "blocks out" many of these E-M waves, UVR still gets through to the earth's surface. Holes in the ozone layer of the atmosphere are one of the known reasons why UVR is on the increase, both in the northern and southern Hemispheres.

UVR is composed of three separate bands (in namometers) from shorter to longer wavelenth:

● *UVC in the 200-290 nm band*

● *UVB in the 290-320 nm band*

● *UVA in the 320-400 nm band*

UVC mainly comes from man-made lamps (mercury lamps, germicidal lamps). UVC causes reddening of the normal skin and eye. It can stimulate production of brown pigment (*melanin*) but not as effectively as UVB.

UVB causes sunburn and also is the more potent type of UVR to stimulate tanning (*melanogenesis*).

UVA causes skin photosensitivity (an abnormal response to various medications). UVA gets deep into the skin and is probably responsible for cumulative skin damage. Most sun lamps and tanning beds produce heaps of UVA.

When skin is exposed to UVR, two processes occur. Firstly, the skin becomes reddened (*erythematous*). Secondly, the skin becomes pigmented (*melanogenesis*). The exact degree of redness and/or pigmentation you get depends on what skin type you are. You can't do much about your skin type—blame your parents if you must. However, you can do a lot to prevent problems associated with UVR exposure to your skin.

Whereas sunburn occurs within a few hours of excessive UVR exposure, skin cancer does not. It takes many years to clock up enough UVR to damage skin cell genes. In turn it takes even longer before these cellular changes are expressed as skin cancer.

Beaches are the sun's war zones. This is where UVR zaps our skin. Sand reflects UV light. Light cloud cover only filters about 20% of UVR. Water doesn't reflect UVR.

In summer 80% of the total daily dose of UVR occurs from 10:00 A.M. to 3:00 P.M. (daylight saving time). No matter where in Australia you are (even Melbourne where it's always cold and wet), mid-day brings the maxed out UVR beast.

Age spots, thinning, wrinkly, and dried-out skin are just some of the signs of sun damage.

Looking like a dried-out prune is bad for the ego. However, melanoma, basal cell and squamous cell carcinomas (cancers) are very bad for your health. After all, death can be fatal.

I don't want to dwell on cancer. The object is not to frighten by describing skin "ulcers" (squamous cell carcinomas) that literally eat into your face, or melanoma that spreads and chokes up vital body organs to slowly cause death. I'm basically interested in giving you an outline of what needs to be done to prevent the problem from occurring in the first place. Each of you has to decide the best method of actually carrying out what's necessary so we can achieve the goal of bringing ourselves from top to bottom of the world skin cancer list.

SEX

I bet you're wondering about this, eh? Well both sexes are equally affected by the sun. However, the way I figure it, it's now time for women to take up the challenge and actually earn their wrinkles, spots and cancers in the surfing arena rather than passively melting in the sand pit. Yes, the same rules apply to girls's skin as they do to guys.

SURF

Unfortunately, surfers are in the box seat for cumulative skin damage. Remember it's your skin. It can happen to you. Damage takes years to manifest itself. Once the damage is manifest, serious skin problems may mean you have to give up surfing. Just think about it, prime of your life with surfing being the force that actually allows you to remain sane (or relatively anyway) while everyone else is fading out. Suddenly, no more surfing and over the edge with the pack you go. Aaaaaagh!

Skin: Sunburn and Skin Types

Burn-out

Dear SURF DOCS,

Lucky me, I'm a 30-something Durban surfer living in Los Angeles. Wave-wise, this place ain't the Bay of Plenty, so I don't find myself surfing as much as I'd like.

My problem is that when the rare swell comes in at Malibu, I find that my white South African skin (Scottish descent) has a rougher time enduring the sun than my now tough skin has enduring these ridiculousy crowded surf spots. Sometimes, even with sunscreen my skin is cooked after just one go-out. Recently, I escaped to the Far North for a surf adventure and I even managed to get a sunburn up there!

What's a white boy like me to do? And, when I do get sunburned, what's the best treatment?

> **BURN-OUT,**
> *in LA-LA land*

■■■■IIII||||

Dear Burn-out,

To begin with, you truly need to understand your skin type; coming to America from another racially-divided country, please don't blanch at that suggestion. The following continuum of skin types is not intended to reinforce racial differences, but rather to help you—and other surfers—to see skin type in terms of sun susceptibility and what to do about it, as surfers.

Skin Type 1: Always burns easy, never tans (very white-skinned, little pigment except for freckles; often red-head and blue-eyed).

Surfers with skin type 1 should surf before 10 A.M. or after 3 P.M. (winter) or 4 P.M. (summer), and not surf in the midday (unless it's the best swell of the year). They should use SPF21 (or greater) sunscreen daily on all sun-exposed areas, and when surfing, also use sunblock (i.e., zinc or pigment-containing creams) on lips, nose, and tops of ears. They should reapply sunscreen and sunblock frequently (hourly if need be). When surfing, they should wear as much as they can to cover their skin, with a wetsuit or lycra, surf caps, surf gloves, and surfing sunglasses. They should get out of the sun when not surfing, and realize that even in the shade they can burn. They should cover up completely whenever in the sun, with long-sleeved shirts, pants, wide-brimmed hat, and sunglasses.

Skin Type 2: Always burns easily, tans minimally (slightly pigmented white skin; often blue-eyed and blond).

Surfers with skin type 2 should surf with the type 1's, mornings and late afternoons, but can tolerate midday sessions for up to about ninety minutes if fully covered by sunscreens and sunblocks, as well as wetsuit, lycra, surf cap, and sunglasses, if feasible. When not surfing, they should still try to avoid being in the sun, and log as much shade time as possible.

Skin Type 3: Burns moderately, tans gradually and uniformly (somewhat pig-

mented skin, with tan, beige, brown, or yellowish color; usually light-colored hair and eyes).

Surfers with skin type 3 should behave as a type 2, but can extend their midday sessions.

Skin Type 4: Burns minimally, always tans well (light-brown and olive-colored skin; darker hair and eyes).

A type 4 can surf anytime, but should still use sunscreens, sunblocks, and protective clothing, particularly in the midday sun. They can log beach time in the sun, but should realize that the sun will still burn and prematurely age their skin.

Skin Type 5: Rarely burns, tans profusely (more darkly pigmented skin, with browns and lighter shades of black; dark eyes and hair).

A type 5 can log serious water and beach time, anytime, but should still use sunscreens on heavily sun-exposed areas.

Skin Type 6: Virtually never burns (black, heavily pigmented skin (except soles and palms); extremely dark eyes and hair).

Endless fun in the sun, truly born to be a surfer.

Burn-out, you sound like a Type 1 kind of guy, perhaps with a smidgen of Type 2 thrown in.

Skin: Sunburn and Skin Types

As for the question of what you—or any surfer—can do if you screw up and get sunburned, early recognition of that fact is essential, so you can take yourself out of the sun and prevent further burning. Granted, some people unawarely put themselves in situations where they get burned, but most surfers know when they're likely to get burned, and have been sunburned so many times before that they can recognize early on when it's happening.

There are subtle signs, long before the skin turns red (which begins 1-3 hours after exposure). There will be an increasing sense of warmth to the skin, leading to it feeling hot (the skin is being cooked). The skin may feel tight, as if it's being stretched.

Most surfers, though, probably aren't aware of the fact that wind intensifies the burning effects of the sun (and also causes its own kind of burn, called *windburn*). Plus, high humidity and water immersion increases the chance of sunburn. Studies have shown that water and heavy sweating wash away the skin's natural sunscreen, something called *urocanic acid*.

With sunburn, the "Little Voice" rule applies. If that little voice in your head asks, "Hmm, are we getting sunburned?," the answer is virtually always "YES." Go in as soon as you hear that little voice; don't start poking your skin to see if it blanches funny and looks red. It's more than likely too late for sunscreen. It's time to go in. Get to shade. You're now into damage control.

After you've turned off the heat (the sun), your next step is to cool your skin. Dowsing or submerging yourself in cool or cold water should help, and will feel good. Keep it up as long as possible. Ice packs will work, too, but be careful not to leave them on too long. No longer than 15 minutes; the skin is already damaged, and freezing it can cause additional damage.

> **Most surfers probably aren't aware of the fact that wind intensifies the burning effects of the sun . . .**

Meanwhile, though, the body's reactions to the burn have begun. Chemical messengers called *prostaglandins* are wailing like fire alarms, causing dilated blood vessels and increased blood flow (what makes the skin look red), as well as triggering pain. The redness and pain will peak at about 12-24 hours after exposure, but you might be able to lessen that reaction if you act soon.

Juice from the aloe vera plant, which grows naturally in many coastal areas (especially in southern Africa, and California), is what many surfers have relied on over the years for treating sunburn.

Aloe is a type of succulent. An aloe plant looks something like a giant upside-down artichoke; if you don't know what one looks like, ask local surfers if there are any growing nearby and to point one out to you.

You need only pick some succulent aloe leaves, break them open, and smear the juice right onto your skin. If there are no aloe plants accessible to you, you don't need to buy the fancy "Contains Aloe!" products. Just get the pure and cheap stuff, sold in most health food stores. The gel form is easier to use than the liquid. Many surfers take aloe on surf trips as part of their first-aid kit. Although aloe hasn't been well-studied, it really seems to lessen the pain and discomfort of a burn, speed up recovery, and reduce later peeling.

If you don't have aloe, vinegar packs will help somewhat with the pain of a sunburn. Just pour vinegar—any kind—on a cloth and drape it over the burned area.

As for medications, taking plain aspirin or ibuprofen will help stop the prostaglandins and somewhat lessen the pain and inflammation, particularly if taken soon after the burn has occurred. Prescription drugs such as steroids (prednisone tablets or cortisone creams) or indomethacin tablets also can make a difference. Indomethacin has been shown to be far more effective than aspirin in treating sunburn.

Most sunburns are only *first-degree* burns, involving the superficial skin lay-ers. There may be small skin blisters 1 or 2 days later, and after a week or so the skin begins to rub off. However, if you begin developing larger blisters almost immediately, and your skin soon begins peeling off in sheets, it means you have had a deeper sunburn, or what is called a *second-degree* burn. *Third-degree* burns are rare from the sun. It's the burnt-toast look, involving all of the skin layers, including the nerves, so you feel no pain. The skin is dead and gone.

The goal, as with all of surf medicine, is prevention—not getting any kind of sunburn.

So, Burn-out, that's the scoop for all you lowly skin types. By the by, we think your name would make a great screenplay title. "Burn-Out." We picture a character-generated action thriller. Maybe starring an ex-Durban surfer. He's being pursued by Quiksilver ad executives. He escapes to a deserted tropical island. He discovers lovely humanoid coconuts (romance sub-plot). There's a perfect wave wrapping around the island. He has his board. Then the real action begins. He forgot to bring sunscreen.

Skin: Sunscreens

Burning to Know

Dear SURF DOCS,

I am a very fair-skinned person and, therefore, at high risk for skin cancer. This scares me. My dermatologist has told me about people my age who are dying of skin cancer. Both my parents, who are also fair-skinned, have had bad cases of skin cancer, which left them with some mean-looking scars.

Sunscreens don't really work well for me. For example, in March, I was in Hawaii, and used sunscreen the entire time. After two days of sun and surf, my body broke out with itchy red bumps. They developed after I'd been in the sun most of the day, and would almost be gone the next morning (until I hit the beach again).

Another example of my problems is this: when I put a sunscreen on my face, it gets in my eyes, making them burn so badly that I can't open them. What should I do, stay out of the sun? Please give me some useful facts.

APRIL
South Florida

■■■■II|||||

Dear April,

Sunscreen is a real hassle sometimes, but for those of us whose skin was not designed to handle the sun, it can literally be a lifesaver. Here are some ideas to help you stay outside and still beat the sun:

● *The itchy red bumps you describe sound like an allergic reaction—probably to your sunscreen but also perhaps to the sun itself. Many people are allergic to PABA, the active ingredient in most sunscreens. Try using one of the sunscreens that doesn't contain PABA (the ingredients are listed on the side of the container). Make sure the one you use is waterproof,*

"**S**unscreen is a real hassle sometimes, but . . . it can literally be a lifesaver."

and use at least Sun Protection Factor (SPF) 15. See Table on pg. 313.

● *To avoid getting sunscreen in your eyes, use a thicker, non-runny, waterproof gel or cream instead of lotion. Put it on at least 20 minutes before you go out in the sun so it has a chance to bond to your skin, before you start sweating.*

● *Some studies have called into question whether sunscreens affect vitamin D synthesis in the skin, leading to more—not less—cancers. This has not been confirmed and seems unlikely to be the case!*

● *Also, it has been found that highly sweat- and water-resistant sunscreens can prevent the skin from sweating, the body's way of regulating heat. This can lead to feeling tired and weak, and eventual collapse (called* overheating syndrome*), but to our knowledge, this has never been reported in surfers.*

● *As for what specific brand of*

sunscreen to use, here are some general considerations when it comes to surfing:

✴ *Blocks out UVA and UVB wavelength (a broad spectrum product)*

✴ *Bonds to the skin effectively, stays on for hours and doesn't get washed away by sweat or surf*

✴ *Doesn't hurt the eyes or irritate the skin*

✴ *Isn't greasy or slippery*

✴ *Doesn't stain clothes or wetsuit*

✴ *Is cosmetically acceptable; easy to put on and doesn't cost a fortune (generic, bulk brands are fine)*

● *Try to avoid being in direct sunlight between the hours of 10:00 A.M. to 3:00 P.M., when the sun is at its peak. The sun is much less damaging in the morning and late afternoon.*

Remember, the closer you get to the equator, the more fierce the sun becomes. Surfers in south Florida and Hawaii have a much higher risk of skin cancer than surfers in Oregon or Tasmania. Because of where you live, April, you'll need to be extra careful.

Skin: Sunscreens

Some Commercial Sunscreens: Active Ingredients, Consistency, Protection Factors, and Resistance to Water

| Trade Name | Type | Sun Protection Factor | | Resistance to | |
		Indoor Solar Simulator	Outdoor Sunlight	Sweating	Water Immersion
PABA sunscreens					
PreSun 15	Clear lotion	15	10	Excellent	Poor
Pabanol	Clear lotion	15	6-8	Fair	Poor
Sunbrella	Clear lotion	15	6	Fair	Poor
PABA-ester combination sunscreens					
Supershade 15	Milky lotion	15-18	6-9	Excellent	Good
Total Eclipse 15	Milky lotion	15-18	9-12	Excellent	Good
MMM What-a-Tan!	Milky lotion	15-20	10	Excellent	Good
PreSun 15	Milky lotion	15-20	8-10	Excellent	Good
Clinique 19	Milky lotion	15-19	7-8	Good	Fair
Sundown 15	Milky lotion	15-20	10-11	Excellent	Good
PABA-ester sunscreens					
Block Out	Lotion/gel	6-8	6	Good	Fair
Pabafilm	Lotion/gel	6-8	4-6	Good	Fair
Sundown	Lotion	8-10	4-6	Good	Fair
Original Eclipse	Lotion	8-10	4-6	Good	Fair
Aztec	Lotion	6-8	4	Fair	Poor
Sea & Ski	Cream	7-8	4	Fair	Poor
Non-PABA sunscreens					
Piz Buin-8 +	Cream	15-20	10-12	Excellent	Good
TiScreen	Cream	16-22	10-12	Excellent	Good
Piz Buin-8 +	Milky lotion	20-22	10-12	Excellent	Good
TiScreen	Milky lotion	16-20	10-12	Excellent	Good
Piz Buin-4 +	Milky lotion	10-12	4-6	Fair	Poor
Uval	Milky lotion	10-12	4	Poor	Poor
Coppertone 4	Lotion	3.5-4	2	Poor	Poor
Physical sunscreens					
A-Fil	Cream	6-8	4-6	Good	Fair
RV Paque	Cream	6-8	3-4	Good	Fair
Shadow	Cream	4-6	2-4	Good	Fair
Reflecta	Cream	6-8	4-6	Good	Fair
Covermark	Cream	6-8	4-6	Good	Fair
Clinique	Cream	6-8	4-6	Good	Fair

* The sunscreens often used by surfers—*Aloe Gator* and *Bullfrog*—compare quite favorably to the above products, and have good resistance to water immersion.

Reprinted from Pathak MA, Sunscreens: Topical and systemic approaches for protection of human skin against harmful effects of solar radiation. *Journal of the American Academy of Dermatology*, 1982:7 (September): 283-312. Used with permission.

Skin Cancer Prevention

Cute and Freckly

Dear SURF DOCS,

I'm proud of the fact that for 14 of my 26 years I've been a hard-core surfer, but lately my skin is really starting to show it. I was bummed last night, at a party, when a chick complimented me on my "cute, freckly, weathered look."

But I don't know that it's anything I can help. I've been using sunscreen pretty regularly, and I don't try to get tan anymore. My mother says it's just how we Irish look when we get older (she's already had two skin cancers!). Is there any hope for me?

CUTE AND FRECKLY
San Diego, California

■■■||||||||

Dear Freckly,

Yes, there is hope—but it will take a different mind set and a more dedicated approach on your part. Despite all the wonderful things the sun provides—how good it makes us feel, the fact that it sustains life on this planet—when you think about it, we're really basking in the glow of the biggest nuclear reaction in our corner of the universe. The sun is an atomic bonfire bigger than a billion Hiroshimas!

Those who take the worst hits from the sun are folks like you, Freckly, people of northern European ancestry, especially the Irish and Scottish. Your ancestors evolved in the frozen north, where the sun is less intense. Their genes slowly lost both the ability to make sun-blocking pigment and the ability to repair the damage from the sun. Freckles are a pitiful reminder of your genetic inability to darken your skin for sun-protection. The "weathered look," which is premature aging, represents poor skin repair from sun damage.

Growing up in a sub-tropical place like San Diego, there's no "luck of the Irish" when it comes to skin damage from the sun. Parents and schools need to take responsibility for helping kids

Skin Cancer Prevention

learn about the sun and how to avoid over-exposure. It's estimated that by age 18, the average American has already received 75% of their lifetime total of sun exposure.

Then, after age 18, when most people begin turning to an indoor worklife, surfers go on adding to their sun exposure, attaining lifetime exposure amounts that are off the chart! For most surfers, or at least the unaware ones, it isn't a question of whether they'll end up with a skin cancer; it's a question of how young they'll be when they get their first one, and how many more will follow.

> "**P**arents and schools need to take responsibility for helping kids learn about the sun and how to avoid over-exposure."

To avoid being one of those statistics, here's what we recommend for all surfers when it comes to the sun:

● **Surf more, sun less.** *If you have all day to surf, keep in mind that midday sun is the worst, early morning and late afternoon the*

best. If you have a choice of where to surf, go with spots with less intense early morning or late afternoon glare and reflection problems. Even ten minutes of reflected sun can burn your face.

● **Dress for the occasion.** *Go for max skin covering if out in the midday. At a minimum, use a surf cap or visored hood to shield your head, face, and eyes (and consider sungoggles as well). If in warm-water climes, don't stop with just a lycra vest, go for something with sleeves—down to the wrist if possible—and a high neck. Those in the know wear full-body lycra/polypropelene suits, which aren't easy to come by in surf shops but are carried as under-wetsuit garments in many dive shops.*

● **Sunscreens and sunblocks.** *Use a waterproof sunscreen of SPF15 or greater. Despite manufacturer's claims, the maximal useful time in the water is about 80 minutes (40 minutes if marked "water-resistant"). Creams and gels are usually better for surfers than lotions and oils, which can make your board slippery. Make sure it screens out both UVA and UVB rays. Use enough: a full teaspoon for the face, about five teaspoons for the whole body (if you're lucky enough to surf naked). Use a sunblock (completely blocks vs. screens the sun) on the most heavily sun-*

315

exposed areas, such as your nose and lower lip (the more common sunblocks are zinc-containing).

● **Check it out.** *Skin self-examination is the call. Currently, one-in-seven Americans will get skin cancer. The risk for surfers is far higher, perhaps three-in-four. Most skin cancers are completely curable if caught in time. Any new skin growth, bump, mole, or blotch should be checked by a doctor.*

● **Live clean, vote green.** *Do whatever you can to stop the destruction of the ozone layer. Surfer's have a special stake in the stratosphere. Educate yourself about CFC's, and avoid releasing more into the atmosphere. Get active in your community, raise a stink. Vote intelligently; help others do the same.*

◎

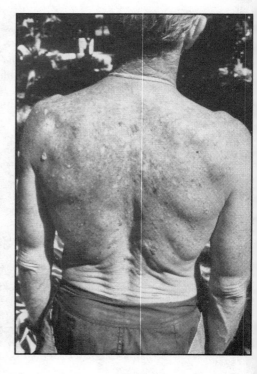

After a lifetime in the sun—*surfer's skin*. He couldn't remember how many pre-skin cancers and skin cancers he'd had cut and burned off. *Beach Photos.*

Pre-Skin Cancer

Actinic Keratosis

Dear SURF DOCS,

I'm 35-years-old and have been surfing for 23 years. For the first 10 years of my surfing life, I surfed a lot. You know the scene, burned nose every summer, peeling down to the bone. It looked cool back then. For the next 10 years, I surfed mostly vacations—summer and Christmas. Last year, I started surfing a lot again, maybe 20 times a month.

I found a scratchy, sensitive spot on my shoulder last year—about the size of a pencil eraser—which kept peeling and never healed, even though months went by. I went to a doctor, and he diagnosed the spot as **actinic keratosis.** It was burned off, using liquid nitrogen. Actinic keratosis, I guess, is cancer of the epidermis. If you let it go and it spreads to the deeper skin layers, things can get really bad.

The doctor was excited to see the spot, and showed it to some nearby medical students, "We don't usually see this until a person is about 50 or so," he said. Great—I've got the skin of a 50-year-old man.

Today, I live and surf in Puerto Rico. Because I am obviously prone to skin cancer, I only surf right before sunset, for about an hour, until it's too dark to see. That's when the harmful UV rays are less strong, as they're coming in obliquely from the setting sun, through the UV-absorbing ozone layer.

My question is, why aren't there sun-suits for surfers (which would protect the surfer from harmful radiation), so we could surf during the day? I'm scared shitless to get a tan now or expose my skin to direct sunlight. I would like to surf in the heat of day, but I'm told that even a sunscreen with a sun pro-

tection factor of 15 or 25 isn't effective enough against the suns rays, when you've already had a "touch" of actinic keratosis.

I don't want to get skin cancer. It sounds bad and with the death of the ozone layer, things are only gonna get worse.

TANNED FOREVER

■■■■IIIIIIII

Dear Tanned,

Most surfers don't yet realize the dangers of the sun. You've gone to the other extreme—it seems like somebody overdid it with the scare story. Don't let "a touch of actinic keratosis" keep you from being a full-on surfer. Here are the facts and what to do.

Actinic keratosis is not skin cancer, but it is considered a pre-cancerous condition. Actinic keratoses are the slightly red, scaly "skin barnacles" that crop up on sun-exposed skin, especially in fair-skinned people who have spent years in the sun. The forehead, bridge of the nose, temples, cheekbone area, rims of the ears, back of the neck and on the shoulders are where they commonly appear. They only rarely progress to cancer, but generally should be removed by a doctor.

Most often actinic keratoses are burned off with liquid nitrogen or an electrocautery tool. Some dermatologists will prescribe a cream to be used (called *Efudex®*), which causes them to scab and eventually fall off. If it is suspected of already being cancer, it may need to be biopsied or surgically removed.

The key to preventing skin cancer: Do not get sunburned. Use high SPF waterproof sunscreen, avoid peak sun hours (10:00 A.M. to 3:00 P.M., in most latitudes), and wear protective clothing.

A sunsuit is a great idea, and, in effect, is already commercially available. For instance, all wetsuits are really sunsuits—they protect the skin they cover from the sun. For warm-water surfing, wear a thin wetsuit (1-2mm) that is long-sleeved and long-legged. As an alternative, full-body lycra suits are now being made for surfing. A leotard with tights would also work. At the least, a t-shirt can be worn in the water; surfers have been doing that for years.

In the future, you'll see more and more surfers protecting their skin from the sun.

And listen—you don't have to become a creature of the shadows. Take care, but if there's a perfect midday surf session to be had, don't feel you can't be part of it—cover up and get covered up!

Skin Cancer and Insurance

Paying for It

Dear SURF DOCS,

At age 36, after 20+ years of surfing, I am currently going through the removal of minor forms of skin cancer. The cancers have been diagnosed as basal cell carcinomas. I'm being treated at a prestigious clinic in La Jolla, and this is why I'm writing to you.

My lifestyle has been surfing first, income later, as I'm sure it is with many other surfers, and the simple fact is, I can't afford the high-priced treatment at this renowned clinic. I'm already in debt from the first carcinoma removal, and I'm scheduled for a second. Although the cost is an estimated $850, by the time the doctor and his plastic-surgeon partner finished with me the last time, the cost had gone from an estimate of $600 to $1,800.

In short, the clinic is putting me in the poor house. I've asked if there's any way people who can't afford treatment can get care adjusted to their income. The answers have been negative. I would appreciate any help on this subject. Long ago, I decided to chase waves rather than dollars, and I hope I can continue doing so.

PATRICK
San Diego, California

∎∎∎∎∎∎|||||

Dear Patrick,

Thanks for your letter. Your situation raises important issues that surfers need to pay attention to. First, the United States is still in the Dark Ages when it comes to providing good health care for its citizens. Unlike New Zealand, Australia, Canada and other countries, we don't have national health care, and

319

only about 60% of the people here are covered by health insurance. Without it, you either end up paying through the nose, or taking potluck at a public clinic.

Until our health system gets its act together, all surfers should make sure they have medical insurance.

Until our health system gets its act together, all surfers should make sure they have medical insurance. Younger surfers may be covered under a parent's policy. College students may be automatically covered under a student health plan, or have to pay a bit extra for coverage (they should check to make sure they're covered over summer break). Employed surfers may be covered through their work, but many hardcore surfers don't have those kinds or regular full-time jobs. If you have to buy medical insurance on your own, expect to pay from $30-100 a month, depending on the amount of coverage, the deductible, and so on.

But you, Patrick, don't have insurance, and you're in a jam. Here are some things to consider:

● *Plastic surgeons charge more then dermatologists. General practitioners (your family doctor) charge the least. Many family doctors do skin cancer removal in their practices.*

● *Plastic surgeons and dermatologists will do a prettier job (with less scarring) if the skin cancer is on the face, but it may be unnecessary (and overpriced) on other parts of your body.*

● *It's possible to get excellent care at a public health facility, such as a county hospital, but you'll have to be aggressive at making the system work for you: finding out who's good, getting an appointment, and working around cumbersome policies and procedures. Public health facilities will charge you, but it's often on a sliding scale, based on how much money you say you make. Very often the same hotshots who work at up-scale hospitals are also on staff at county hospitals. The care you receive will be every bit as good; the carpets just aren't as plush.*

Finally, don't forget that preventing a skin cancer is a lot cheaper than treating one.

Skin Cancer: Melanoma

Learn from Mikel

Dear SURF DOCS,

I am 41-years-old, and have been surfing seriously since 1959.

The first sign of any problem began in May 1988 when I noticed a lump under my right armpit. Due to normal preliminary blood tests and the fact that I appeared to be perfectly healthy, my family doctor's initial opinion was that I had a localized infection, causing my lymph glands to swell in that area. He prescribed antibiotics, to be taken for 5-6 weeks. During this time the lump grew steadily. My doctor referred me to a surgeon, who performed an biopsy and determined that I had malignant melanoma.

In most cases of melanoma, an asymmetrical discolored mole is an indication that something is wrong. To my knowledge, I had no mole which could've been considered the "primary" site. The doctors believe my melanoma may have started on my right arm or possibly my shoulder, remaining undetected during that stage, going into spontaneous remission and developing later in my lymph nodes.

On July 14, I had 34 lymph nodes removed from my right armpit (four were malignant). With only three months to adjust to this devastating chain of events, another tumor was discovered in my right shoulder near my clavicle bone. Since surgery is the best and most effective way of treating melanoma at this time, I elected for another procedure to remove the second tumor. While preparing me for surgery the doctors ordered a routine CAT scan of my upper body, including my head, and—to my horror—discovered two more tumors in the left hemisphere of my brain. Although the surgeries would be risky, it was decided after

Sick *Surfers* ASK THE SURF DOCS & Dr. GEOFF

days of deliberation that all the tumors could be removed. The shoulder surgery was performed first, followed by brain surgery 3 weeks later.

The doctors felt radiation treatment to my shoulder and brain following the surgeries would increase my chances of winning my fight with the disease. I have had to endure almost 6 weeks of these treatments, the loss of my hair and a complete change in lifestyle. I am feeling well enough physically to get back in the water, but the emotional battle I wage against this disease inhibits my motivation to do so. Statistically my prognosis is grim; however, with a loving family, good friends and so much to live for, I will continue to fight this battle.

My main purpose in telling this story is to warn my fellow surfers of the dangers of overexposure to the sun. Recent scientific research suggests that with the decrease in the Earth's ozone layer there will be a dramatic increase in cases similar to mine. Melanoma, once a disease affecting older people, is now showing up in those as young as 20. Please don't make the mistake of thinking it won't happen to you. Use sun screen products and avoid overexposure whenever possible.

In retrospect, thinking about my years of surfing and the fun I had in the water, it's hard to say whether I'd trade those good times for my disease. You, however, have the opportunity to make the choice that I no longer can. Protect yourself.

MIKEL
Santa Cruz, California

∎∎∎∎∎∎∥∥∥

Dear Mikel,

On behalf of surfers everywhere, thank you for your letter. Your advice is outstanding and, coming from you, is far more powerful than if it came from us surf docs. Unfortunately, you have had to learn about melanoma the hard way. What, though, should every person, particularly surfers, know about melanoma? In addition to the information in your letter, the following is what we consider essential.

There are over 100 different kinds of cancers, and melanoma is but one of them. Whereas most cancers take upwards of 15 to 20 years to develop, melanoma can grow in half that time, or less. Its full name is "malignant melanoma," but most people call it the "black mole" cancer. Melanoma is considered to be a form of skin cancer, although, as with you, Mikel, it may appear in non-skin locations.

322

Skin Cancer: Melanoma

Skin cancers are classified as being melanoma or non-melanoma. The non-melanomas are the garden variety skin cancer: 500,000 cases per year in the U.S.; they are frequent in older people; common in sun-exposed areas; take many years to grow; begin as raised, scaly, red bumps; are easily treated; and are highly curable. The melanomas are a whole different story: only 25,000+ cases per year in the U.S.; they can strike people of all ages; are not always sun-exposure related; can grow rapidly; have a varied appearance; are difficult to treat; and are not always curable.

Melanomas develop from melanocytes, which are highly specialized cells that produce melanin. Melanin gives your skin color and allows you to tan. (The region of the South Pacific where there are particularly dark-skinned islanders is called Melanesia.) Melanocytes are found in places other than the skin, for instance the eyes, mouth, and brain, so there can be non-skin melanomas—but they are rare.

Whites have the highest incidence of melanoma, but it does occur in Blacks. Australian Whites have an extremely high incidence, due to their largely English-stock skin type and high-sun exposure, largely coastal life style. And among Australians (or, for that matter, Americans), those who are surfers must be seen as being at extremely high risk for melanoma.

The most at risk area is the site of a prior, severe, blistering sunburn—and the younger you were when you were burned, the worse. Combined with our society's increasing number of in-the-sun life styles, the now apparent gradual depletion of the ozone layer is thought to account for the increasing number of melanomas. It was once a rare disease, but its incidence has doubled every ten years for the past thirty years. By the year 2020, one in every hundred people will be developing melanoma at some time in their life. In surfers, it may be one in fifty—unless we take radical actions now.

Other factors are significant in causing melanoma, including genetics and inherited traits. It can "run in the family," but this only accounts for about 10% of all cases. More common is something called *dysplastic nevi syndrome*. "Nevi" is the medical term for moles. Most everyone has already developed between 10 and 40 normal moles on their body by the time they are in their 20s. Moles don't usually start anew after you are an adult.

Dysplastic nevi syndrome has to do with moles that usually appear after you are an adult. They are usually larger than normal moles (i.e., wider across then a pencil-eraser), asymmetrical (not perfectly round or one-half doesn't match the other half), have irregular edges, and are often multi-colored.

Check out your own moles; say something to your buddies if you think they've got some weird moles. If the mole's appearance or growth pattern is anything like that of a dysplastic nevi or a melanoma, don't hesitate—go straight to a dermatologist and have it looked at. Be especially mindful of a mole, however small or normal-appearing, that appears in a prior severe sunburn site. No matter how normal it may look, it may already be a melanoma—all melanomas start by looking small and normal.

Your letter underscores the fact that once a melanoma appears, it isn't always obvious what it is, particularly to a general or family physician. Sometimes they aren't noticed or taken seriously until they are widely spread throughout the body. Even after it is widespread, there are often no symptoms. You may feel fine, at most a little tired, until it begins to choke off an organ such as the brain. Melanocytes are derived from the nerve tissue from when you were an embryo, and retain the ability to grow and spread as rapidly, and to similar places, as when you were just weeks old.

The treatment for melanoma is complicated. If it hasn't spread deep into the skin, or to other parts of the body (including the lymph nodes), there is a 90%+ chance of being cured of it by having fairly straight-forward surgery.

If it has spread, as with you, Mikel, treatment with chemotherapy or radiation therapy is sometimes used, but with varying success, and cure rates of under 50%.

Two profound facts to keep in mind about the treatment of melanoma:

1. **Melanoma is one of the few cancers that has the potential for spontaneous remission, that is, suddenly disappearing, even if it is widespread and has failed to respond to treatment.**

2. **The reason melanoma occasionally spontaneously disappears is thought to be due to the immune system, making melanoma one of the most promising cancers for successful treatment by immunotherapy (the use of natural, biological substances that heighten or correct the immune system). Immunotherapy is the hottest thing going in the cancer world—much like thrusters were for surfing in the '80s. Your doctor should give you information on the research centers that are doing cutting edge treatment research on immunotherapy and melanoma.**

Finally, and to non-surfers this question may seem ludicrous, but to hard-core surfers it will make incredible sense: Can the desire to surf add to one's will to live? Can the desire to keep surfing increase the chances of surviving a horrible disease like cancer? We surf docs believe that to be true. Keep surfing, Mikel; keep living.

See inside front cover photos.

Sleep

Pillow Surfing

Dear Dr. GEOFF,

Everybody's health conscious today. I stayed awake until four, five every morning trying to figure out what was wrong with me. Finally I figured out what was wrong—I wasn't getting enough sleep . . . Oh, I'd doze off for eight or nine hours . . . but after that I'd just lie there tossing and turning. It got so bad, I couldn't even go back to sleep after the alarm went off . . . hmmmmm

Seriously though, have you any ideas on how to get to sleep quicker?

B.H.
Wammeroo, Western Australia

∎∎∎∎∎∎∎∎∣∣∣

Dear B.H.,

Sleep is very much in the thing amongst various medical specialities these days. The Europeans started to push it back in the '50s and over the last 10 years or so it has become a real growth industry for research.

Sleep, or rather disorders of sleep, is something that bothers all of us at some time or another. One pommie is recorded in the medical literature as not having slept for over 10 years. (He still continues not to sleep even after a court settlement for the car accident that apparently caused his problem.)

Researchers say that a biological clock dictates sleep.

This tic-toc in the brain is very sensitive to body temperature. As the body temperature lowers, adjustments to electrical rhythms within the brain take place. These cause dampening down of the "awakening" centers of the brain. A temporary electrical short circuit if you like.

Of course, many factors can stuff up this delicate little clock and its associated circuits. Having to work night shifts, consistent all night raging, crossing time zones as part of overseas air flights, stress, depression and nasty little brain problems such as infections and tumors being just a few of the circuit breakers.

Also, some people's clocks are on say, 20 or 26 hour cycles. Compare this with the traditional 24 hour clock cycle and you can imagine the chaos.

Time spent sleeping is another major variable. Some people really "need 10 hours," others get by with "only 4 hours." The amount of sleep needed changes as we age and circumstances change.

In the same way as watchmakers are able to repair your trusty old spring loaded time piece, various medical techniques are available to repair (or at least modify) your biological clock. These days they have sleep labs which can really zero in on your problem.

However, you have to first decide how bad the problem really is. In particular, is it interfering with your lifestyle? Alternatively, can you use the extra time spent not sleeping to your advantage?

Having decided that it is a serious problem, go see your Doc and discuss the problem with him to make sure there is nothing significantly medically wrong. If your doc only gives a prescription for sleepers, tear it up.

The best step is to learn psychological techniques of sleep induction which some doctors or psychologists are trained to teach.

If it's still a problem after all this, then take up night surfing. At least it's not crowded and you can pick your own wave.

Other common causes of sleeplessness include:

● *Sleep apnoea/snoring—which can make people feel very tired and "washed out," particularly when first awake in the morning (sleep labs excel at picking this up)*

● *Being constantly over-amped after doing too much "high adrenalin" sporting activities (e.g., surfing)*

● *Drugs—particularly alcohol, cigarettes, Valium (and other benzos), speed, cocaine or marijuana*

● *Traveling through time zones, or what is called jet lag. (The best approach for treating jet lag is to expose yourself as quickly as possible to the daylight sun in your new time zone. That will reset your bio clock.*

● *Shift work*

One of the most delightful causes of sleeplessness is "surfed-out insomnia," from surfing say, 6 to 8 hours in one day, which so dramatically alters your body chemistry that it somehow keeps you from sleeping. You'll sweat a lot, toss and turn, and are constantly thirsty, and not very hungry. But even though you're not asleep, you'll be dreaming of all those great waves you got.

Smoking Cigarettes

Dying to Know

Dr. Geoff saith:

A few weeks ago, I had the privilege of meeting a group of mega-stars of the future (a group consisting of two gals and 10 guys from the Australian National Team). It was interesting to get their perspective of health and to try and answer some of their questions. Mark Richards was also there adding his perspective on nutrition (very finger-lickin' suspect) and telling it like it is when describing his various sporting injuries over the past few years.

I noted that about one-third of these hotties smoked. They were all, however, interested in the effects of cigarettes, especially in relationship to sporting performance. I would like to share with my readers the following information.

Smoking *is* most definitely a health hazard. It is, however, a slow death rather than a *dramatic* event such as heroin O.D. Nonetheless, thousands of young kids (and in particular an alarmingly increasing number of young females) are right now setting the stage for later misery. Heart disease, clogging of leg arteries, strokes and lung cancer are being nurtured by the smoking habit.

THE TOBACCO LEAF

Many hundreds of biologically active substances are contained in tobacco leaves. Tobacco smoke is a mixture of vapor and liquids. Tar is the name given to this gunk. It makes up about 40% of cigarette smoke and varies from 3 to 40 mgs. per cigarette, depending on the cigarette brand.

Investigations have identified some 254 chemicals including aromatic hydrocarbons and phenols. While surfboards also contain chemicals from these two groups, it would be a clever surfer who could make surfboards from cigarettes!

Both aromatic hydrocarbons and phenols in various forms can cause cancer. They also irritate the nose, throat and chest just in the same way surfboard chemicals do. However, it is nicotine and carbon monoxide (CO) that affect the heart and blood vessels (the pipes carrying blood to various parts of the body).

NICOTINE

Smoke from an average cigarette contains 1 mg. of nicotine. 60 mgs. of nicotine given intravenously (mainlined) will kill a person. Only 4 mgs. can produce alarming effects in the occasional smoker such as faintness, giddiness, racing thoughts and fast heart rate.

This is because nicotine has effects on certain parts of the nervous system. Small doses make certain areas of the nervous system more sensitive; larger doses lead to a loss of sensitivity and reduction of normal response. At the same time, nicotine releases adrenaline and noradrenaline with effects on blood pressure and heart rate.

For the smoker, the actual response depends on the algebraic sum of stimulant (+) and depressant (-) effects, in turn depending on nicotine dosage. Dosage in turn depends on the type and numbers of cigarettes smoked and smoking methods.

After one or two cigarettes, heart rate and blood pressure rise, the amount of blood being pumped by the heart increases, and blood flow to the skin and various organs decreases. Some of these changes occur in normal people when exercises are commenced. However, if such changes occur without exercises (i.e., when just smoking) it leaves less reserve for exercise and activity itself. Performance is therefore limited.

Within the blood itself various chemical changes occur, including concentration of free fatty acids, a tendency towards the blood thickening and therefore clotting more easily, and an increased stickiness of the platelets (these are the cells of the blood involved with part of the clotting mechanism).

These effects make the blood thicker and it therefore flows much more slowly. This in part leads to arteriosclerosis or hardening of the arteries (just in the same way a rusting of pipes is more prominent when water flows less quickly).

CARBON MONOXIDE

Everyone knows *not* to be in an airtight enclosed room with an open fireplace. Carbon monoxide is formed and the concentration of this poisonous gas gradually increases if no circulation is allowed. Carbon monoxide poisoning can have a permanent effect on the brain, because of damage to certain brain cells.

Cigarette smoking contains about 2% carbon monoxide. As a result of inhaling this poisonous gas the blood contains less oxygen. Also, the available oxygen is not released from blood into various organs as efficiently.

As all of you know, oxygen is vital to cells, allowing them to efficiently burn their fuels (sugars). This is particularly so for muscles, brain, and heart. Anything which reduces efficiencies of these organs impairs athletic performance.

VERY INTERESTING, BUT WHAT'S THIS GOT TO DO WITH HEALTH?

A number of studies both overseas and within Australia have shown the following:

● *Death from heart disease and stroke (where part of the brain dies) is twice as common in smokers as non-smokers.*

● *It is even more dramatic in the younger age groups (particularly 30-50 years old).*

● *The more cigarettes smoked per day, the greater the death rate. For example, men under 45 years of age who smoke 20 cigarettes a day have been shown to have up to 15 times increased death rate of non-smokers.*

● *Giving up cigarettes does lead to a reduced risk of heart disease. After five to ten years of abstinence the risks of death return to those of non-smokers.*

● *Women are now smoking earlier as well as smoking more cigarettes and this increased smoking trend is dramatically increasing deaths from lung cancer in women. What was once a relatively uncommon cancer in women is now becoming quite a significant cause of death in the younger female age groups.*

WHAT CAN YOU DO ABOUT GIVING IT UP?

Absolutely nothing if you're not motivated to do so. Why people are smoking more at an earlier age is just not understood. Obviously a number of factors including group pressures, advertising, parental attitudes and many other factors play a part. Perhaps it's a tendency towards loss of self-respect and therefore loss of respect for one's own body.

However, I personally respect my body and know that it has a certain limit as well as life-span. I personally don't want it screwed up by some unnecessary outside substance so that I can't keep surfing. I guess it depends on the individual as to whether they wish to adopt a similar philosophy.

For those hooked on the habit, the best and easiest method of quitting is simply to stop on your own. Nicotine gums and patches are for those few people who can't hack the 47-72 hours of nicotine withdrawal. There is no doubt some formally organized stop-smoking programs work. The Adventist program seems to be a particularly good one (it's got nothing to do with religion, so don't worry). Various community health centers run programs which appear to have good successes. Hypnosis can help some people. Relaxation training is also a useful adjunct.

Remember, we reap what we sow. The more the body is cared for, the more faithful years of service it will give. In particular, the more years of surfing available for your enjoyment.

Surfing and Smoking? You know the famous annual South African surf contest, "The Gunston 500"? Did you know that Gunston is a cigarette company? The South African surf magazine *Zig Zag* sells their entire back cover of each issue to Gunston for their cigarette ads. One of their ads shows James Jones locked-in on a big wave with the caption "Men rate Gunston great!" and in the trough of the wave is a large pack of Gunston cigarettes.

Stingray Sting

Doing the Shuffle

Dear SURF DOCS,

Last summer, after a fun glass-off session at my favorite beach break, I was walking (not shuffling) to shore in knee-deep water when I felt a sharp pinch on the back of my ankle.

"Pesky crabs," I thought, hobbling up to the sand. That's when I saw the circular puncture wound with blood streaming out. Instantly, I began experiencing a whole new concept in excruciating pain.

By the time I'd driven home, the pain had spread up my leg as far as the knee and it hurt so much I was way beyond tears.

One of my surf chums suggested soaking the foot in the hottest water I could stand. That reduced the pain somewhat, but not completely. Then somebody else said the lifeguards use vinegar. That had no effect whatsoever. Another

surf buddy recommended elevating my foot and applying an ice pack. The ice burned worse than the sting, so I went back to soaking in scalding water.

Finally, an ancient copy of Camping in Baja California *prescribed "cover your whole body in hot wet rags and drink an entire bottle of tequila." Right.*

Even medicos at the emergency room where I got a tetanus shot the next day didn't have a clue how to effectively treat the pain of a stingray sting.

So, what's the scoop? Will shuffling your feet really help to avoid stings or simply help you painfully stub your toes?

DAVID
San Diego, California

■■■■■||||||

331

Dear David,

Despite stories of white-knuckle pain, stingray stings aren't commonly thought of as serious surf injuries, but they should be. There are over 1,500 *reported* stings per year and while most cleared up in a couple of miserable days, some resulted in serious infections and even death.

Calling it a "stingray attack" isn't quite fair. We're the attackers; the stinger is the ray's defensive weapon, used to make a getaway when something pins or traps them. Following the classic advice to shuffle your feet through shallows is the best way to avoid getting stung, the ray just wants a chance to get the hell out of there.

Footwear isn't the answer, unless you wear motorcycle boots. The stinger is a bony barb mounted under a sheath of skin near the tip of the tail. The barb can be a couple of inches long and has a serrated edge, like a kitchen knife.

When pinned, the stingray whips its tail up, plunging the barb with blinding speed into whatever is directly over it. Glands along the barb pump venom into the wound and the surfer instantaneously feels a searing, sharp pain.

The venom is a protein that usually kills only the tissue around the sting, but if the venom is injected into a nerve, vital organ, or blood vessel, its effect can be catastrophic.

Three goals in treating a sting are:

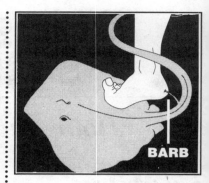

1. **Deactivating the venom and treating its effects.**

2. **Caring for the wound and preventing infection.**

3. **Relieving the pain.**

Deactivating the venom is possible because it is *broken down by heat*. The best thing to do is to plunge the foot into as hot water as you can stand **as soon as possible.** (The venom is already working.) Don't burn your skin—get a thermometer and keep the water right at a safe limit say 112°F (80°C). Stay in it for an hour, continually adding hot water.

Ice, vinegar, alcohol, piss, and other popular remedies are useless. Even elevating the injured part, usually a good idea for an injury, is not helpful and can cause the venom to spread.

Generalized (whole body) reactions are not common, but they can be very serious. Watch for pale, clammy skin; weak, rapid pulse (over 100 beats per minute); rapid or labored breathing, and/or hives. If any of these appear, get the victim to a doctor immediately and be prepared to do CPR if necessary.

As for wound care, the first step is to add a squirt of an antibacterial solution (Betadine®) or some mild soap to the hot water you're soaking in. The mud that stingrays lie in is loaded with bacteria and a sting is very likely to get infected. Once you're through soaking, rinse the wound out with *gallons* of clean water. Watch for pieces of the barb to come out (they usually aren't left in).

Generally it's best to leave these wounds open, although the serrated

> **" . . . shuffling your feet through shallows is the best way to avoid getting stung . . . "**

edge of the barb can cause a gaping cut that may need sewing. If you have a puncture wound with just a small hole, be sure it can drain, otherwise it'll get infected. Soak the wound in clean warm water two or three times a day. Watch closely for signs of infection: redness,

pus, swelling, and/or increased pain. You need antibiotics if the wound is especially jagged or dirty, if you are a long way from home, or if the wound starts to look infected. Get a tetanus shot if you haven't had one within five years. Cover the wound with a loose gauze dressing.

The pain of a sting can be shattering. Give pain medicine right away; don't wait until the pain is out of control. Acetaminophen (Tylenol®) ibuprofen, or aspirin can help if that's all you've got, but stronger drugs like codeine or oxycodone (Percodan®, Percoset®) are better. If these don't do it, get to a doctor for treatment with even stronger injectable drugs, like meperidine (Demerol®), pelhidine, or morphine. Infiltrating the area with a local anaesthetic agent (e.g., 1% plain lidocaine) can also help to reduce the pain. Alcohol won't relieve the pain until you drink to the fall-down-pee-in-your-pants-maybe-stop-breathing stage.

If the stung person isn't getting back to normal after 36 hours, get to a doctor. As you found out, though, many physicians don't know much about stingray injuries. Be prepared to educate them.

Stonefish

Excruciating Pain

Dr. Geoff saith:

These slow moving, super-camouflaged brutes love the warm shallow waters of the Indian and Pacific Oceans. Their 13 lovely dorsal spines contain a toxin guaranteed to bring tears to the eyes of the bravest Valley Cowboy. Stonefish camouflage is so good that even local natives get stung. So a little White-eye hot off the plane has no chance of seeing one before it's too late.

When molested, or trodden on, their spines become erect and pressure from the unsuspecting foot strips back the skin from over the spines and in they go.

Prevention is the best cure and wearing good quality sand shoes when walking through shallow areas is a reasonable compromise. At least your surfing performance is not as limited as when wearing combat boots!

If you tread on one, the pain is immediate and excruciating to the point of producing a frenzy. Even with treatment the pain lasts for some weeks—although nowhere near as bad as when first stung.

As the toxin is destroyed by heat (at least to some extent), immersion of the affected part (usually the foot) into hot, *not* boiling, water produces some relief. Thorough cleansing with salt water also helps. Cold packs, or the use of burning chemicals (potassium permanganate or gun powder!) is ***not*** recommended.

The use of a crepe bandage and limb immobilization—as for sea snake bites—while traveling to the nearest hospital, may also be helpful.

Strong analgesics, if obtainable, are also recommended. Don't O.D. on these.

An antivenom is available (produced in Victoria) but whether your friendly local hospital has some is another matter. Luckily, at least in the Pacific Islands, the antivenom is freely available—even in remote places. (For example, the Australes Islands.)

Stonefish

Those readers priding themselves on using non-Western medicine may be interested in traditional Tahitian stonefish sting (Raau puta nohu) remedies:

● *Two almost-ripe fruits of the morinda citrifolia linne (a shrub found over all islands of the Pacific and Indian Oceans) are halved. The upper half of one is rubbed against the lower half of the other so the juice is exuded. Rub the sting with each of the two sections.*

● *Grate a kernel of hutu (Barringtonia Asiatica Kurz—long used by natives to poison fish and make them easy to catch) and half a coconut. Mix, wrap in a cloth and an auti (Liliacea family) leaf. Roast and apply hot.*

Perhaps some of the more enlightened readers are now getting the message as to why learning some local lingo and doing some basic homework on local flora and fauna can be a worthwhile exercise.

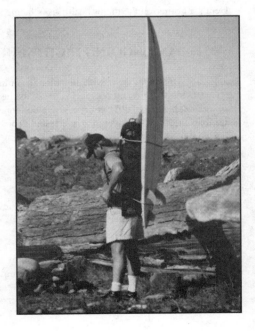

Ready to travel? *Beach Photos.*

Surf Travel
Medicine

1993

*E*very surfer takes surf trips; it's part of being a surfer. Most beginning surfers start with short trips up or down the coast, and as they get better and their hunger for waves grows, they soon find themselves going greater and greater distances for better and better waves. Sooner or later—if all goes as planned —they find themselves *really* out there, where no surfer has gone before. The process of safely getting to that place is the essence of surf travel medicine.

Here's a primer on the major health risks facing serious surf travelers, as of mid-1993.

AN ONGOING NIGHTMARE: MALARIA

The situation remains grim with malaria. It continues to kill millions of people every year, and there is still no vaccine. Plus, the parasite that causes malaria, called *Plasmodium*, has many different types, and continues to develop resistance to drugs faster than they can be developed and tested. Things are actually getting worse as stable rainforest ecosystems are destroyed, leaving mosquito-ridden wastelands in their place.

The drug mefloquine (Lariam®) is still recommended to travelers for prevention of malaria, but resistance has already been reported in parts of Thailand. Resistance will likely follow in other Southeast Asian countries, including Indonesia. Look for other drugs to be recommended in the future, but in the meantime, mefloquine is still the best drug to use.

For almost every malarial country in the world, including Indonesia and Southeast Asia, the recommendation is to take mefloquine: one 250 milligram tablet weekly, starting one week before leaving, then weekly through your trip, and continuing weekly for a full four weeks after leaving the malarial country.

Surf Travel Medicine

Not all pharmacies carry mefloquine, so call beforehand. You will need a prescription. Mefloquine is a pricey drug, about $7.00 per pill, so you may be tempted to skimp on how many pills you buy, and maybe not take those final four doses. Avoid temptation! Owing to the peculiar life cycle of malaria, you need those extra doses. Taking it weekly is essential; the earlier recommendations for mefloquine called for taking it every two weeks, but cases of malaria occurred with that dosing.

As for starting the drug a week before you leave, that's not because it takes a week to work (it starts working within a day); that way if you happen to have a bad reaction to the drug, you can go to your doctor for an alternative medication.

Mefloquine has been thoroughly studied, for instance it fared extremely well in a European study of 140,000 travellers. Still, it's a heavy drug when used at higher doses to treat malaria. Expect no problems if used short-term (less than a year) for prevention. The only common side effects are mild stomach upset and dizziness (one person told us that mefloquine gave him the weirdest dreams he'd ever had). Keep in mind that mefloquine shouldn't be taken by pregnant women, kids under 30 lbs., or by people with epilepsy.

Mefloquine isn't needed for all malarial countries; you can still safely use the older anti-malaria drug, chloroquine (Aralan®), in a few places, including Central America and southern Mexico. The antibiotic doxycycline (100 mg. capsule taken daily) is an effective alternative to mefloquine, but it makes some people extra-sensitive to sunlight. Surfers need to be extra-careful with sun exposure anyway, so with proper use of sunblock and protective clothing, doxycycline is a reasonable alternative (plus it may help prevent traveler's diarrhea). Some countries recommend malarial prophylaxis with daily use of a drug named proguanil, but it has not been shown to be as effective as mefloquine.

The official word on Bali is that it has no malaria, but we continue to hear reliable reports to the contrary. Plus, given that most surfers going to Bali end up going to known malarial islands such as Lombok, Sumbawa, and Java, we recommend that all surfers going to Bali take malarial prophylaxis.

In the struggle to figure out the right drug to prevent malaria, it's often forgotten that the best protection is simply to avoid being bitten by a mosquito. Have a contest with your surf buddies to see who can get the fewest bites. The loser is really the loser.

The malaria-carrying mosquito mainly bites at night, especially at dusk and dawn, so:

1. **Cover up with clothes when mosquitos are around.**

2. **Use mosquito repellent containing a high proportion of the chemical DEET.**

3. **Stay inside screened areas from one hour before sunset to an hour after dawn (a recent study showed that mosquito nets impregnated with the insecticide permethrin are particularly effective).**

Surfers who groove on dawn and pre-sunset go-outs are in a real dilemma because that's when the mosquitos are at their hungriest. Mosquitos won't usually be out in the lineup, unless the offshores are blowing hard, but they can be in close to shore, and for sure they'll be on the beach waiting for you. If it will be more than a minute or two between the water and your bure or tent, leave a stash of insecticide and clothes right where you get out of the water, and put it all on immediately. Prevention is the key.

Wherever you're going, don't rely exclusively on the information presented here. Things change too fast with malaria. The Centers for Disease Control (CDC) in Atlanta have a great hotline with up-to-the-minute information on malaria and other tropical diseases. The number is (404) 332-4555. It's a voice-mail type thing, where you keep getting choices and keep pushing buttons, and after what feels like forever you finally find out what you want to know. Bear with it, the information is excellent and up-to-date. Call before leaving on a surf trip to any tropical or near-equatorial country.

THE SCOURGE: CHOLERA

Cholera is a disease caused by a toxin produced by a bacteria, *Vibrio* cholerae, that sometimes turns up in raw fish and shellfish. Cholera is a true plague, slowly creeping around the world, wiping out people wherever it goes. No really good vaccine has yet been developed for it, and antibiotics are of little use.

Cholera is at present raging through the slums of South and Central America, and has worked its way up into Mexico. It caused over 6,000 deaths in 1992. A disease that shouldn't exist, much less kill anyone, cholera is a disease of poverty and is completely preventable with simple hygienic measures such as clean drinking water and proper sewage disposal. Life-saving treatment is also simple, requiring neither drugs nor sophisticated equipment.

Surf Travel Medicine

Cholera spreads quickly through crowded urban slums, places where the water, soil, and food are contaminated with human shit. Even in cities where cholera is rampant, the rich are mostly unaffected. Tourists eating in nice restaurants and drinking bottled water are also largely "immune." During the first year of the present epidemic only six American tourists came down with cholera.

Surfers are probably at higher risk for contracting cholera than the average tourist, because they're often traveling on a shoestring budget and have a refreshing tendency to go native. But even in the midst of a cholera zone, prevention is simple, the same as preventing travelers' diarrhea or dysentery. The rule is: BOIL IT, COOK IT, PEEL IT, OR FORGET IT. Drink boiled or bottled water, avoid ice (unless you know the water was treated), and send back any food not still hot from a thorough cooking or boiling. Don't bother to try cholera vaccine, it doesn't work well enough.

If you become infected, say from eating contaminated ceviche or drinking funky water, it only takes 12 hours to 5 days for the symptoms to appear. Cholera kills by dehydrating you, from a gushing diarrhea that wrings you dry in a matter of hours. Untreated cholera is fatal about 50% of the time; with good treatment it's almost never fatal. Treatment is simple, and absolutely essential, consisting of replacing the lost fluid by oral rehydration (drinking gallons of properly prepared liquids).

The recipe for Oral Rehydration Solution is:

Starting with uncontaminated water (boiled or bottled), **for every glass (8 oz.) of water, add 2 teaspoons of sugar, 1/4 teaspoon of baking soda, and a pinch of salt.** And then keep guzzling, to where you're at least matching the amounts you're squirting out.

Oral Rehydration Solution is recommended worldwide for severe diarrhea by the World Health Organization, and it really works. It will save a life, especially if started as soon as symptoms appear. Often, people with cholera seem to vomit everything up, but if you just keep powering oral rehydration, enough will get through. File the recipe away in your head and remember that oral rehydration may keep you from dying of dehydation from any bad diarrhea, whatever the cause.

The CDC Hotline for cholera hot spots is the same number as for malaria: (404) 332-4555. Check it out.

BREAK-BONE DISEASE: DENGUE FEVER

Dengue fever is a strange disease caused by a mosquito-borne virus. Surfers are at higher risk for dengue than most travelers: it occurs almost exclusively in coastal towns of Southeast Asia (including Indonesia and the Philippines), Africa, and the Caribbean. Recently it has cropped up in Florida. There is work on a vaccine to prevent it, but it is not yet proven to be safe and effective.

Sometimes called "break-bone fever," dengue causes intense joint, bone, and muscle pains, along with headache and fever. It's like a really bad flu. The symptoms generally last 3 to 7 days, often climaxing in an all-body rash, then it's over. A viral disease, there is no antibiotic or drug to treat dengue, other than taking medications such as Tylenol (acetaminophen) for the fever and aches.

For the traveling surfer unlucky enough to get dengue, the big problem is in telling it apart from malaria. If it's malaria, you'll want to cut your trip short and get to where you can be treated. If it's dengue, you'll probably be able to just ride it out where you are (much to the relief of your surf buddies). The way to tell the difference is that malaria symptoms tend to occur in patterns or cycles, with the fever often coming abruptly at night (with a severe shaking chill afterwards), often every 3rd night, and not a lot of symptoms in between (other than feeling weak), while dengue symptoms keep up for the whole course of the illness. But that distinction isn't foolproof. If in doubt, bail. Also, there is a rare complication of dengue you should be watchful for, widespread internal and external bleeding, which necessitates immediate medical attention.

As with malaria, to prevent dengue is to avoid mosquito bites. Unlike the mosquito that carries malaria, the dengue-carrying mosquito also bites during the day. Pesky critters, those mosquitos—such disease carriers! And here's yet another . . .

SURE-FIRE BRAIN DAMAGE: JAPANESE ENCEPHALITIS

Another weirdo viral disease carried by mosquitoes, *Japanese encephalitis* (JE) is on the rise in almost every Asia country, except some western Pacific islands, including Japan and the Philippines, where it is uncommon (don't ask us why it's called Japanese Encephalitis if it doesn't actually occur in Japan). Unlike dengue fever, JE is mainly a rural disease; the mosquito that carries JE has a great fondness for pigs. It's also seasonal, occurring in most locales only in the rainy months. The one big exception is Indonesia, where it is year-round.

JE is a heavy disease: a third of those who get it have bad flu-like symptoms that eventually get better; another third have permanent brain damage; and the other third end up looking like extras in the "Scanners" films, and all die. There is no good treatment.

Despite the grim statistics, JE is not yet a big problem for travelers: only five U.S. tourists have gotten the disease since 1981. It turns out that only a small percentage of mosquitos in a given area carry the virus, and only one out of fifty people bitten by JE virus-carrying mosquitos get the disease.

However, there is an effective vaccine against JE, and surfers going to rural epidemic JE areas should use the vaccine. Again, call the CDC hotline, (404) 332-4555, for current vaccine recommendations. As with malaria and dengue fever, the best protection against JE is to avoid mosquito bites.

NOT MELLOW, YELLOW: HEPATITIS A AND B

Hepatitis A abounds in the Third World coastal villages traveling surfers typically spend time in. Again, it tends to be a disease of poverty and poor sanitation; you're most likely to get it from unwashed fruits and vegetables, or contaminated water. Luckily, a shot of gamma globulin before leaving on your trip will probably protect you. The longer you're away, the bigger the dose (the more-than-three-months dose is a real pain in the butt).

Recently, a vaccine has become available against hepatitis A. It appears to be safe and effective, but is not yet widely recommended in the U.S. If you're a hard-core grunge surf traveler, it would be highly recommended to get the hepatitis A vaccine.

The more dangerous hepatitis, B, requires a different strategy. If you're a health worker, into unsafe sex, the type who still thinks shooting drugs is cool, or if you just don't want to get the damn disease, then you should consider becoming vaccinated against hepatitis B. It's effective and safe, so much so that it is now a standard childhood vaccine along with polio, measles, and all the others.

THE OLD STANDBY KILLER: ACCIDENTS

The overall leading cause of death to travelers is accidents. In a study of travelers to Mexico, accidents accounted for over 50% of deaths, compared to 7% of all deaths in the U.S. Those Mexico travelers, for instance, had a ten-times higher rate of drowning (usually associated with alcohol use), and a three-times higher rate of airplane crashes (mostly small aircraft). As for car crashes, you're about ten-times more likely to be in a crash in a Third World country, ranging to twenty-times higher in countries like Guatemala. The rate is probably still higher in places like Indonesia.

For surfers, fifteen-foot Pipeline is definitely safer than the average motor bike ride out to Uluwatu from Kuta Beach. Even though the Indonesian government requires helmets be worn, don't be fooled into thinking you'll be safe, particularly the way some surfers go about it, riding with a surfboard slung under their arm.

Consider the case of San Francisco surfers, Jeff and Dennis, on surf safari in Indonesia. On the way back from Ulu, Jeff crashed his motor bike and radically crushed his ankle. The next day, after visiting Jeff in the local hospital, Dennis managed to crash, too, ending up with a huge spike of glass crammed into his wrist. He went straight to the airport and got on the next plane to a better hospital (in Perth). Jeff eventually had to escape to a hospital in Hong Kong.

Don't learn these things the hard way. Successful surf travelers travel safely.

SURF TRAVEL MEDICINE

Ideally, if you have a health provider who is a surfer, they'll be keyed into your special health travel needs. Whomever you end up seeing, it might be a good idea to bring along this synopsis. If you don't have a regular doctor, the quickest and easiest way to get all of your pre-travel shots and vaccinations is to go to a travel medicine clinic. Most big cities and universities have them. Check in your phone book under "Travel," looking for names like "Travel Clinic" or "Travel Health."

There are just a few other routine health matters to check on before you travel. Are you up-to-date on your regular vaccinations? This would include:

● *Tetanus booster every 10 years*

● *Consideration of a measles booster if born after 1956*

● *Being sure you have protection against German measles (rubella) for all women*

● *Checking to see if you need a polio booster*

● *A periodic skin test for tuberculosis*

● *Keep in mind prevention of venereal disease, including AIDS. Bring and use condoms.*

Finally, don't forget, one sure way to learn all you'd ever want to know about exotic illnesses is to take an extended vacation in a Thailand jail for smuggling heroin.

Surf Wax Munchies

Eat It

Dear Surf Docs,

Every time I purchase a bar of wax, I notice a warning the manufacturers put on the paper that comes with it: "WARNING: Do not eat or chew."

Why not? It tastes great and it's less filling. I've been chewing wax ever since I started surfing, and nothing happens to me.

DR. JEKYLL

∎∎∎∎∎∎∥∥∥∥

Dear Dr. Jekyll,

Do you like chewing on dirty chemicals? Because that's what you put in your mouth every time you succumb to the surf wax munchies. We assume you're not swallowing the wax, which would *really* be bad. But you should also know you are absorbing chemicals very efficiently, even just chewing, both through your gums and when you swallow saliva.

The basic ingredient of surf wax is paraffin wax, a synthetic substance, but the type used in surf wax is usually food grade (meaning it can be used in or on foods). For instance, the same type of wax is used as a candy bar additive, and to put a shine on supermarket apples. Beeswax, or a beeswax-like substance, is also added to give the wax pliability. Some of the dyes are the same as those used to color soft drinks.

Thus endeth the (possibly) food-grade part of surf wax. Now we get to the Toxic Avenger goodies.

All surf wax is softened by petroleum-derived products such as Vaseline®, so we don't lose our nipples when paddling out. Bottom line: You're sucking on a thicker, slightly cleaner grade of motor oil, Dr. Jekyll.

Also, surf wax scents don't come from vanilla beans, bananas or mint leaves, they come from factories.

343

They're totally synthetic. In addition, some waxes have plastic in them for temperature control. Chalk-up another petroleum-derived ingredient.

Finally, synthetic rubber or petro-chemical resin is added to increase the stickiness factor. John Dahl of Wax Research reckons that of all the ingredients, these two might be the most unhealthy to ingest. The fact is, though, nobody really knows about the long-term effects of chewing or eating surf wax because it's only been around for about 25 years. And no one is actively researching the subject. That sounds like a long time, until you realize it took the medical establishment nearly 50 years to prove cigarettes were coffin-nails.

. . . surf wax scents don't come from va-nilla beans, bananas or mint leaves, they come from factories.

We Surf Docs, though, have recommended use of surf wax to temporarily cover broken, sharp teeth resulting from an injury to the mouth.

In addition to not wanting you to eat these chemicals, wax-makers like Zog of Sex Wax fame put those warnings on their products because the machines used to make them aren't necessarily clean. They don't have to be. Surf wax *isn't* food.

So, just because nothing's happened to you yet doesn't mean it won't if you keep chewing wax. Anyway, why eat more chemicals than we already do? You might find yourself turning into Mr. Hyde . . . and he died an ugly death.

Surfboard Manufacturing Risks

A Grim Line-Up

Dear SURF DOCS,

I am 40-years-old, and concerned about the long-term effects of working with polyester resin and polyurethane foam.

I was involved in surfboard manufacturing in Southern California during the sixties and seventies, and will always be involved in a certain amount of surfboard repair, including grinding out a fin now and then.

Just about every aspect of surfboard building and ding repair seems potentially hazardous, from foam dust to resin and catalyst. I have never seen anything written about the long- or short-term effects of using these materials, but there must be something on the subject by now. Thanks for any information you can come up with.

JOHN
Washington State

■ ■ ■ ■ ■ ■ I I I I I I I

Dear John,

The hazards of surfboard repair and manufacture comprise an area which has only recently begun to get the attention it deserves. For decades, boards have been shaped and glassed in whatever space could be scammed—often in cramped quarters without adequate ventilation. Your concern over the potential harm caused by surfboard materials is well-founded. As it turns out, a number of the materials used to make boards are potentially dangerous. Since virtually every serious surfer makes or fixes boards at some point, it is important that all surfers learn to do it safely.

345

A quick run-through of the process of making a board. First, a polyurethane foam blank is cut and sanded to the right shape. Then the blank is wrapped in fiberglass cloth, which is saturated with polyester resin, with catalyst added. The board is sanded, and another layer of resin (with catalyst) applied. At this point, the board is either polished, or a gloss coat or resin is applied.

Here are the hazards in the process:

1. **Polyurethane foam dust from shaping can irritate the airways, especially in sensitive—allergic— people. The long-term effects of breathing in foam dust aren't known, but anything that irritates the airways over a long period of time can cause chronic lung problems—sometimes, even cancer.**

2. **All types of resins are mostly styrene, a toxic chemical, which evaporates easily, saturating the air around the work area. Styrene is irritating to the lungs, airways and skin. Long-term exposure can cause liver disease and, again, even cancer.**

3. **The catalyst used most commonly contains methyl-ethyl ketone peroxide (MEKP), which irritates the hell out of airways, skin and eyes. MEKP is also a suspected carcinogen, and has been linked with two types of blood cell cancer.**

4. **Fiberglass cloth is hazardous stuff. Composed of tiny fibers, it can be irritating to the skin when the fibers lodge in pores, causing the itching every glasser has experienced. Breathing the dust may be the real hazard. Fiberglass was recently placed on a list of suspected cancer-causing agents.**

" . . . realize that these long-term effects are generally caused by heavy exposure over a long period of time."

This is a grim line-up, but before you take your glassing supplies to the nearest toxic waste dump site, realize that these long-term effects are generally caused by heavy exposure over a long period of time. Making surfboards can be nonhazardous, and it is pretty easy to achieve safety. Nobody should have to work under the conditions that have traditionally prevailed among surfboard makers. Here are some minimal guidelines for a safe environment:

● *Work only in a well-ventilated area—make sure there are at least two openings (for air flow-through), and use a fan to keep air moving.*

Surfboard Manufacturing Risks

People who work with resins on a regular basis should wear a regulator mask with a replaceable filter cartridge. Make sure you understand how the mask operates, and when to change cartridges.

● *Wear a filtering mask (available at most hardware stores) when sanding or handling cloth. Those who do this a lot need more heavy-duty equipment.*

● *Wear rubber or latex gloves when working with resin, catalysts or cloth.*

● *If anything gets in your eyes, flush it out with gallons of clean water—don't rub. Wash off anything that gets on your skin immediately. Itchy fiberglass can be removed by using a gel facial mask (in the cosmetic section at the drugstore)—peeling off the mask will pull out the fibers.*

By taking the proper precautions and not cutting any corners, your surfboard work will be clean, and the risks to your health nil.

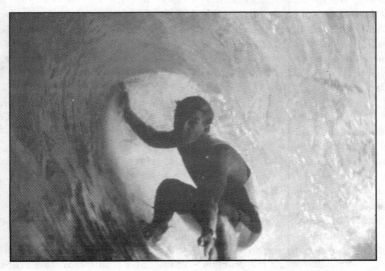

Locked in with the SMA. Western Oz. *Photo courtesy of John Small.*

Tendinitis: Muscle Overuse

Stand Up Stiffies

Dear SURF DOCS,

I'm 30-years-old and have been surfing for four years, the last couple being the most intense. Last season, one of my elbows began aching if I surfed for more than 3-4 hours. The pain would be gone the next day. It has gradually worsened, now both elbows are stiff and ache after surfing 1-2 hours and the pain lingers for two to three days.

The pain is most pronounced in my motion to stand on the board. It's that quick push-up that gives me a sharpish pain. It progresses to a constant ache right at the underside of my elbow and the inside of my arm. Needless to say, this gets in the way of my surfing.

I've seen a sports medicine doctor, and he diagnosed the problem as "triceps tendinitis." He gave me a prescription for some incredibly high-priced drug called "Naprosyn" (naproxen)—39 bucks for 40 tabs.

The drug does work. I take it twice day, ice my elbows after a surf, and I can stay in the water for as long as I like, with the pain 99% gone—but now I feel a slow-burning ache in my elbows all the time. I'm still surfing a lot.

I plan to surf until it's too cold, then give my elbows a rest until spring. My questions are these:

1. Have you run across this problem with other surfers?

2. Am I causing further and maybe permanent damage to my elbows by continuing to surf while using a drug that relieves the pain, but doesn't cure the problem?

Tendinitis: Muscle Overuse

3. **Are there any other treatments you recommend?**

4. Am I fucked for life?

CRAIG
Massachusetts

■■■■IIIIIII

Dear Craig,

Nope, you're not fucked for life, although you could have a chronic problem on your hands if you don't take care of it. Your doctor's diagnosis sounds accurate, and Naprosyn® (naproxen) is an effective drug, but it is surprising that you weren't given further instructions on how to deal with tendinitis. It is common in surfers, although the shoulder is a more common location than the triceps.

Everyone talks about tendinitis, but what is it? Tendons are what attach muscles to bone. The tendons run in sheaths filled with lubricating fluid. When you strain or overuse the tendon, you heat things up and dry out the fluid. Without sufficient fluid, your tendon is like a piston going up and down in a cylinder without oil. The hot tendon becomes inflamed, which causes more damage. With continued overuse, the vicious cycle of pain and inflammation puts you in a downward spiral that sends you to a doctor and keeps you out of the water.

The two parts in dealing with tendinitis are:

1. **Treating the inflammation**

2. **Preventing strain and overuse**

Naprosyn® (naproxen) is effective at reducing inflammation, but ibuprofen and aspirin works just as well (believe it or not) for a fraction of the cost.

Watch out for narcotics (i.e., codeine and percodan). They simply cover up the pain, allowing you to blissfully trash yourself. Anti-inflammatory drugs (like aspirin, ibuprofen and naproxen) reduce pain by reducing the inflammation which causes damage and pain. By properly using anti-inflammatories, you're not just covering up the pain, you're preventing it. Although you can still over-do it, anti-inflammatories may allow you to surf out the season without further damage.

The next step is to prevent this from happening again by stretching your shoulders and elbows daily. Check out Bob Anderson's book *Stretching* (Shelter Publications, P.O. Box 279, Bolinas, CA 94924). Yoga is a good way to do this, too.

Be especially careful to warm-up before surfing. When the surf season is over, continue stretching and begin gradual strengthening exercises. You want to accomplish two things:

● *Increase the strength of the triceps muscle itself*

> **. . . prevent this from happening again by stretching your shoulders and elbows daily.**

● *Increase the strength of all the muscles used to hop up on your board—this will take some of the strain off your triceps*

Your sports medicine doctor can help you come up with a good program, or you can ask a physical therapist. Conscientious effort in the off-season may make next year's surfing trouble-free.

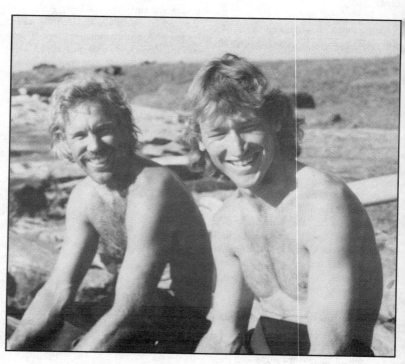

He's-no-limey, SMA loyalist Bill Heick (left) and the esteemed Dr. Kevin Starr. *Beach Photos.*

Tendinitis: Surfer's Elbow

Overuse Injury, in N.Y.C.?

Dear SURF DOCS,

I am 37-years-old and have developed tendinitis in my left elbow, there seems to be a bone chip, as well. The doc advised me to rest my arm, but after three months it's worse than before. I've stayed out of the water, but I'd like to keep surfing. Will I damage my arm by doing so?

STEVE
New York City

■■■■■IIIIII

Dear Steve,

Tendinitis is an overuse injury caused by overdoing a repetitive motion. These injuries are all too common in surfers, because surfing involves a lot of repetitive motion, and partly because we tend to ignore our limits when the waves are good. Shoulders are the part of the body most often affected, with elbows coming in second.

Doctors often tell people with overuse injuries just to rest, but that's really not enough. Healing and prevention require an active approach.

What you have sounds like *surfer's elbow*, a form of tendinitis similar to tennis elbow. It can be caused by the way you paddle, the strain of hopping up on take-off, or even by the motion used in waxing your board. Surfer's elbow usually heals without any problems. Understanding what's going on and what to do about it will get you back in the water as soon as possible.

All overuse injuries are similar, and tendinitis is a good example. When you overstress the tendon (the fibrous cord that connects muscle to bone) it becomes damaged, and inflammatory chemicals known as *prostaglandins* are

351

released. The resulting inflammation is what you experience as pain and swelling.

Given a chance, the healing process happens in three stages:

● *First, inflammation increases the flow of blood to the area and begins sending repair materials to the injured site.*

● *Second, new protein fibers are laid down to replace the broken ones.*

● *Finally, the new fibers are linked and woven together to complete the repair.*

If the damage continues (and sometimes even if it doesn't), you can get stuck in the first stage of healing, and still have pain and inflammation. Initially a good thing, this inflammation then becomes destructive and prevents further healing.

Our guess is you've been stuck in that first stage of healing for a long time. Your bone chip may, in fact, have developed as a result of long-term, low-grade tendinitis.

The real experts on overuse injuries are the Olympics' sports trainers. When Olympic athletes develop tendinitis, their trainers have several things to consider:

1. **The cause of the problem (they need to analyze the style of** the athlete's performance in a particular sport, then suggest subtle changes).

2. **How to treat the problem.**

3. **How to keep the athlete from getting out of shape while healing**

The trainers first approach the problem by classifying the type of pain the athlete has. This serves as their guideline of how severe the injury is, and exactly what kind of treatment is needed.

"Doctors often tell people with over-use injuries just to rest, but that's really not enough. Healing and prevention require an active approach.**

Dr. James Puffer, from UCLA and head physician for the U.S. Olympic Team, divides the pain of overuse injuries into four types, and recommends a building-block approach to treatment:

● **Type One** *pain happens only after activity, and is typical of early* *endinitis, when it's most easily healed. For this type of pain Dr. Puffer recommends cutting back about 25% in your activity, applying ice to the affected area afterward, and doing stretching and strengthening exercises.*

● **Type Two** *pain comes while you're still exercising, but doesn't restrict your performance. For this kind of pain, follow the same recommendations for those for* Type One, *but cut back your activity by 50%, and use an anti-inflammatory medication such as aspirin or ibuprofen.*

● **Type Three** *pain occurs during activity, and is severe enough to restrict your performance. It requires complete rest, applying ice to the affected area, using anti-inflammatory medications until the inflammation goes down, and stretching and strengthening exercises. Some doctors also treat* Type Three *pain with injections of anti-inflammatory steroids.*

● **Type Four** *pain is there all the time, activity or not, and is evidence of chronic, severe tendinitis. With this kind of pain you should follow all the previous recommendations, but sometimes surgery is needed to repair the damage.*

You will notice that for most cases of tendinitis, activity—not complete rest—is recommended. Full healing is often actually slowed down by complete rest. Your level of pain should be the guideline for the amount of activity you pursue. Start slowly, increase gradually, and back off if it hurts.

We think you probably have *Type Two* pain, which means you shouldn't have stopped surfing—just cut back and try to change what might be causing the problem. With tendinitis in the elbow, check out your paddling stroke and the way you hop up on the board on take-off.

If you practice good self-care, chances are you won't need to have surgery for your bone chip.

Now, about the surf in New York City . . . ?

Testicular Injuries and Cancer

Nuts to You

Dear SURF DOCS,

A good surfing buddy of mine has got what you docs call "testicular cancer." He's not an old guy, and was healthy and surfing lots. But a while ago his board bashed him in the nuts, and he noticed a bump on one of his balls that never went away.

Well, he finally went to a doctor, and they sent him straight into the hospital! The next day they cut off his bad nut and told him they'd also found cancer in his lungs, so they'd have to give him chemotherapy, too!

They say they think they can cure him. Is that possible? How did he get it?

FLATHEAD
Humboldt County, California

■ ▮ ▮ ▮ ▯▯▯

Dear Flathead,

Thanks for writing—your letter gives us a chance to lay out the facts on a subject we've long wanted to write about. It's not a cancer that you hear much about, but, believe it or not, *testicular cancer is the number one cancer in surfers*.

This frightening fact has little or nothing to do with the actual act of surfing, but directly reflects the profile of most surfers: young, white males. Testicular cancer is the most common cancer of men between the ages of 15 and 35. It's actually more common in young men than breast cancer is in young women. For some reason, black males

354

rarely get it. There are parts of Africa where a case of testicular cancer has never been reported—and when they do, it's usually after the age of 60.

Perhaps the scariest fact is that the incidence of testicular cancer is rapidly increasing, with a two- to four-fold increase over the past 20 years (no one is sure why). The highest incidence is in young white professional men in the San Francisco Bay area!

Before you white surfer boys go for preemptive neutering, you should know the good news about testicular cancer: it is one of the most curable of all cancers.

The curability of testicular cancer is one of the great "miracles of modern medicine." Prior to 1974, 90% of testicular cancers were fatal, but in that year a new form of chemotherapy came along—a drug called *cisplatin*—and the cure rate jumped to over 90%, even if it has spread to the lungs! And apart from losing a testicle to surgery, and having to endure a few weeks of chemotherapy (and sometimes radiation therapy), a man can then expect to lead a normal sex life and still have kids.

So, Flathead, it sounds like your friend's doctors are treating him correctly, and, yes, he will almost certainly be cured.

As for what causes testicular cancer, no one is sure—so there isn't really a way to prevent it. For instance, it isn't a cancer that seems related to how good or bad your diet is, or how much exercise you get. However, some things are known about it.

It's thought that most testicular cancers take years to grow. And, a traumatic blow to the testes, such as from a errant surfboard, has not been proven to be a factor. Such trauma would, however, perhaps lead to noticing a lump that had been silently growing there for months (if not years).

> **. . . you should know the good news about testicular cancer: it is one of the most curable of all cancers.**

This is not to say that surfers shouldn't worry about being struck in the balls by their boards! Many surfers have had severe, permanent damage to one or both testicles from such an occurrence. The usual story is of not quite making a take-off on a good-sized wave, free-falling in a still standing position, having the board slip-up sideways between the legs, and then being slammed in the nuts by the rail when your board keeps you from penetrating the wave's face.

It is definitely a good idea for surfers to wear whatever they can to shield their genitalia from trauma: close fitting swimsuits or those with built in supporters or shields, athletic cups, and wetsuits all provide added protection. This notion may seem strange or excessive to some surfers, but, until recently, that was the case with wearing surf helmets, too.

Having an "undescended testes" tops the list of risk factors for testicular cancer. In about the seventh month of fetal life, the testes move from an ovary-like position in the abdomen, down the groin, and into the scrotal sack. If they get hung up along the way and don't fully make it into the scrotum, it's said to be an undescended testes. Your risk is lowered to normal if the testes are surgically brought down before the age of eight, otherwise you are 20 to 50 times more likely to get testicular cancer.

Your risk for testicular cancer may be higher if your mother received radiation or took diethylstilbesterol (DES) when she was pregnant with you. Testicular cancer is rarely hereditary.

An odd risk factor is if you wear jockey shorts (higher risk) versus boxer shorts or no underwear at all (lower risk); bathing suit-type or use of a wetsuit has never been studied. It's thought that jockey shorts keep your balls warmer, making them more likely to develop cancer. The distance from the heat of your body is thought to be the difference. This theory is borne out by the fact that, statistically, the left testicle

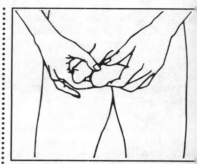

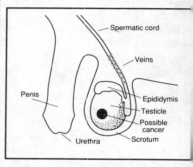

Testicular Self-Examination. Illustration reprinted with permission from Barbara Bates, MD, *A Guide to Physical Examination.* J.B. Lippincott Company, Philadelphia, PA. 1974.

hangs lower than the right (ask any good tailor), so it isn't kept as warm as the right testicle, and correspondingly it only has 47.7% of testicular cancers.

Tobacco and alcohol don't appear to be related to testicular cancer; nor venereal diseases (gonorrhea, syphilis, herpes, chlamydia).

Testicular Injuries and Cancer

It is recommended that all men—especially those between 15 and 35—regularly examine themselves for signs of testicular cancer. The earlier it is found, the better—early detection is the key. *Testicular self-examination* (TSE) is simple to do:

1. The best time to examine your testes is after a hot bath or shower (when the testes hang lower). Do it while standing or lying down. It only takes about one minute, and should be done at least once a month. It doesn't hurt, and it isn't "playing with yourself." It's an intelligent thing to do.

2. Gently roll each testicle between your thumb and fingers, being sure to examine the entire surface area of each testicle. What you are feeling for is any change or difference in your testicles. Don't press hard—cancer rarely begins inside the testicle. Feel over the smooth outer surface of each testicle. Imagine the testicle as a grape, and you are delicately feeling over its surface. Feel for size, shape, consistency, sensitivity to pressure, and compare the left to the right testes (the left testicle is often slightly larger than the right).

3. A cancer of the testes most often begins as a painless, iso-lated, pebble- or pea-like bump on one testicle. Occasionally, a person with testicular cancer has a dragging or aching sensation in the groin or scrotum, but pain is a late symptom.

4. Be aware that the majority of testicular changes are not cancer; for instance a recent painful swelling is likely to be inflammation or infection. Your self-exam should be refined enough that you can feel the spermatic cord (a thin hard cord that suspends each testicle), and the epididymis (a soft, gum-wad sized sperm-collecting structure cupped around each testicle where the spermatic cord attaches).

5. If you detect any change in your testes, go see a doctor. Don't delay, even if the surf is good.

Titty Rash

Nip Pull

Dear Dr. GEOFF,

I have just started surfing and it seems that I have a disadvantage because I'm a girl. My problem is my chest, my titties, if you don't mind me saying so. I have created a very bad rash on both of my titties, which has forced the skin to go hard and brittle. It causes a bit of embarrassment on Saturday nights and I want to keep surfing too.

Yours faithfully,
GEORGY

▮▮▮▮▮❙❙❘❘❘

Dear Gorgeous Georgy,

It's great to see women getting into surfing at long last. As I've been saying for years, I can hardly wait until such time as at least 50% of surfers are women. It will certainly help to get a little bit more perspective into the sport.

A number of women have a similar problem to yourself, namely breast irritation, especially of the nipples. Both the skin and the nipples are sites of irritation which is essentially brought about by mechanical rubbing of the rough surface of the surfboard deck (and the wax on it) against the tender skin of the breast and nipple through the bikini or t-shirt. Men also get the same problem through *direct* skin contact.

The solution that most surfers seem to find is to wear a suitable wetsuit (or vest in the summer). Using Vaseline on the skin of the breast or nipple under the wetsuit will also help.

358

Warts

Toadman's Blues

Dear Dr. GEOFF,

I've got this problem with warts. They are all over my bloody hands! They range in size from the head of a pin to the head of a bloody roofing nail. Most of them seem to be around the joints (knuckles, wrists, etc.) but there's a huge crop just down from the wrist on my right arm. Some are really cracked and dry (the big ones) and yet others are just round and smooth. There are also a couple on my right palm which are below the skin level. They have only been spreading in the last couple of months or so. I've also recently found a young crop on my forehead above my right eye. I should also state that 90% of these warts are on the right side of my body. I've used a special wart burning acid but they grow back in a big group or grow back twice as big.

Can you give us some advice on where they come from, why I've got heaps, will they subside, will more pop up and mainly what is the best way to get rid of them? I work as a landscape laborer and occasionally nick the tops off the big ones and they bleed for ages. Some get quite painful when doing monotonous and tedious work, also after a long surf they turn white and very soft. I am twenty years of age and am exposed to the elements (sun, wind, etc.) if that is any help. They are popping up at the rate of two to three a fortnight, either in little groups or solo efforts and I am starting to stress. My hands look like a breeding ground for the little buggers, so all information will be comforting. I hope I have given you enough information and will greatly appreciate your advice.

Yours stressingly,
CRAIG THE TOADMAN

Dear Craig,

Human papilloma virus (HPV) causes warts. There are at least seven different forms of this highly contagious virus which can cause different forms of warts.

Our body's immune system plays a part in controlling warts. This is best illustrated when kids first begin school. Within the first few years it would be a rare kid who didn't get at least a few warts. These mostly disappear as the child gets older and presumably the immune system becomes more mature and able to deal with the wart virus.

In later years warts may occur under periods of extreme physical or emotional stress.

You have given a good description of your warts. They sound like plain or flat warts. Trauma seems to be playing a part in the spread of your warts. This is in fact quite a common occurrence, especially for flat warts.

A number of different methods, both physical and psychic have been tried in the management of warts. Most methods work mainly because in otherwise healthy people, the body gets rid of HPV by itself within about three months or so.

Some of the methods used include:

● *Covering with a sticking plaster*

● *Paints, pastes and creams*

● *Formalin*

● *Diathermy*

● *Freezing*

● *Excision*

● *Psychic healing*

SELF-TREATMENT

You are going to have to follow this treatment for about 12 weeks and be very patient.

● *Wash the warts with hot soapy water and soak for 5 minutes*

● *Dry with your own towel*

● *Use pumice stone to rub off hard, dead material on top of the wart*

● *Use whatever particular paste, ointment or solution you have decided on as specifically directed*

"**A** number of different methods, both physical and psychic have been tried in the management of warts."

Warts

Various forms of salicylic acid/ trichloracetic acid are the commonest types of proprietary topical agents used.

In your case, one of the major problems is that as a landscape gardener you are constantly injuring your hands. As indicated above this might be an added factor in causing your warts to spread. If possible, the warts should be covered with sticking plaster. Wearing protective gloves might also help.

Should this regimen not work, cryotherapy (i.e., the use of freezing agents such as liquid nitrogen) is often effective. The interesting thing about this form of treatment is that freezing/ thawing can be shown to stimulate the body's own immune system to the wart virus.

Psychic healing is an unusual phenomena, and often works better than other therapies. Wart charmers and wart buyers are to be found in most societies. In Tokyo there is even a wart shrine. I am aware of a lady who buys warts. She actually gives the person ten cents for each wart! I've seen a couple of truly miraculous cures by this method. Just think, treatment which actually gives you a cure and some money.

Surgical treatment is mentioned mainly to condemn it. It is painful, leaves scars, and in at least 30% of cases, recurrence occurs (this level of recurrence being higher than just about any other method).

There are more specialized methods using up-market (i.e., expensive) drugs including 5-Fluorouracil, Interferon, and Idoxundine. Referral to a skin specialist (dermatologist) is recommended for these methods.

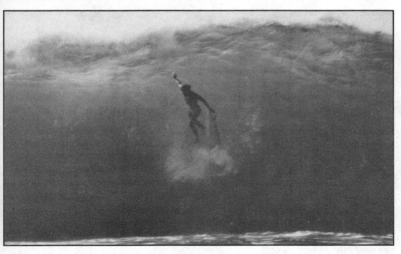

Oops! *SMA Photo.*

Wetsuit Allergy

A Rash Conclusion

Dear SURF DOCS,

I recently had an allergic reaction to a new wetsuit. My neck, armpits, arms, hands and groin area got irritated and swollen. I hurt and itched like hell. I went to my doctor the following morning, and she gave me some Benadryl® (diphenhydramine) capsules, and a cream called Symenol® (flucinolone). The irritation got better after a couple of days.

My problem is, I've used the wetsuit again, and the reaction recurred—even worse the second time.

I called both the shop where I bought the suit and the manufacturer to see if I could give it back, but they said no way. Great! I bought their wetsuit, got a giant rash, and they say there's nothing defective about their suit! Now, I'm stuck with $200 worth of rubber and can't even use it!

I'd like to know if there's something you could tell me about what's causing my problem, and how I can stop it. Should I not use the wetsuit at all?

I've never had anything like this happen to me—please help.

PATRICK
Malibu, California

P.S. A rash guard didn't help at all.

▪▪▪▪▮▮▮▮

Dear Patrick,

It sure sounds like you've had an allergic reaction. You're pissed off because you have a new wetsuit and can't use it, and the guys at the surf shop think it's a perfectly normal suit.

The good news is, we called the manufacturer for you, and they said they'd be happy to take the wetsuit back. As for figuring out what went wrong, knowing more about allergic reactions might be the key.

Some things—like poison oak—cause a reaction in many people, while other things, (wetsuit glue) affect only a very few. You can be allergic to a substance on first contact, or suddenly develop an allergy to something you've been around all your life. What's more, allergies can disappear as suddenly as they appear.

Steroid creams like Symenol® and antihistamines like Benadryl® can decrease the swelling and itching, but what's most important is to figure out what's causing the reaction, and how to avoid it.

In your case it does seem your new wetsuit is the problem. Given the sudden appearance of a new rash with a new wetsuit, it's unlikely that you've developed a rash to something in all wetsuits. It's more likely that you're sensitive to some chemical used in the manufacturing process of your particular suit. Wetsuit makers are constantly trying out new processes and compounds and it takes only a trace of a chemical to trigger a reaction.

Trying to figure out exactly which chemical is causing the reaction probably isn't worth the hassle. You'd have to round up a list of all the chemicals used to make that particular batch of wetsuits, then find an allergy specialist willing to test you for reactions to the things on your list. The testing is laborious and expensive—it's also not very reliable.

We'd suggest simple measures. First, wash the suit out with a gentle detergent, you may be able to remove a surface chemical (the fact that your rash guard didn't help may mean it was something on the surface of the suit dissolving through the lycra). Then, try wearing the suit in a swimming pool or tub to rule out the possibility that the rash was caused by something in the seawater that was held next to your body by the suit. Finally, borrow and try some other suits with different nylon and neoprene to see if they also cause a reaction.

If, after trying the above suggestions, it still seems your new suit is the culprit, don't keep trying to use it. Call up the manufacturer again and tell them your doctor said you'd had an allergic reaction to their suit. It's in their best interests to investigate allergic reactions to their products. The manufacturers we talked to after receiving your letter said they'd willingly take a suit back, in this situation. You may have to bypass the customer service department and talk to someone in research and development—that's what we did.

Yours is the third apparent case of wetsuit allergy we've heard about in the last six months. We'd like to hear about any others. This may be more common than anyone thinks.

Wetsuit Pimples

Wetsuit Folliculitis

Dear SURF DOCS,

I've been surfing for many years and have only recently developed what I think is an unusual reaction to my wetsuit: pimples. I've never had this problem before and fortunately it only occurs around my neck. I wear an O'Neill "Heat" suit that has a smoothie neck lining which doesn't even give me a rash. I rinse it in fresh water after using it to keep it clean. I've neglected to mention that I'm a girl and (luckily) lack the hairier, coarser neckline of a male, and have been furnished with a more soft, supple, and, unfortunately, in this case, sensitive neckline. Could my gender be the deciding factor, or is this a non-discriminatory problem?

PIMPLED POLLY
Newport Beach, California

▌▌▌▌▌▌▏▏▏▏

Dear Polly,

It sounds like you've got what we Surf Docs call *wetsuit folliculitis:* inflamed hair follicles caused by a wetsuit rubbing against the skin. O'Neill isn't at fault, any brand can do it. Despite advertising claims to the contrary, wetsuit material—whether neoprene ("smoothie") or nylon—is pretty coarse stuff (bear witness the need for "rash guards"). To understand the cause, treatment, and prevention of wetsuit folliculitis, you first need to know a little human biology.

Our animal descent really shows through for both men and women when it comes to the generous number of hairs we have down the back of our neck. Every hair grows from out of a pit, which is called a *hair follicle*. The walls of the hair follicle contain sebaceous glands, which produce oils that keep hair and skin shiny and supple. The oils normally ooze out of the follicle along the shaft of the hair, then spread across the skin.

Wetsuit Pimples

When something tight-fitting, which is largely inflexible and relatively rough-surfaced, such as a wetsuit, rubs and catches the hair, the skin around the hair follicle becomes irritated. This leads to inflammation and swelling. The swelling can block off the opening of the follicle, so that the oils produced by the sebaceous glands are trapped inside. That's when you've got a pimple.

To make things worse, the body tries to break down the oils with enzymes, which leads to toxic fatty acids—and more swelling. It's a vicious cycle until the follicle opens up.

When we surf, our near constant head movements and paddling motions are constantly pulling and stretching the wetsuit across our necks and shoulders, which is the most common site of wetsuit pimples. The smoothie wetsuit may glide more easily over your skin, but it would still catch on the hairs of your neck and lead to folliculitis.

The treatment of wetsuit folliculitis involves decreasing the inflammation and unclogging blocked follicles. For the inflammation, use hydrocortisone 1% cream (available over-the-counter in the U.S.), three times a day. The blocked follicles will be opened up by the nightly use of benzoyl peroxide gel, (also over-the-counter). You don't need the maximally strong stuff (10%); low-strength (2.5% or 5%) would be kinder to your skin. Also, begin using a gentle soap at home, such as Dove® or Neutrogena®. Oatmeal-type soaps are also useful.

. . . necks and shoulders, the most common site of wetsuit pimples.

Wearing a rash guard or even a t-shirt will shield your hair follicles and help prevent other skin problems, such as rash. Peel down and get out of your wetsuit as soon as you leave the water. Shower right away. If there isn't a shower at your beach, bring a gallon of water. Also, applying a dose of hydrocortisone right then may preempt inflammation.

You'll be stoked to know that you aren't a victim of evolutionary sexual discrimination. In fact, it's quite the opposite: males have larger and coarser hairs and are more likely to get wetsuit rash than females.

Wipeout Techniques

Sub-Marine

Dear SURF DOCS,

My friend, Mondo, totally shreds, so I'm stoked he's teaching me how to surf.

But last week, he was out at the jetty, went for an aerial, lost it, and went over the falls upside down. He came up bleeding and spitting out teeth, and had a big ding on the nose of his board. He's like, "Hey, shit happens, it's karma!" But I don't even believe in karma. I wipe out all the time. I haven't gotten anything worse than a bruise yet, but I'm scared there's worse to come. Gimme some tips on how to survive a wipeout.

KARMA SHMARMA
Half Moon Bay, California

▮▮▮▮▮▮▯▯▯

Dear Karma Shmarma,

Wipeouts are inseparable from surfing. True, the better the surfer, the fewer the wipeouts, but even the best surfers in the world wipeout now and then. In fact, if a surfer isn't occasionally wiping out, it means they're not exploring the limits of the wave and of their own surfing.

For beginning surfers, unless related to Moses, first attempts to stand and ride a wave are usually lessons in wiping out. So, for all you grem's out there and surfers like Mondo, who failed "Wipeout 101," here are the basics on wiping out stylishly and safely (i.e., methods to save more than face).

The most common time for a wipeout is on the take-off, usually from being too slow to stand-up and having your feet land off-center and slightly too far forward on the board. As you then enter the face of the wave, you'll either pearl or lose control trying to bottom-turn. Plop!

Wipeout Techniques

Wiping out while actually riding a wave is less common, and depends more on how chancey you are in your wave positioning and maneuvers. If you're up and riding, even a giant close-out can be safely managed without a wipeout, by gliding over the back before it fully closes out or by straightening out and riding in with the white water.

You'd be surprised how much control you have when it comes to wiping out. Choose when, where, and how you will fall. It can make all the difference if you control a wipeout by bailing early or delaying falling by one or two seconds.

The basic principle of a controlled wipeout is first to direct your board shoreward and away from you (or anyone else) and then to penetrate the surface and get under or through the back of the wave. This kind of control only comes with practice and wave knowledge.

If you've ever learned how to snow-ski, you'll remember when you began to learn how to control falling, usually by sitting backwards. And once you'd mastered that maneuver, it became easier to ski and you began taking more chances, confident you could always fall safely. Surfing is the same. Once you've learned how to do a controlled wipeout, you'll more quickly become a better surfer.

The four biggest dangers in a wipeout are:

1. **The lip**

2. **Your board**

3. **The bottom**

4. **Other surfers**

The highest risk wipeouts involve the lip; it removes your ability to control your wipeout. The best you can do is cover your head and face with your arms and hands and hope you aren't thrown too hard, don't get slammed by your board or into the bottom, and aren't held down too long. For most beginners, the waves they are learning in don't have much in the way of a lip or curl, so the lip isn't usually so critical. For hotties, though, an aerial is a lip-taunting maneuver from start-to-finish, and the wipeout and injury rate is probably higher than for any other maneuver in surfing.

Most injuries in surfing involve a surfer's own board whacking them during a wipeout. Beyond the obvious strategy of trying to fall as far from your board as possible, preferably with the board beachside to you, the chance of being injured by your board can be minimized by:

1. **Using a longer leash, at least one to two feet longer than the board so it won't stay with you during the wipeout (also, avoid stretchy leashes which zing the board back at you)**

2. **Eliminating sharp points on your board (use a rubber or sili-**

con nose guard, avoid pin-tails and swallow-tails)

3. **Blunting the tips and trailing edges of the skegs (just grab some sandpaper and sand them down —it won't affect their performance one bit!)**

Helmets should be required equipment for all beginning surfers, at least until they have a better sense of where their board is during a wipeout. For instance, a board that has flown up in the air may come down on their head. More experienced surfers usually have a pretty good idea where their board is, even during a wipeout. After a wipeout, all surfers should come back up to the surface slowly, with an outstretched hand to ward off their board if it is flying down or being zinged back by the leash.

The least common but most serious surfing injuries, such as spinal cord injuries and fractures, involve wiping out and striking the bottom. It really doesn't make much difference whether it's sand, rock, or coral bottom, they're all hard and can break your neck. The obvious rules are:

1. **Know how shallow it is where you are surfing**

2. **Know your abilities**

3. **Choose your risks accordingly**

No beginning surfer should surf where it's so shallow on the take-off that if they wipeout they are practically guaranteed to strike the bottom. It's too great a risk even for more advanced surfers, unless accustomed to making better than 90% of their take-offs. A helmet can lessen the risk, but is no guarantee.

Ironically, smaller waves break in shallower water than larger waves, so, in fact, surfing larger surf is actually safer when it comes to avoiding the bottom. Every surfing-injury study done to date has shown that smaller surf yields larger numbers of injuries. In larger surf, you have more time and space in which to control your wipeout. Whatever your height, head-high waves probably are about the safest-sized surf.

There are also many wipeout-related injuries involving other surfers, usually where two surfers wipeout together, or where a surfer crashes into a surfer who is paddling out or in the impact zone, having wiped out on the wave before. Again, the idea is to control your wipeout to fall away from the other person and to have a safety-proofed board. The more crowded the conditions, the more dangerous. Use a helmet.

As for other in-water hazards, such as rocks or coral sticking out of the water, jetties, piers, logs and other submerged objects, it all comes down to ability, awareness, and being prevention-minded. Surfing with poor vision (needing vision correction), poor visibility (riding into the sun or its' reflection, or in misty and foggy conditions), and in low-light (i.e., dawn and near dark, or night-surfing) dramatically amplifies the risk of blindly slamming into water hazards. Helmets become essential.

In general, keep your eyes closed and protected during a wipeout. If it's a long hold-down, and you're not sure which way is up, only open them after the wave starts to let up (unless you have contacts on) to see where the surface is. Wearing some kind of a wetsuit—a flotation device—even if only a vest in warm water, practically will guarantee that you'll float back up after a wipeout, even if you do nothing to try to get to the surface.

Many surfers fear wipeouts because they think they'll run out of air. This almost never happens. Most wipeouts last less than ten seconds. The dreaded two-wave hold-down (i.e., being held underwater for 30 or more seconds) is so rare that you can ask 100 surfers in a row and not find a single one who has ever experienced it. Just be sure you are in good aerobic shape and be careful not to exert yourself during a session, whether while paddling or riding a wave, to where you can't at any moment hold your breath for at least 30 seconds.

Then, if you're facing a wipeout, get in a good breath and enjoy it. Don't fight it. Relax. Conserve your strength and breath. Go for the ride. Really, you have no choice; it has you, at least for the time-being. If it helps any, try to remember that there is no other moment in surfing when you can more fully experience the power of a wave than during a wipeout. Wipeouts can be sacred.

TYPE OF WIPEOUT	CONSIDERATIONS
Small Wave	Try to get back over the top of the wave; don't dive through the bottom—it may be too shallow
Large Wave	Penetrate and go deep, avoid the lip
On Take-off	Try to jump backwards and avoid being pulled over the falls; failing that, try to free-dive to the bottom (in bigger surf)
Mid-face	Use your board as a platform to push off from to try to punch through the face and get out the back of the wave
Bottom of Wave	Avoid skipping over the surface—get some part of your body to penetrate; make sure your board is shoreward and to the side

Sick *Surfers* ASK THE SURF DOCS & Dr. GEOFF

TYPE OF WIPEOUT	CONSIDERATIONS
In the Pit	Dive backwards, under the lip—don't let it come down on you
In the Tube	Push through the back, dive forward (if your board has a nose guard), or sit back—push your board well away from you
Backside	Pivot back into the face, or try to dive towards the shoulder
Beach Break	Beware of varying bottom depths, especially after storms; straightening out is often easier and safer
Point Break	Narrow zone of power, on a diagonal down the point; the shoulder and shoreside are where the wave lets up most quickly; beware of rocks
Reef Break	Varying bottom depths; wave can break, start to let up, and then intensify and break again (the longest hold-downs)
Coral Reef	Suddenly gets shallow; try jumping backwards into the white-water; never fall face first; wear booties/reef walkers, and helmets
Thick Kelp	Shield your face (can hurt you), but keep your elbows out so your arms won't become tangled up against your body
Lobster Trap Lines, or Caught on Bottom	Immediately pull your leash off (use both hands, you may only get one chance)
Logs, Single Large Rock	Don't fall between the object and the wave, try to dive over it
Pier, Jetty	Hold onto your board and keep it in front of you, as a cushion
Surfer/Swimmer Ahead	Go low, bail early, or straighten off to avoid them; don't try to squeeze high on the wave to get by them (recipe for disaster)
Heading into Heavy Local	Pray for death
Tandem Surfing	A wild sexual opportunity—KARMA SU(rf)TRA

XTRA: For Mothers, Surf Widows, and other Co-Surfies

Surf Today to Surf Tomorrow

If you are a mother and your beloved Jack or Jackie lately has announced his or her intention to take up surfing, or if you are a co-surfer fretful type, having now read through this book you may be thinking that your loved one, the surfer, is destined for a body bag (or trash heap). Ergo, this post-note.

Worry not! Surfing truly is safe. Surfing takes place in a soft, liquid environment. Not on pavement (skateboarding, roller-blading, bicycling), not on hard ice-snow (skiing and snowboarding), not high above the ground (hang-gliding, parachuting, bungee-jumping), and not on a field of monsters intent on tearing your head off (football, rugby). Surfing takes place amidst the surf, a lovely natural form of energy, the waves, in a unique space where neither ship, machine or man otherwise goes.

Compared to the American public, the Australians have a far better understanding of surfing. In Australia, surfing is seen as essentially safe and healthy. The expectation is that most Australian kids will at some point try surfing, and in practically every Australian school, amounting to hundreds of thousands children every year, the principles of ocean safety are taught.

Although this book outlines in gritty detail seemingly endless health risks faced by surfers, the list is in fact quite finite and easily contained in this small book. It would have been a mere booklet if surfers were mindful of the following simple precautions.

THE TOP 10 LIST OF SURFING SAFELY

10. Be a good swimmer. *The minimum prerequisite for surfing is an ability to swim 1000 meters in less than 20 minutes.*

9. Know how to bodysurf (or bodyboard). *It will teach you almost everything you need to know about waves—catching them, diving under them, understanding their power.*

8. Choose a safe surfboard. *Eliminate sharp points on the tail and nose (apply a plastic or rubber tip to the nose), blunt the tips and trailing edges of skegs. Use soft-foam surfboards to learn on.*

7. Wear a leash. *This will prevent the board from striking other surfers, and keep a flotation and rescue device (your board) nearby. Also, if you were knocked unconscious and sank, you could be found and retrieved by pulling you up by your leash.*

6. Wear the right wetsuit. *Make sure it fits properly and is thick enough to prevent hypothermia. In warm-water climates wear at least a wetsuit vest to avoid wind-chill. A wetsuit serves as a flotation device; it's hard to sink and drown when wearing one.*

5. Protect your head, ears, and eyes. *Wear a surf helmet, and/or wetsuit hood, and/or earplugs (prevents* Surfer's Ear*). Wear sunglasses when on the beach, and consider surf goggles in the surf, or use a brimmed wetsuit hood or surf cap to shade your eyes. Consider tinted contact lenses.*

4. Protect your skin. *Wear water-resistant sunscreen (SPF15 or greater) and sunblock, to prevent skin cancer and premature aging of the skin.*

3. Study and ocean and choose safe surfing conditions. *Avoid surfing in crowds, over shallow reefs and sandbars, and after drinking alcohol. Know about currents and how to get out of a rip.*

2. Become a barefoot doctor. *Know in-water rescue techniques and CPR. Be prepared for medical emergencies, especially on surf trips.*

1. Surf today to surf tomorrow.

Surfing Organizations and Associations

Surfer's Medical Association (SMA)
P.O. Box 1210
Aptos, CA 95001-1210 USA
Phone and FAX: (408) 684-0916

*SMA has a part-time staff person who takes messages and returns calls.
Expect to leave a message. If you have a medical emergency or are in need
of an immediate referral, please be advised that this is not a service provided by the SMA. See pages 276-79 for information on joining the SMA.
All surfers interested in surfing are welcome to join.*

Disabled Surfer's Association (DSA)
Box A14, Enfield South
NSW 2133 Australia
011-61-2-642-7243

National Association of Surfing Attorneys (NASA)
1642 Great Highway
San Francisco, CA 94122 USA
Phone: (415) 664-NASA
FAX: (415) 664-6273

*Formed in 1993, this organization is modeled after the Surfer's Medical
Association.*

Surfer's Environmental Alliance (SEA)
1642 Great Highway
San Francisco, CA 94122 USA
Phone: (415) 665-7008
FAX: (415) 665-9008

Surfrider Foundation
122 South El Camino Real, #67
San Clemente, CA 92672 USA
1-800-743-SURF

For health and surfing information as well as updates on travel medicine be sure to read the **Surf Docs** Column in *Surfer* Magazine (P.O. Box 1028, Dana Point, CA 92629 USA) and **Dr. Bob** in *Tracks* (P.O. Box 746, Darlinghurst, NSW 2010 Australia).

Sick Surfer?

Send your letters to:

Surf Docs
c/o *Surfer* **Magazine**
P.O. Box 1028
Dana Point, CA 92629

Replies will be limited to those published.

Index

Index

Index

Index

Index

Index

Index

Index

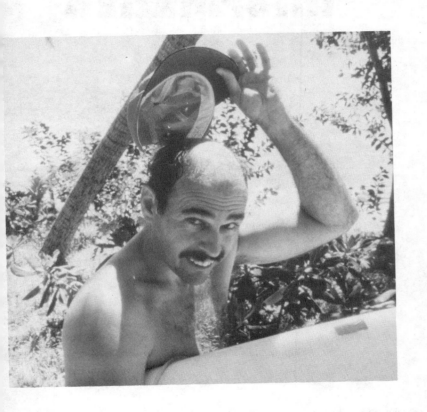

Ordering Information

Bull Publishing Company
P.O. Box 208
Palo Alto, CA 94302-0208 USA
Toll Free (sorry, U.S. only): 1-800-676-2855
(415) 322-2855
FAX: (415) 327-3300

Want additional copies of *Sick Surfers Ask the Surf Docs and Dr. Geoff* for yourself, your friends, your surf club? Just drop us a note or give us a call . . .

Discounts are available for your surf clubs:

10-49 copies	10% discount
50-499 copies	20% discount
500+ copies	25% discount

_____ copies of *Sick Surfers* . . . @ $12.95 each _____

CA residents add 8.5% tax _____

Shipping ($3.00 1st book; 75¢ each additional) _____

TOTAL ENCLOSED _____

We accept checks, Visa or MasterCard:

Visa/MC number _____ Exp. _____

Signature _____ Phone (____) _____

Name _____

Address _____

City/State _____ Zip _____